Health, Nutrition
and Economic Crises

HEALTH, NUTRITION, AND ECONOMIC CRISES

Approaches to Policy in the Third World

Edited by

David E. Bell
Michael R. Reich

The Harvard School of Public Health

AH *Auburn House Publishing Company*
Dover, Massachusetts

Library of Congress Cataloging in Publication Data

```
Takemi Symposium on International Health (2nd : 1986 : Harvard
  University School of Public Health)
   Health, nutrition, and economic crises : approaches to policy in
 the Third World / edited by David E. Bell, Michael R. Reich.
       p.   cm.
   "This volume is a result of the Second Takemi Symposium on
 International Health, held on May 20-22, 1986, at the Harvard School
 of Public Health in Boston, Massachusetts."--Pref.
   Bibliography: p.
   Includes index.
   ISBN 0-86569-170-3 : $28.95
   1. Medical economics--Developing countries--Congresses.
 2. Nutrition--Economic aspects--Developing countries--Congresses.
 3. Medical policy--Developing countries--Congresses.  4. Nutrition-
 -Government policy--Developing countries--Congresses.   I. Bell,
 David E., 1919-   . II. Reich, Michael, 1950-   . III. Title.
 RA410.9.D44T35 1986a
 362.1'09172'4--dc19                                       87-30834
                                                              CIP
```

Printed in the United States of America

Preface

This volume is a result of the Second Takemi Symposium on International Health, held on May 20–22, 1986, at the Harvard School of Public Health in Boston, Massachusetts. The Symposium brought together distinguished participants from around the world to discuss the effects of economic crises on health and nutrition in poor countries and to explore the policies that might mitigate the adverse consequences of economic adjustment. The Symposium considered a set of papers prepared in advance, many of which were later revised to reflect issues raised in the discussions. The revised papers are presented in this volume, along with an introductory chapter by the editors.

The meeting was organized by the Takemi Program in International Health, which was established at the Harvard School of Public Health in 1983. The Program is named in honor of the late Dr. Taro Takemi, an eminent Japanese physician and President of the Japan Medical Association for more than a quarter of a century. In its various activities, the Program seeks to carry forward Dr. Takemi's objectives of health improvement based on the application of economics to medicine, greater equity, and more attention to environmental concerns. It gives particular emphasis to issues of mobilizing and allocating resources for health. As part of the Program an international conference is held every two years, alternating between Tokyo and Boston, as a reflection of the ties across the Pacific and the concerns on both sides for international health.

This Symposium was co-sponsored with UNICEF, the Ford Foundation, and the Institute for Seizon and Life Sciences in Tokyo. Their support is gratefully acknowledged. It made possible the conference as well as the preparation and publication of the materials in this volume.

For their untiring assistance, Laurie Shepard, former Program Coordinator of the Takemi Program, and Naomi Pierce, editor at Oelgeschlager, Gunn & Hain Publishers, are warmly thanked.

Contents

Part II. Approaches to Food and Nutrition Policy

Part III. Approaches to Health Policy

List of Tables

List of Figures

Chapter 9: Epidemiology of Hunger in Africa

Chapter 10: Towards Basic Human Needs

Chapter 11: A Public Health Approach

Chapter 12: Health Policy Responses

Chapter 14: Drug Supply and Use

Chapter 16: User Fees and Health Financing

About the Editors
and Contributors

Jere R. Behrman is the William R. Kenan, Jr. Professor of Economics at the University of Pennsylvania. He also is co-director of the Center for Analysis of Developing Economies and of the Center for Household and Family Economics; Associate Director of the Lauder Institute of Management and International Studies, and member of the Population Studies Center and the South Asian Regional Studies Department at the University of Pennsylvania. He also has been a consultant or researcher for a number of international and national organizations. His research and extensive publications have focused on economic development, including extensive work on macroeconomics and on health and nutrition determinants. He is co-editor of the *Journal of Development Economics.*

David E. Bell is the Clarence Gamble Professsor of Population Sciences and International Health, Director of the Center for Population Studies, and Chairman of the Department of Population Sciences at the Harvard School of Public Health. He received his M.A. in Economics from Harvard University and holds honorary LL.D.'s from Pomona College, Harvard University, the University of Vermont, Notre Dame University, and the University of North Dakota. His research interests include population and public policy, economic development, and the organization of international research and development of health problems of developing countries.

Elisabeth Benjamin is a candidate for an M.Sc. at the Harvard School of Public Health's Health Policy and Management Program with a concentration on international health. Currently she is working as Health Planning Officer for Catholic Relief Services in the Philippines.

Mayra Buvinic is Director of the International Center for Research on Women and past President of the Association for Women in Development. Among her best-known publications are *Women and Poverty in the Third World* (Johns Hopkins University Press, 1983) and "Women's Projects in the Third World: Explaining their Misbehavior" (*World Development*, May 1986). Dr. Buvinic holds a doctorate in social psychology from the University of Wisconsin, Madison and a degree in psychology from the Catholic University of Santiago, Chile.

Lincoln C. Chen is the Taro Takemi Professor of International Health at the Harvard School of Public Health and the Director of the Takemi Program in International Health. Dr. Chen was the Ford Foundation Representative for India, Sri Lanka, and Nepal. He received his M.D. from Harvard Medical School and his M.P.H. from the Johns Hopkins University. His numerous publications address issues related to maternal and child health, nutrition, and population policy.

Flora Chu is a medical consultant for the Program on Technology and Health Care at the Institute for Health Policy Analysis, Georgetown University Medical Center. She studies health policy issues, particularly concerns related to the emergence of new medical technologies and the appropriate use of existing technologies in clinical practices. Dr. Chu is the author or co-author of several publications and reports on topics related to technology assessment. She received her B.A. in biology from the University of Pennsylvania and her M.D. from the University of Maryland at Baltimore.

Adrian Griffiths is the co-founder and Director of Research of the Health Management Institute, Geneva, an international consulting group. He was formerly on the faculty of the London School of Hygiene and Tropical Medicine of the University of London, and then head of health management and economics at the Sandoz Institute for Health and Socio-Economic Studies, Geneva. He teaches at the University of Geneva and sits on the editorial boards of several journals in the fields of health and public finance. He is the author of numerous publications in the fields of health management and financing, pharmaceuticals, and epidemiology.

Richard Jolly has been Deputy Executive Director (Programmes) in UNICEF since 1982, and previously served as Director of the Institute for Development Studies in Sussex, England. He has lived and worked in Kenya, Uganda, Zambia, and Madagascar and has served as a consultant to many other countries and international agencies. He has written or contributed to many publications, including *Planning Education for African Development* (East Africa Publishing House, 1969), *Redistribution with Growth* (Oxford University Press, 1974), *Disarmament and World Development* (Pergamon, 1978 and 1985), and *Adjustment with a Human Face* (Oxford University Press, forthcoming). Dr. Jolly is a graduate in economics from the University of Cambridge and earned his doctorate at Yale University.

Andrew M. Kamarck Is President of Asclepius Corporation. He worked at the World Bank for twenty-nine years, as Economic Advisor on Europe and Africa, Director of the Economics Department, and Director of the Economic Development Institute. On leaving the World Bank in 1979 he became Associate Fellow, Harvard Institute for International Development. His books include *The Economics of African Development* (rev. ed. 1971), *The Tropics and Economic Development* (1976), *Politica finanziaria degli alleati in Italia* (1977) and *Economics and the Real World* (1983). Dr. Kamarck has a B.S. in economics and a Ph.D. in political economy and government, both from Harvard.

Yukio Kaneko is a Professor of Economics and Dean of the Graduate School of Economics at the Hiroshima University of Economics, Japan. He previously taught at Waseda University and Chuo University, both in Tokyo. His research interests include the theory of development economics, econometric modeling and economic policy formulation, and he has written numerous papers and books on these topics in both Japanese and English. Professor Kaneko earned his doctorate in economics at Kobe University.

Joanne Leslie is a public health nutritionist at the International Center for Research on Women, where she co-directs the Center's Program on Women's Work and Child Welfare. She is the author of many publications, and recently co-edited a book entitled *Food Policy: Integrating Supply, Distribution, and Consumption*. Dr. Leslie has an M.Sc. and D.Sc. from the Johns Hopkins School of Hygiene and Public Health.

Margaret Lycette, Deputy Director of the International Center for Research on Women, is an economist who specializes in low-income housing, small enterprise credit, and vocational training. Ms. Lycette directs the ICRW's major technical services work with the Agency for International Development. A graduate of Boston University, Ms. Lycette earned an M.A. in economics at the Johns Hopkins University and is now a Ph.D. candidate in that program.

Leonardo Mata is Chief of Microbiology at the Institute of Health Research (INISA), University of Costa Rica, and has recently served as visiting professor in the Department of Population Sciences, Harvard School of Public Health. Professor Mata specializes in microbiology, nutrition, food hygiene, and epidemiology. He has consulted to several international agencies, including UNICEF and the World Health Organization. He won the UNESCO Science Prize in 1980 and is the author or co-author of numerous articles and reports in his fields. He earned his M.Q.C. degree in microbiology and clinical chemistry from the University of Costa Rica and holds M.S. and D.Sc. degrees in tropical public health from the Harvard School of Public Health.

Koh'ichi Nidaira is Associate Professor of Economics at the Hiroshima University of Economics. His research and teaching focus on public economics, development economics, and applied economics. He earned his master's degree in economics at Waseda University, Tokyo.

Takateru Ohse is a consultant to the Japan Association for Tropical Medicine. He has worked as Professor of Public Health at the National University of Taiwan and as the Head of the Parasitology Department of the Atomic Bomb Casualty Commission's Hiroshima Laboratory, U.S. Atomic Energy Commission. He has also worked with the World Health Organization, the United Nations Economic Commission for Africa, and the government of Ethiopia. Dr. Ohse earned his M.D. from the Keio University Medical School in Tokyo.

Seymour Perry is Deputy Director of the Institute for Health Policy Analysis at Georgetown University Medical Center, where he holds dual appointments as Professor of Medicine and Professor of Community and Family Medicine. Dr. Perry spent fourteen years at the National Cancer Institute in cancer research, becoming deputy director of the Division of Cancer Therapy. Then, as Associate Director of the National Institutes of Health, he played a key role in initiating the NIH Consensus Development Program, the first formal assessment program for medical technologies in the executive branch of the government. In 1978, Dr. Perry became the first Director of the National Center for Health Care Technology, an agency created by Congress to assess major medical technologies. In 1985, he was elected to a two-year term as the first President of the newly formed International Society of Technology Assessment in Health Care. He serves on numerous advisory and editorial boards and is a member of the Institute of Medicine of the National Academy of Science.

Per Pinstrup-Andersen is Professor of Food Economics in the Division of Nutritional Sciences and Director of the Cornell Nutritional Surveillance Program at Cornell University, Ithaca, New York. Prior to his current position, Professor Pinstrup-Andersen was Director of the Food Consumption and Nutrition Policy Research Program at the International Food Policy Research Institute in Washington, D.C. His research and extensive publications focus on economic analyses of various aspects of food policy.

Michael R. Reich is Executive Director of the Takemi Program in International Health and Associate Professor of International Health in the Department of Health Policy and Management at the Harvard School of Public Health. His research and teaching activities focus on the political economy of health policy. He has numerous publications on environmental policy, pharmaceutical policy, and other health issues. Dr. Reich received his B.A. in molecular biophysics and biochemistry, M.A. in East Asian studies, and Ph.D. in political science, all from Yale University.

S. W. R. de A. Samarasinghe is Senior Lecturer in Economics at the University of Peradeniya and Associate Director of the International Centre for Ethnic Studies in Kandy, Sri Lanka. Dr. Samarasinghe spent the academic year 1985–1986 as Takemi Fellow in International Health at the Harvard School of Public Health. He has published widely on themes in political economy and development studies in relation to Sri Lanka. He graduated from the University of Ceylon, Peradeniya, Sri Lanka, with a B.A. in economics and obtained his Ph.D. in the same subject from Cambridge University, England.

Donald S. Shepard is Associate Professor of Operations Management and Operations Research at the Harvard School of Public Health and Research Associate at the Harvard Institute for International Development. His publications and reports include studies of the cost-effective analysis of immunizations and oral rehydration therapy for the Agency for International Development, the World Bank, and the World Health Organization in Indonesia, Ivory Coast, Honduras, the Gambia, and Ecuador, and projections of costs and financing of hospital and primary health care services in Honduras and Rwanda. Dr. Shepard holds an M.P.P. and a Ph.D. in public policy from the Kennedy School of Government at Harvard University.

Lance Taylor is Professor of Economics at the Massachusetts Institute of Technology. He has been active as a development economist since

1968 and has worked as a consultant or visiting professor in more than twenty countries, including Mexico, Brazil, Egypt, and India. His most recent book is *Structuralist Macroeconomics* (1983), and he is currently coordinating a project to analyze the experience of eighteen developing countries in adjusting to external shocks for the United Nations World Institute of Development Economics Research in Helsinki. Professor Taylor earned his Ph.D. in economics at Harvard University.

C. Peter Timmer is Professor of Development Studies, At-Large, at Harvard University and a Faculty Fellow at the Harvard Institute of International Development. He previously taught at Stanford University and Cornell University. At Harvard, Professor Timmer first was affiliated with the School of Public Health and then the Business School. He holds B.A., M.A., and Ph.D. degrees in economics, all from Harvard University.

1

Introduction and Overview

David E. Bell and Michael R. Reich

For roughly the first thirty years after World War II, the international economic climate for developing nations was favorable, with rising international demand for their exports and ready sources of borrowed capital. Over the last dozen years, drastic changes have occurred in the international economy, with powerful adverse effects on many poor countries. These international shocks have shaken Third World economies already severely stressed by resource shortages, limited technical and managerial skills, low levels of capital investment, and high rates of population growth.

To deal with the economic shocks of recent years, developing countries have had to make a series of major policy adjustments—including currency devaluations, cuts in government expenditures, and reductions in imports—frequently under external pressure from international lending agencies and from private banks. These adjustments have often resulted in lower economic activity, higher unemployment, and lower real wages. In sum, countries sought to restore the basis for long-term economic growth through changes that brought real short-term setbacks.

This volume examines the impact of these economic adjustments on health and nutrition in developing countries and identifies policies that might minimize the resulting human costs. The authors include economists and experts on health and nutrition from a variety of disciplines.

The purpose here is not to review economic policies as such; the nature of the international economic pressures and the policy responses

1

appropriate to them merely form a backdrop. Instead, the main objectives were to ask how health and nutrition in poor countries have been affected by international economic crises and to explore possible policy adjustments—especially in health and nutrition policies but also in economic policies—to protect and promote the health and nutritional status of disadvantaged populations.

This overview chapter summarizes some of the central findings and conclusions of the book. The subject is novel, and the attempt to bring together persons of widely varying disciplines and backgrounds was, as always, only partially successful. Nevertheless, we believe this is a lively and provocative first effort that provides a useful basis for both action and further study.

The chapters in this volume follow a four-step set of questions:

1. What have been the origins and magnitude of the economic adjustments required of developing countries, and are these conditions likely to continue in the future?

2. What effects have economic adjustments had on the nutrition and health of people in developing countries?

3. What policies would be most useful in minimizing the adverse impact of economic adjustments on food and nutrition?

4. What policies would best promote public health in the face of economic constraints and crises?

Questions 1 and 2 are discussed in the section on economic adjustment; question 3, in the section on food and nutrition policy; and question 4, in the section on health policy.

Origins and Magnitude of Economic Adjustments

Lance Taylor (Chapter 2) summarizes the several external shocks that have confronted developing countries over the past dozen years. These have notably included:

Violent swings in oil prices: up in the 1970s, down in the 1980s;

A slowing rate of economic growth in industrialized countries since the mid-1970s, and severe economic recession at the beginning of the 1980s, which resulted in low prices and decreased demand for the exports of developing countries; and

Overambitious borrowing by developing countries, abetted by unrestrained lending by international financial institutions, especially by private banks in industrialized countries.

The effect on many developing countries was a double bind: they lost export earnings at the very time their debt obligations were high and rising. Consequently they had no choice but to cut back on domestic investment and consumption to reduce imports and thereby to free up the foreign exchange needed to pay debt interest and amortization. Borrowing countries sought and received stretched-out schedules for repaying debts, but only after agreeing to undertake severe adjustments at the behest of lenders consortia with the International Monetary Fund and the World Bank participating. The effects of the adjustments on domestic economic activity and employment were often drastic, and real wages in many countries dropped sharply in the early 1980s.

There were important differences among countries. Oil producing countries faced different circumstances than oil consumers. Foreign debt was concentrated in some of the large Latin American countries that were given very large loans by a number of prominent U.S. banks. Despite these differences, however, the general picture holds. The late 1970s and early 1980s were a period in which international economic circumstances greatly exacerbated the hard central task of developing countries—to lift the income levels in their countries and to spread the higher incomes more equitably.

This is the bleak picture that Taylor paints. Two of his conclusions stand out. Why has this occurred? "At root, the poor growth perform- ance of the developing countries [in this period] is caused by the economic slump of the industrialized world." And what of the future? "Given their debt situation and poor external prospects, developing countries will have to undertake massive belt-tightening in the foresee- able future."

This view of the difficult situation faced by developing countries is generally accepted, but many persons note differences in economic circumstances and policy responses among regions and among coun- tries. Saburo Okita, for example, asked to comment on Taylor's chapter, emphasized the important regional differences in the nature and sever- ity of the economic adjustment problem. Okita sees the African picture as "alarming," with complex interactions among environmental deterio- ration, declining per capita food production, rapid population increases, and stagnating economic growth. In Latin America, the debt burden increased rapidly in the late 1970s and early 1980s, and special measures to alleviate the debt burden will be needed to restore economic health. Asia, in Okita's view, presents a brighter picture than the other two regions, with stronger growth and smaller debt burdens in China and India and especially in Korea, Taiwan, Hong Kong and Singapore (the so-called Newly Industrializing Countries). He expresses the hope that lower interest rates, price stability and cheaper energy costs in industrial- ized countries "will eventually stimulate growth of the world economy."

S. W. R. de A. Samarasinghe's case study of the economic adjustment process in Sri Lanka (Chapter 3) shows that opportunities for positive adaptation exist for some countries. His chapter describes in careful detail a set of adjustments introduced by the Government of Sri Lanka in 1977, including major modifications in exchange rates, sharp reductions in government expenditure for food subsidies, and increased reliance on market forces to guide investment and output. This program was aimed, in Samarasinghe's phrase, at "adjustment with growth" and depended on the simultaneous provision of a large amount of foreign aid. The adjustment program achieved considerable success in stimulating output and employment while redressing the balance of payments deficit, and it demonstrates the considerable range of policy initiatives developing countries can take if they can attract the necessary international assistance.

These qualifications do not alter the fundamental observation that the recent slow economic growth and recession in the industrialized countries have sharply reduced the economic opportunities for developing countries. The resulting short-range adjustment problems for many poor countries are of major magnitude and have substantially complicated their long-range goal of achieving advances in economic welfare.

Effects of Economic Adjustments on Nutrition and Health

The liveliest difference of view expressed in the volume is in response to the question: how severe have been the impacts of economic adjustment on health and nutrition? Richard Jolly (Chapter 4) argues that adjustment policies have had strongly adverse effects on the health and nutrition of poor people in developing countries. Jolly cites evidence that real per capita incomes have fallen in each year of the 1980s in many countries, especially in Africa and Latin America, and that the proportion of children who are moderately or severely malnourished has increased in several African countries in the early 1980s. Using data from a UNICEF study, he argues that the effects of adjustment in many cases have fallen disproportionately on the poor and vulnerable, with the most serious impact on children. Jolly criticizes efforts that focus only on the economic problems of poor countries and ignore the "human dimension" of adjustment policy. And he calls for a new policy of "adjustment with a human face," which would "combine the basic economic elements of adjustment policy with conscious efforts to ensure that the basic nutrition and health and education needs of the entire population are satisfied."

Jere Behrman (Chapter 5) presents a contrasting perspective on the effects of economic adjustment policy. After a careful analysis of the theoretical and empirical evidence, he concludes that while economic adjustment policies "certainly have some negative impact . . . the coping capacities of societies, households and individuals apparently often have been substantial so that the demonstrable impact on health and nutrition has been surprisingly limited." Behrman stresses the conceptual and empirical problems that create uncertainties in assessing effects on health and nutrition and argues that "any conclusion must be tentative at this time."

Both views have been supported strongly by observers in the two worlds of economics and public health. Certain points of special importance deserve mention.

Economic adjustment programs affect health and nutrition in two main ways: by reducing the incomes of poorer groups in the population and by reducing the nutritional and health services provided by government.

With respect to reduced incomes, there is no doubt that most economic adjustment programs, because they deliberately seek to cut back consumption, imports, and investment, will also reduce incomes for many poor people. In some cases, however, incomes of some of the poor may benefit. For example, low-income farmers may benefit if food imports and/or food subsidies are cut and food prices therefore rise.

Lower incomes for poor people do not automatically result in sharp reductions in nutritional and health status. Their impact on health and nutrition may be limited by both institutional and individual responses. Governments may seek, as part of the overall adjustment process, to protect food supplies for the poor, as the Government of Sri Lanka tried to do, with only partial success, in the case described by Samarasinghe. Moreover, as Behrman notes, families may adjust their purchases of food to protect levels of consumption, by shifting to cheaper, less desirable products which may still maintain nutritional intake.

With respect to the second avenue of impact, via government budgets, economic adjustment programs typically seek to reduce government expenditures as one means of lowering domestic demand and freeing resources for export. Reducing government expenditures may affect nutrition and health in two ways. One is by reducing government food subsidies. Such subsidies often benefit middle- and even high-income families, in which cases their reduction will not affect the poor. But food subsidies may be of great benefit to poor families, and unless these are maintained (as they were in part in Sri Lanka) the effects could be serious.

The second possible effect of reducing government budgets is through lower health expenditures. Behrman cites evidence that reductions in health sector budgets have been smaller on average than reductions in other sectors. Nevertheless, any reductions in the already limited health services for the poor in developing countries could be damaging.

The present state of the evidence makes it very difficult to estimate the actual effects of lower incomes and reduced budgets. Problems in measuring or demonstrating the effects arise from incomplete data, complex social interactions, and the recency of the economic crisis. Much better information is needed, particularly data from continuing surveillance of the health and nutrition status of people, especially children, by income classes. Until such data are available, it is not possible to assert confidently how severe are the impacts of economic adjustment on health and nutrition.

Several qualitative conclusions are warranted. First, economic adjustment programs, by affecting the incomes and services available to the poor, will to some extent adversely affect their health and nutrition. Second, planners need to take into account the probable consequences of economic adjustment programs for the nutrition and health of the poor—even if the level of impact cannot be precisely predicted. Third, a variety of buffering responses can be used by governments and families to limit the adverse impact. Fourth, there is every reason to encourage national and international policy-makers to aim at "adjustment with a human face." Fifth, policies to achieve "adjustment with growth" are clearly desirable, even though they may not be feasible in all cases, and foreign assistance to that end can have major benefits in welfare terms.

Options and Alternatives for Food and Nutrition

What can be done to minimize the adverse impact of economic adjustment on food and nutrition in developing countries? The six chapters addressing this question present a wide variety of options and alternatives. Four major conclusions may be drawn.

First, low-income households can be protected to some degree through food price subsidies or food distribution programs. Per Pinstrup-Andersen (Chapter 6) describes a wide variety of programs in a number of countries that use different methods and concentrate on different commodities. He shows that food subsidies and distribution programs can indeed contribute significantly to the real income of the poor, citing evidence from Sri Lanka, Egypt, Bangladesh, Kerala State (in India), Mexico, the Philippines, and elsewhere. Food price subsidies and distribution programs may, therefore, have a useful place in protecting low-income families against the adverse effects of economic adjustment programs. It is not easy, however, to design them in ways that will simultaneously reach the most needy groups, fit within tight budgets, and attract continuing political support.

Food price subsidies have often proven to be very expensive as a proportion of government budgets, running as high as 15–20 percent of total budget outlays and contributing to budget deficits and inflation. The reason for the high cost of food subsidies is usually that they have been designed to benefit broad groups in the population; Pinstrup-

Andersen notes that "very few of the existing food price subsidy schemes are targeted to low-income households." Targeting to particular low-income groups, therefore, is appealing as a means of reducing budget costs without negative effects on the poor.

Targeting, however, is difficult to achieve. The necessary information to identify poor households with members at risk of malnourishment is not easily available, particularly because different groups of the poor will be affected differently by economic crises and adjustment. Inflation may erode the value of food supplements, as happened in Sri Lanka. Pinstrup-Andersen says that a program narrowly targeted to particular groups of the poor "is likely to have little political support . . . and if implemented may have a short life."

Second, direct food subsidies and distribution programs are not by themselves a sufficient response to the food and nutrition problems that accompany economic adjustment. C. Peter Timmer (Chapter 7) describes the complex web of relationships that constitute the food system of any nation, linking together food consumption patterns, the food production sector, domestic and international food prices and markets, and the national macroeconomic policies that affect the food system. Timmer argues that developing countries will need to take a variety of actions, some broadly aimed and some narrowly targeted, to minimize the effects of economic adjustments on the food intake of poor consumers. Successful policies "to alleviate the likely energy deficits among the poor . . . will almost certainly not be restricted to narrow sectoral interventions designed to deliver more food to hungry people. A reduction in hunger, even in the context of macroeconomic crises, will most likely come from a coordinated effort involving many sectors." The set of policies to be chosen will depend on the specific characteristics of each country. In some cases, the effects of exchange rate devaluations on the nutrition of the poor may be more powerful than the effects of food distribution programs, and the two approaches—along with others—must therefore be coordinated.

This major judgment has important practical consequences: it means that policy makers for health and nutrition need strong working links with policy makers for food and agriculture and economic planning. In most governments, these links are far from strong enough. Timmer urges greater use of food policy analysis, to understand and coordinate the intersectoral connections that affect the nutritional status of the poor.

The third conclusion from this set of chapters is the need to design economic adjustment policies that will aim at long-run as well as short-run objectives. Andrew Kamarck, for example, argues (Chapter 8) that even if the immediate effects of economic crisis in Africa were satisfactorily dealt with, formidable long-term "climatic, medical, political and sociological problems" would remain. It is thus not sufficient to attack only the immediate elements of the crisis; the underlying obstacles to economic and social progress must be challenged at the same time. A policy such as the United Nations Program of Action for African Economic Recovery and Development, 1986–1990, which places major emphasis on improving the opportunities for women farmers, will have its strongest impact over the longer run. By adding to the competence and resources of Africa's women farmers, the level of rural incomes and welfare will be lifted, and African economies will be made more resistant to future economic crises. To achieve these objectives, the tilt of government policy needs to be shifted from urban to rural populations, a difficult change involving real political risks.

Pinstrup-Andersen makes a similar point. While food subsidies and transfer programs may be helpful in correcting acute problems, he argues, "Enhancing the capacity of the poor to generate sufficient incomes to meet their requirements for food and other demands is the most appropriate long-term means to meet welfare goals." Therefore, "although some of the appropriate activities, such as investment in employment-intensive industry, education, [and] cost-reducing technology . . . may have a pay-off for the poor only in the longer run, it is important that macroeconomic adjustments are designed to achieve such long-run poverty reductions. Transfer programs to correct acute problems should not be used as an excuse for not following a development strategy aimed at the alleviation of poverty and malnutrition. For example, the large reductions in public investment in primary education in many countries during the last ten years are likely to have severe negative effects on future income-earning capacity of the poor."

This advice to maintain strong emphasis on the longer-term processes of economic development, even while wrestling with the urgencies of crisis, is surely sound although difficult to achieve. It carries major policy implications both for governments of developing countries facing economic adjustments and for international aid agencies wishing to help them. As Takateru Ohse points out in Chapter 9, the methods used for agricultural development can have devastating consequences for ecologically fragile arid areas, as has occurred in Africa. In some areas, shortening the fallow period between cultivation cycles has resulted in damage to soil fertility, loss of water retention capacity, widespread erosion, and irreversible desertification. Large-scale irrigation development projects have also produced unintended consequences, in the spread of water-associated endemic diseases, notably malaria and schistosomiasis.

Yukio Kaneko and Koh'ichi Nidaira (Chapter 10) emphasize the importance for economic development strategies to take into account basic human needs. They recommend a focus on increasing the productivity of the poor, in order to reduce absolute poverty and malnutrition over the long run. Such a focus, in their view, would require new indicators of advances, spanning food, education, health, sanitation, and water supply.

The fourth important conclusion from these chapters is that good nutrition is far more than a matter of supplying sufficient food. Leonardo Mata (Chapter 11) cites two powerful reasons why poor nutritional status may result even in the presence of adequate food supplies. The first is infection: "Infected children may not accept food, even of the best quality." The second reason is the lack of knowledge about nutritious foods and about good food handling among family members, principally mothers. During exclusive breast-feeding of babies, until they are about six months of age, "human milk generally provides the calories and nutrients needed for optimal growth. Thereafter, food supplements should be given in adequate composition and amount to support growth. Many people do not know enough about feeding mixes of sufficient nutriture and caloric density [and cleanliness] for good nutrition and growth."

Mata calls this needed knowledge "maternal technology." He points out that many mothers have been raised in "societies that have not permitted them to acquire an understanding . . . of the ubiquitous fecal contamination of food and environment and other threats to child nutrition and survival." On the other hand, he notes that "many women in villages and city slums possess effective maternal technologies, and their children thrive well despite the odds and hardships."

Measures to cure or prevent infections, especially in children, therefore, and measures to promote good maternal technologies, must accompany concern for sufficient food supplies in seeking to raise the nutritional status of poor families. These measures need to be respected both in short-run programs of economic adjustment and in longer-run programs of economic development.

Options and Alternatives for Health

What can be done to achieve the best possible health outcomes in developing countries in the face of economic constraints and crises? The five chapters that address this question were designed to approach it from different points of view. Together, they present a strong and consistent set of observations and conclusions.

A first group of conclusions from these chapters concern the connections between medical and non-medical factors in improving health status. Lincoln Chen (Chapter 12) writes that the health of populations is determined both by "the productivity of health care systems . . . [and] the health impact of social, economic, political, and environmental factors." Moreover, "changes wrought by economic crisis may exert impacts on both health care systems and non-medical factors. It is possible that changes in non-medical factors may have far greater health consequences than changes in the health system per se. Health policy responses, therefore, cannot be dissociated from policy changes in other sectors."

In his comparison of the health status and health systems of India and China, Chen finds two major factors that explain China's substantially better health achievements. First, while the per capita level of gross national product is similar, China's per capita health expenditures are three times those of India. Second, China has achieved substantially greater decentralization of health facilities and of the mobilization and control of resources applied to health. Neither of these differences stems mainly from policies within the health sector; both derive instead from the overall set of political attitudes toward social programs and the overall pattern of responsibility and action for rural change. Health policy analysis, therefore, "must consider the broader political economy of the society."

The connections between health and non-medical factors apply also to the family, which Chen calls "the central production unit for health." He notes that "many studies have shown that even if environmental and economic variables are controlled, some families are consistently better, and others poorer, health achievers." In Chapter 13, Joanne Leslie, Margaret Lycette and Mayra Buvinic explore the conditions that families, and particularly mothers, face in achieving health for their children, and the choices they must make in doing so. Poor women carry heavy burdens of work: household responsibilities, child care, and income-generating activities. They must weigh carefully the time and income costs of health care activities, reflecting the connections between health and non-medical factors.

The structure of the delivery of health and nutrition services thus can greatly affect their accessibility and ease of use for women. The availability of day care may increase women's employment options while promoting health and nutrition care for children. Leslie et al. point out that different health care activities have different time costs and time savings for women. Immunizations, family planning, and some curative drugs are quite efficient: their time costs are low and they offer substantial future time savings through decreased child illness and increased child spacing. On the other hand, oral rehydration therapy, growth monitoring, and improved weaning practices cost women considerably more time and promise smaller future time savings through decreased child illness.

Second, these chapters discuss several ways in which economic crises and adjustments can affect health adversely. Adrian Griffiths (Chapter 14) documents the significant reduction in drug supplies that has occurred in the great majority of developing countries that import most or all of their drugs. This reduction results directly from cuts in government budget allocations for health, and from decreased foreign exchange allocations for imports. Moreover, Griffiths points out that reducing government health budgets may result in more than proportional reductions in drug imports, because bureaucracies usually react to budget cuts by protecting staff and decreasing non-staff items, including drugs, disproportionately. It is clear that in times of economic adjustment, poor countries need policies to protect the supply of necessary drugs.

A similar point is made by Seymour Perry and Flora Chu in Chapter 15 on medical technologies. At present, in most developing countries, large quantities of medical equipment and supplies must be imported. Such imports are vulnerable, like drugs, to stoppage or cutbacks when government budgets and foreign exchange for imports are reduced as part of economic adjustment programs. These financial limitations can also exacerbate the "frequently occurring problem" of inadequate servicing and maintenance of medical equipment in poor countries.

From another angle, Leslie et al. describe how economic crisis can add to the multiple demands poor women face in developing countries. In normal times, women must not only manage the family household and supplement the family's income through farm or non-farm production, they must also fill a central role as promoters of family health. They are responsible for recognizing the signs of illness in family members, offering treatment and care, and where necessary investing the time and energy to reach the nearest clinic, wait for service, and obtain and administer medication. Economic crises and adjustments typically increase these demands. Women will have to work more hours to compensate for lower wages, adjust to shorter hours and larger fees at health clinics, and make do with smaller amounts of less nutritious foods. Furthermore, the effects of economic crisis and adjustment on poor families may be perpetuated from one generation to the next, as daughters may be held out of school to take care of younger children so that mothers can work more to maintain the family's income.

All of these chapters all reflect the bleak reality of how economic crises disrupt the lives of poor families in developing countries. But the authors also make clear that the scale of the impact is uncertain. The common problem of scarce data blocks accurate measurement of the health effects of economic adjustment. In addition, the recent economic crises have occurred against a background of long-term trends significantly beneficial to poor families. For example, as noted by Leslie et al., the long-term trend in education has been strongly upward in developing countries: "female primary school enrollment rates have more than doubled in sub-Saharan Africa since the 1960s." And the long-term trend in mortality has been sharply downward. These improvements have been highly uneven, since poorer people in poorer countries have benefitted least, but they have been real. The recent difficulties in many cases therefore represent pauses and setbacks in long-term trends of improvement. Nonetheless, in designing economic adjustment programs, protective policies are clearly necessary if health conditions are to be maintained in times of economic adversity.

A third set of conclusions from these chapters emphasizes the need to do more in times of economic crisis than simply to adopt protective health policies. If health policies were in good shape for normal conditions, then it might be enough to design modifications for times of crisis. But this is far from the case. The health policies of developing countries need improvement not just to mitigate the consequences of short-run economic crisis, but also to achieve better results within the severe economic constraints that will persist for the next few decades. The two sets of policies are inextricably connected, and it may be possible in some instances to use the spur of crisis to achieve improvements needed for the longer run.

Griffiths, for example, notes that a considerable range of improvements are needed for developing countries to deal sensibly with drugs: more accurate prescription and more efficient use of drugs; more economical procurement, storage, and transport of drugs; policies to reduce the large numbers of marginally useful drugs that unnecessarily absorb scarce foreign exchange and consumer income; and a variety of others. All these steps will help the longer-run task of providing the best drug supply at the least cost for the health needs of developing countries. They will also assist a country in meeting the effects of possible economic crises.

The complex links between policies for times of crisis and policies for the longer run are well illustrated in Chapter 16 by Donald Shepard and Elisabeth Benjamin. They argue strongly for the introduction or strengthening of user fees as a means of mobilizing financial support to pay the recurrent costs of health services. Shepard and Benjamin point to the persuasive evidence from many countries that people are able and willing to pay, especially for tangible items like drugs. They also note, however, that the introduction of user fees for public sector health services can encounter administrative and political obstacles. Arrangements must be made for those who cannot afford to pay. In many countries there will be opposition on principle to fees for service in the public health sector. Moreover, if fees are charged, users may demand more reliable services from health providers.

Nevertheless, Shepard and Benjamin make a strong case that user fees will permit more health services to be provided with less burden on public revenues. Where such fees exist, they can "insulate health services from contractions in government budgets resulting from economic crises." Thus they can be a valuable contribution to maintaining health services in times of economic adjustment. But the installation of user fees may be easiest when they are linked with improvements in quality or access to care. Consequently, user fees should be introduced before a crisis occurs, not during it. The guideline is clear: health policies for times of crisis are likely to work best when based on solid policies in place for the longer run.

Conclusions

The chapters in this volume demonstrate the rich implications for policy in bringing together economists and public health experts, both in considering policies for times of economic crisis and policies for the longer pull. The interactions among these specialists will be more valuable when more data, especially on health and nutrition, are available. Toward this end, the development of better surveillance and monitoring information is urgent.

Second, many ways already exist to improve the planning by economists and others to take account of the effects of economic adjustments on health and nutrition. Both economic adjustment programs and health and nutrition programs could be adapted to achieve more humane and less damaging results during economic crises, while still allowing the necessary shifts in balances of payments, budgets, and other economic circumstances. Many modifications in standard policy, however, would encounter a common obstacle to change in developing countries: the needed changes would benefit the less powerful but could threaten the more powerful.

Finally, this book throws fresh light on the structural difficulty in today's world that international economic forces tend to work out their effects in one-sided ways. The banks in rich countries that made unwise loans have suffered little; the adjustments have fallen in overwhelming measure on the people in poor countries. Yet few systematic correctives for this problem seem in view.

PART I

ECONOMIC ADJUSTMENT: EFFECTS ON HEALTH AND NUTRITION

2

Macro Effects of Myriad Shocks: Developing Countries in the World Economy

Lance Taylor

How developing countries are inserted into the global economy is a topic of long-standing debate. Its intensity sharpened over the past decade with the successive shocks that hit the system—the oil price jumps of 1973 and 1979, interest rate increases that began in 1979, a steady deterioration in primary commodity terms of trade since the mid-1970s, the debt crisis of 1982, and the very recent reductions in interest rates, oil prices, and the strength of the dollar. The latest events are the only ones that can be read as economically favorable to the Third World, but as we will see, even their promised benefits may be small.

This chapter reviews the evidence regarding effects of the shocks and theories about how worldwide economic change in general is transmitted to the poor countries. The discussion is mostly from outside a national economy, since Behrman's chapter in this volume reviews the scene inside very well. Together, the two chapters cover both global and national macroeconomics as they impinge on the open economies in the Third World.

We begin the discussion with a synopsis of the economic developments over the past fifteen to twenty years that have been especially important for countries of the Third World. Issues specifically related to their external debt situation are taken up next. The discussion then turns a bit more theoretical, presenting an overview of the standard global macro model. This model is then applied to illustrate the range of

17

output growth prospects that may face poor countries over the next few years. I will discuss how they responded to external shocks in the recent past. Finally, implications for domestic health and nutrition are briefly drawn.

Global Macroeconomics

An impressive growth performance by developing countries was rudely interrupted in the early 1980s. More generally, external economic forces acting upon the Third World have changed dramatically over the past quarter century. These events can be organized in terms of a simple global macro model. The theory is set out in Section 3, while we present an introductory quantitative assessment here.

The prime mover in the system is the North—the main source of demand for exports from lesser developed countries (LDCs). Growth in the Organization for Economic Cooperation and Development (OECD) countries, a group of industrial nations, was fairly steady in the benign 1960s but fluctuated violently in the 1970s and 1980s in the wake of the oil price shocks of 1973 and 1979. A deeper trend was the decline in productivity growth in the industrialized economies. Productivity increases started to slow several years before 1973 and have yet to recover.

The terms of trade (or relative prices) between developing country imports and exports—the key determinants of their short-run trade account—followed a complicated trajectory. They hit a long-term peak after the first oil shock but went down violently following the second and remained low through 1985. This long trough has led some observers to detect a permanent deterioration in Third World export prices—an old theme discussed in more detail below. The factors influencing the terms of trade are complex—cycle and growth in the OECD countries, supply changes, and the strength of the dollar (since most primary commodity prices are denominated in that currency)—and forecasting long-term shifts has proved impossible in the past. However, for the immediate future, there are few signs that the terms of trade will strongly recover. Five to ten years of low prices are an ominous portent for Third World primary commodity exporters.

The sudden rise in external debt of the developing countries was the most publicized economic event of the late 1970s and early 1980s—the "crisis" which began in 1982 still dominates financial markets. The maneuvers of the major creditors and debtors—"money center" banks and countries like Brazil, Mexico, Argentina, and the Republic of Korea—have been amply documented in the press. The plight of smaller, poorer borrowing countries is less well known. Many owe 2 percent or more of their gross national product (GNP)—up to half of their annual flow of imports of capital goods—in interest obligations alone. Their future possibilities for growth, highly dependent on the deployment of imported machinery and equipment, are correspondingly dim.

The situation in the not too distant past was more favorable than it is today. In the two decades between 1960 and 1980 the developing countries made impressive economic progress. As shown in Table 2.1, developing market economies grew at 5.2 percent per year between 1961 and 1973 and at a still solid 3.8 percent between 1974 and 1980. These rates were above those of the developed market economies in the same periods, and substantially higher than the historical speed of expansion of the now industrialized countries.

This achievement has been put in jeopardy by the world recession that began in 1980 (the strong economic performance of the United States in 1984–85 notwithstanding). As Table 2.1 shows, the story of the 1980s is slow or negative growth tempered by a mild recovery in

Table 2.1
Population, GDP Per Capita, and GDP Growth Rates by Major World Regions

	Popu-lation (millions)	GDP per Capita in 1980	Growth Rates of GDP (percent)						
			1961–1973	1974–1980	1981	1982	1983	1984	1985
Developing Market Economies	2160	546	5.2	3.8	1.3	0.4	0.2	3.3	2.5–3.5
Africa	440	459	6.1	4.3	−0.2	−0.6	−0.5	2.1	1.0–2.0
East and South Asia	1248	251	4.8	6.0	6.6	3.5	5.5	5.7	3.0–4.0
West Asia	124	1593	7.3	5.1	−3.5	−4.6	−1.3	1.2	2.0–3.0
Western Hemi-sphere	349	1343	4.8	6.0	0.7	−1.4	−2.6	2.6	3.0–4.0
Developed Market Economies	763	6347	4.9	3.2	1.4	−0.2	2.5	4.6	2.0–3.0
Selected Countries									
Ivory Coast	8	322	7.6	6.7	1.4	−3.8	−4.2	−2.2	2.0
Kenya	16	420	7.1	4.8	3.9	1.6	3.8	0.9	2.0
Sudan	19	410	0.9	9.0	3.2	4.2	−2.1	−2.4	−8.0
Zambia	6	560	3.9	0.3	6.2	−2.8	−2.0	−1.3	2.0
Egypt	40	1001	4.7	9.4	7.8	5.9	5.4	5.2	3.0
Turkey	45	1470	6.2	4.6	4.4	5.0	3.7	5.8	4.0
Sri Lanka	15	270	4.2	4.8	5.8	5.1	5.0	5.0	4.0
India	673	240	3.6	4.1	5.8	2.9	7.7	4.5	4.0
Bangladesh	89	130	2.0	6.1	5.9	1.1	2.9	4.5	4.0
Thailand	47	670	8.0	7.5	6.3	4.1	5.9	6.0	5.0
South Korea	38	1520	9.0	8.6	6.9	5.5	9.5	7.9	6.0
China	977	290	7.1	5.4	4.9	7.7	9.6	14.0	11.0
Brazil	119	2050	6.9	6.8	−1.6	0.1	−3.2	4.5	7.0
Mexico	70	2090	7.7	6.2	7.9	−0.5	−5.3	3.5	1.0
Peru	17	930	4.5	2.4	3.9	0.4	−10.9	4.8	2.0
Jamaica	2	1040	4.9	−2.6	2.5	1.0	2.0	−0.4	−4.0

Source: United Nations, World Bank.

1982–84 which may have tailed off in 1985. The few bright spots include India and China among the poorer countries, East Asian middle income economies, and Brazil in mid-decade. For the rest of the Third World the recent record has been bleak.

At root, the poor growth performance of the developing countries is caused by the economic slump of the industrialized world. Longer-term prospects are uncertain. The main short-run problems the poor economies face in their external relationships are (a) a reduction in world demand for their export products (particularly agriculture commodities and minerals) stemming from slow growth in OECD economies, (b) an adverse shift in the terms of trade, caused by several factors and perhaps a sign of a downward trend, and (c) an increase in payment obligations for amortization and interest on outstanding debt, made especially acute by extremely high interest on floating rate debt since 1980. Longer-term handicaps include a reduction in foreign aid and complete revulsion of the private banking sector from loans to the Third World since 1982.

Factors (a) through (c) have played havoc with the external current account deficits of the non-oil developing countries, which rose to around $100 billion in 1980–81, but fell back to $50 billion or less thereafter. If their *trade* account after interest and other "factor payments" are subtracted from the current deficit, poor countries were running a historically unprecedented surplus of $15 billion by 1984. These changes after 1982 are directly related to the slow growth rates shown in Table 2.1. We will see below that a time-tested method to improve the external account is to reduce the internal level of economic activity. This is exactly what foreign exchange constrained economies have done. They have also made extreme efforts to increase the exportability of their products and reduce import coefficients. As discussed later, a study sponsored by the United Nations shows that in the period 1978–81/82, twelve of fourteen countries that suffered adverse external shocks increased their ratios of exports to GNP. The mean (median) increase was 3.0 (2.9) percent—a remarkable achievement (Helleiner, 1986). Eight of the countries also reduced import ratios. However, there was generalized reduction in gross capital formation in the study's sample countries after the second set of worldwide economic shocks in the late 1970s. Such a decrease in investment did not occur after the first oil shock in 1973, as the solid growth rates of the developing countries until 1980 testify. Further improvements in "tradeability" and adequate growth will be impossible unless the investment cuts are restored. The problem is that the surest way to improve the current account by economic contraction is to limit import-intensive capital formation. A vicious circle appears—cutting investment to improve the current account in the short run makes potential foreign exchange shortfalls more severe in the future. Many economies are on this self-destructive treadmill.

External Debt

The growth in foreign debt of developing countries has gone hand in hand with their deteriorating trade position—rapid expansion while countries ran current account deficits in the 1970s and an abrupt halt as trade accounts were forced into surplus after 1982. The year 1981 is a useful reference point. It immediately preceded the Malvinas/Falklands War and the Mexican crisis which ushered in the current international capital regime. Net debt in fact continued to grow through much of 1982, but its expansion after the events surrounding Mexico in August largely took the form of rollover advances by banks to cover interest obligations only. Hence, 1981 gives a good snapshot of the end of a bygone era.

Data on the evolution of long-term debt (maturity period exceeding one year) from public and private sources owed by representative countries and regions appear in Table 2.2. The analysis that follows concentrates on these numbers, but it should be recognized that developing countries have substantial short term obligations as well—estimates of total debt for all countries in the World Bank's Debtor Reporting Service in 1981 were $470 billion long-run and $145 billion short-run. The usual simplifying assumption—implicitly accepted here—is that short-run debt is tied to trade finance and can be expected to roll over so long as trade flows are not disrupted.

Three conclusions follow from Table 2.2. First, the share of debt from public sources in GNP declined for many middle income countries (especially in Latin America) that "graduated" from foreign assistance programs in the 1970s. However, obligations to foreign, public creditors rose sharply in smaller, poorer countries. A hidden feature of the debt crisis takes the form of the extremely high obligations (as shares of GNP and exports) to both public and private creditors of many of the poorest countries of the world. Some of the major recipients of public loans are in Asia and the Western Hemisphere, but Table 2.2 shows that African countries in the 1970s rapidly caught up. Their situation became more difficult in the 1980s as overseas development assistance and other official credits stagnated in current dollars and fell in real terms. According to World Bank data, overseas development assistance from OECD countries and other official capital flows in *current* dollars were 1980, $32.6 billion; 1981, 32.1; 1982, 35.1; 1983, 32.5; 1984, 32.2.

Table 2.2

The Evolution of Debt for Selected Countries, 1970–81 (% of GNP)

	Public Sources				Private Sources			
	1970	1976	1981		1970	1976	1981	
Turkey	14.00	8.02	15.44		0.66	0.72	8.50	
Yugoslavia	7.04	7.28	6.31		2.50	1.29	2.22	
Syria	10.57	13.10	13.74		2.40	2.31	0.72	
Indonesia	23.66	15.86	11.47		3.04	10.97	6.81	
India	14.17	14.48	10.11		0.61	0.33	0.41	
Korea (Rep.)	7.12	12.17	11.93		13.77	12.53	18.99	
Malaysia	5.98	6.44	6.53		3.84	8.09	12.25	
Pakistan	17.52	43.21	29.29		1.72	1.78	1.81	
Philippines	4.07	6.17	8.69		4.74	5.62	10.45	
Singapore	7.34	6.55	3.97		0.68	5.42	6.24	
Thailand	4.45	4.06	7.89		0.50	0.91	6.45	
Burma	3.50	6.69	24.62		1.10	0.90	5.16	
Sri Lanka	11.02	16.12	29.21		2.77	3.25	6.67	
Bangladesh		26.04	34.26			1.63	1.31	
Nepal	0.23	3.15	9.94		0.10	0.04	0.00	
Algeria	10.41	7.06	5.98	(1980)	9.79	0.64	30.41	(1980)
Gabon	19.81	7.46	11.87	(1979)	7.28	28.41	32.95	(1979)
Nigeria	4.88	1.92	1.40		1.22	0.14	5.21	
Egypt	18.63	29.52	39.15		5.44	6.43	7.76	
Cameroon	11.06	12.59	19.37	(1979)	1.07	6.11	11.81	(1979)
Ethiopia	7.86	13.41	17.89		1.61	0.46	1.66	
Ivory Coast	9.65	9.48	10.40	(1979)	7.49	15.49	25.83	(1979)
Kenya	14.20	17.12	20.06		5.24	2.83	13.28	
Zimbabwe	5.82	1.32	3.10		9.56	2.84	11.38	
Zaire	5.08	23.07	47.72		11.51	40.89	25.82	
Africa, Lesser Developed Economies:								
Malawi	27.77	35.42	35.40		10.36	8.58	17.40	
Sudan	13.41	20.44	19.31	(1978)	2.30	12.76	11.89	(1978)
Tanzania	11.88	31.03	26.01	(1980)	7.46	1.51	1.56	(1980)
Argentina	2.89	2.21	1.55		5.64	6.01	6.94	
Brazil	4.10	2.90	2.51		2.97	8.31	12.76	
Chile	14.15	19.18	4.31		10.64	12.80	9.15	
Colombia	15.21	11.52	7.07		2.45	4.40	6.53	
Ecuador	9.31	6.33	6.46		3.67	5.41	17.98	
Mexico	3.30	2.97	2.22		5.72	14.95	15.57	
Peru	5.99	9.99	15.56		7.77	17.39	14.12	
Venezuela	3.14	1.70	0.53		3.12	7.69	16.26	
Bolivia	25.99	20.03	20.53	(1980)	20.00	16.24	18.04	(1980)
Paraguay	13.76	10.68	8.50		5.05	3.25	4.36	
Uruguay	5.79	6.91	2.71		5.19	11.18	8.56	
Carib. & Central America:								
Costa Rica	9.75	12.69	33.95		3.89	9.53	36.63	
Domin. Rep.	13.62	8.58	10.68	(1980)	0.65	4.19	7.18	(1980)
Guatemala	2.85	4.66	7.90		2.74	0.15	0.00	
Jamaica	3.80	10.75	31.73		7.18	18.41	17.05	
Nicaragua	14.18	17.16	47.79	(1979)	5.83	18.57	29.01	(1979)
Panama	8.88	16.50	16.40	(1980)	9.67	38.04	49.90	(1980)
Trin. & Tob.	5.17	2.94	2.53	(1979)	6.44	0.90	7.87	(1979)

Source: Data on debt from the World Bank and on GNP (deflated by current exchange rates) from the International Monetary Fund.

Flows from OPEC countries fell from $9.7 billion in 1980 to $6.8 billion in 1982. This slowdown in foreign aid efforts marked a significant reversal in a trend of growth that began in the 1950s.

Second, debt from private sources increased rapidly for most countries. The South Asian region lagged in this process, but the ratio of private credit to GNP rose sharply elsewhere (especially in Africa and the Latin American/Caribbean zone). Ratios of private debt to GNP or exports are higher for many smaller countries than for the major debtors (Brazil, Mexico, Korea, etc.). The same is true of interest obligations, since all developing economies pay floating, current interest rates on the bulk of their private debt.

Third, these observations suggest that countries which borrowed heavily from private sources fall broadly into two groups. At one extreme, some small, open economies took enough credit to raise their debt/GNP ratios by large increments. Such increases are especially notable in African and Western Hemisphere countries, hit hard by external shocks. For most of the poorer economies, recourse to foreign debt is best seen as an attempt to cushion the decade's adverse developments in trade.

Larger borrowers in absolute magnitude had smaller increases in their private debt shares of GNP. One can argue that their borrowing was of a more discretionary nature as well. They were offered large loans and chose to take them. Some of the larger Asian economies and a few from Africa either were more prudent or did not get as much access to Eurodollar credits. They started out with lower private debt ratios and increased them rather less.

Without losing sight of immediate problems, it makes sense to place the debt issue of the 1980s against a long-term background, to ask whether secular or merely conjunctural forces underlay the crisis that began in 1982. The natural time of reference is the "long" 19th Century that culminated in World War I. During that period, foreign capital flows originated largely in Britain, France and (later) Germany. Now developed economies were the major debtors, with annual inflows ranging up to 10 percent of GNP and one-half of capital formation in peak years in Canada, Australia, and the Scandinavian countries. Poorer nations, many still colonies, also received some international investment. By 1914, Latin American, African, and Asian countries accounted for 43 percent of outstanding foreign capital (Kuznets, 1966).

Flows diminished drastically in the decades between the wars, including the depression years. In 1913 prices, international capital movements in the early 1900s were on the order of a billion dollars per year. On average, annual flows dropped to $100–200 million between 1920 and 1940 and then recovered to about three billion (seven billion in current dollars) in the late 1950s. By that time the United States had emerged as the major creditor.

There were also changes in forms of finance. Long term bonds originating in London and Paris were the chosen vehicle in the 19th century. Private bondholders predominated, and the issues were usually tied to investment projects in recipient countries—to this day trolley cars in Rio de Janeiro are called "bondis" in honor of a long-forgotten British loan. After 1945 there was a shift toward direct foreign investment and (especially) official donations and loans, which accounted for over one-half of annual flows in the late 1950s.

The process of bond finance was by no means tranquil. Numerous scholars have detected cycles of capital flows to different parts of the world, with a time period of decades. Kindleberger (1985) observes:

> . . . the bond market experienced spurts of lending—for Latin America in the 1820s, the United States in the 1830s, for Latin America again in the 1850s, Canada from 1900 to 1913, Latin America and Australia (plus Germany) in the 1920s—but . . . foreign lending to a particular area died away between spurts . . . it is perhaps fair to say that after a boom in lending to LDCs followed by default, *European capital markets lost interest for roughly 30 years before lending again.* (Emphasis added.)

If the historical pattern holds, the current trough in private lending may persist for about a decade before beginning another upswing, though of course individual countries may get access to capital markets in the meantime—again consistent with historical experience. Also, it is worth noting that the major vehicle for the lending episode of the 1970s was different from the one in the 19th Century—syndicated Eurocurrency (mostly Eurodollar) loans from banks as opposed to bonds. Bank credits were extended at floating interest rates, tied to the London Interbank Offered Rate or LIBOR. After a spell of being low or negative in the middle of the decade, real interest rates rose sharply after 1979. How much of the increase was due to restrictive OECD monetary policy and how much to revulsion from developing country loans on the part of banks is not clear. If revulsion was the key factor, the shrinkage of loans in the 1980s bodes ill for developing country borrowing for the rest of this century.

North-South Interactions

The numbers just presented on growth, trade, and debt show the intricacy of the South's role in the global macroeconomic system. There are other complications, explored in this section. We begin with a summary of the "standard" North-South model and go on later to ask in quantitative terms how much the South is likely to benefit from changes in the key variables—the interest rate, the strength of the dollar and growth in industrialized countries. There is a wide range of possibilities, not all favorable by any means.

Development economists have long pondered the role of the South in trade and thirty years ago sketched a model framework which in successive elaborations arrives at a plausible description of the world system. The initial approximation is that poor countries are hewers of raw materials and drawers of oil for the rich. Old trade patterns persist, imposed by colonialism and developing countries' own lack of technical mastery when they were integrated into the global economy last century. Developing countries export commodities whose sales at best expand as rapidly as the industrial countries' aggregate demand. To a large extent, prices of LDC exports are denominated in dollars, and they fluctuate widely relative to prices of goods exported by rich economies. Since developing economies in the aggregate are small compared to the OECD, their own output fluctuations only weakly influence economic conditions in the developed world.

This view of the developing countries' international plight dates back at least to Prebisch (1959) and Nurkese (1959); in modified form it is advocated by Lewis (1980) as well. It is clearly an oversimplification, if only because the major debtors are newly industrializing countries (NICs) which have learned to export goods with higher demand and supply elasticities than the primary commodities envisaged by Prebisch. Their success shows that developing economies are not so tightly constrained by their external economic history as the model suggests—there do exist autonomous paths to sustained growth.

If we ignore such possibilities for the moment, then the model is driven by growth in the First World—it needs the corresponding theory. One option is to assume that investment is determined by available saving as in Kaldor (1976); alternatively, growth may be determined by investment along Keynesian lines as in Taylor (1981). In the latter case, better terms of trade for developing countries will stimulate their demand for imports and feed back into export-led growth in the rich countries. In the Kaldor version, industrial countries will grow more slowly as their imports become more costly. Either way, the response will be weak, and growth in the overall system will largely depend on what happens in the North.

This simple structure requires elaboration before it can be applied to the world of the 1970s and now. First there were the oil price shocks. It is simplest to follow Taylor (1981) and treat OPEC not as part of the south but as an independent agent with control over its own product price (a simplification that made more sense for 1973 than it does after more than a decade of energy substitution and new oil discoveries). A rise in the oil price for a Keynesian North will reduce aggregate demand. A cumulative process can ensue which will lead to slower growth in both North and South until a new steady state is reached. Such a scenario did not unfold in the 1970s, largely because of the resource transfer to the South that led to the buildup of debt. The contractionary effect of the shocks was present but overwhelmed until late in the decade by other events. Thereafter, especially for the non-NICs, its impact became clear.

A second event—and the major blow to the poorer developing countries—was deterioration of their terms of trade. Price fluctuations for primary commodities are complex, involving supply, demand and OECD business cycle effects. According to indexes constructed by the IMF (1984), non-oil commodity prices deflated by the United Nations manufactures price index recovered strongly in 1976 and 1977 after the first oil shock but declined steadily from 1978 on.

Explanations for the deterioration differ. First, there is the old structuralist idea that developing countries' terms of trade are likely to suffer a long-term decline for several reasons—low income elasticities implying slow growth of demand for primary products in the North, an international market structure in which technical progress leads to lower export prices in the South and higher real wages in the North, the diversity of Southern economies which makes it impossible for them to form cartels (except for petroleum producers in their brief decade of glory) to hold up prices by restricting supply.

The arguments sound plausible, but empirically it is difficult to find long-term trends in the terms of trade (Evans, 1979; Spraos, 1983). The history since World War II is mixed—a historical high after the Korean conflict, fluctuating decline until the mid-1970s when there was another peak, and a steady decrease since. Even from the IMF, Chu and Morrison (1984) observe that "The long-term downward trend in real commodity prices from 1972 to 1982 has been more than twice the trend from 1957 to 1971. In addition, primary commodity prices during 1972–82 were more than three times as unstable as they were during 1957–71 . . ." Fleisig and van Wijnbergen (1985) add econometrically a seven percent negative annual terms of trade trend in 1970–84. At long last, Prebisch's (1950) 35-year-old prediction may be coming true. Or it may not—future trends are unknowable in any operational sense.

A second set of factors affecting the terms of trade centers around trend and growth in the OECD and the strength of the dollar. Regarding the latter, many authors point out that a fall of the mark, say, will drive up the perceived cost to German importers of a commodity whose price is fixed in dollars. That price will decline relative to world inflation, and if the good in question is exported by a small country, its terms of trade will worsen. In the early 1980s many primary exporters were hit hard by this phenomenon; they benefitted from a depreciating dollar in the late 1970s. Econometric estimates of the terms of trade elasticity with respect to the average dollar exchange rate range between one-half and one. (The economists's "elasticity" concept relates percentage changes—if the elasticity is one-half, a 10 percent weakening or devaluation of the dollar will increase the terms of trade by 5 percent.)

Extra Northern growth will of course increase both price and volume of Southern exports. The magnitudes of the effects are controversial. In a well known defense of the "muddling-through" strategy for resolution of the debt crisis (or for—on Panglossian lines—the unavoidable desirability of the poor countries' paying off the banks), Cline (1984) uses a marginal elasticity of LDC export values with respect to OECD growth of three. More sensible econometrics, e.g., Marquez and McNeilly (1986), virtually cuts Cline's number by half. As illustrated below, the difference matters. To enable poor countries to export enough to cover their debt burdens, Cline requires 3 percent annual OECD growth; Marquez and McNeilly require 4.3 percent.

Countries that borrowed heavily—the NICs mostly—were hit harder by interest rate increases than by deteriorating terms of trade. Real rates were low (or negative, depending on the inflation index one uses) throughout most of the 1970s. There was an upward spike in 1979, and only very recently have real rates begun to decline. As usual, economists have more than enough explanations for this one set of events. They include:

First, a dedicated and largely successful effort by the U.S. Federal Reserve to thwart inflation by tight monetary policy. In this scenario, dear money drives up interest rates and reduces activity enough to make cost-based price pressures go away. Providentially, high interest rates draw in enough capital from other OECD countries and OPEC to finance large American fiscal deficits in the 1980s. The dollar appreciates to ratify the trade deficit required to absorb the transfer, and the United States' inflation rate thereby falls. Concurrent deregulation of financial markets and lagged pressures by rentiers to keep their real income flows up after a long period of low real rates combined to support the Fed's policy stance.

Second, in flow terms, there was an OECD fiscal and/or investment imbalance. Government spending net of tax-*cum*-transfer receipts rose, or else there was a burst of private investment demand in the early 1980s. These scenarios from van Wijnbergen (1985) and Blanchard and Summers (1984) respectively—presuppose that interest rates go up in response to *flow* excess demands for loanable funds. They are dubious on theoretical grounds, since after all one aspect of the Keynesian revolution was an emphasis on determination of interest rates in markets for asset *stocks*. Stock-based explanations of the interest rate excursion have not shown up in the recent literature.

Third, in line with the arguments presented above, there was clear revulsion from loans to developing countries after 1982. Explicit credit rationing was a consequence, but high world interest rates as banks searched for safe havens in which to place assets was another.

In sum, one has a series of explanations for a single set of events, without any clear means to distinguish among them. The situation leaves perspectives for the future decidedly unclear. The uncertainty is crucial for developing economies, as can be illustrated with a simple set of calculations.

The Range of Prospects

There are enough complications in the model just sketched to render all quantitative predictions of North-South economic interactions dubious. Nonetheless, econometricians have not been daunted by the task. They have concentrated on export earnings of the debtor countries and on the effects of interest rate changes on the current account. Their goal is to forecast changes in debt volume over the medium term. This approach leaves out all the complexity of the Prebisch-Nurkse view of North-South interaction and runs from current account changes to guesses about shifts in the volume of debt. The possibility that loans may simply dry up from the supply side is not taken into account.

The main linkages go through export volumes, terms of trade, and interest costs. Dramatically lower petroleum prices in the late 1980s could also affect the picture, but more by stimulating OECD growth than by cutting developing countries' import costs. In mid-1986, growth rate projections for the OECD were approaching three percent annually in 1986–87, up from previously lower levels as forecasters factored the oil price reductions into their models. As we will see shortly, there would be beneficial effects on the LDCs, but perhaps not beneficial enough.

The key stylized fact is the dependence of most poor countries on primary product exports with income-inelastic First World demand—in his Nobel Prize Lecture, Lewis (1980) talks about a quantity elasticity between 0.8 and 0.9. With the emergence of the NICs, which are heavily indebted but export income-elastic manufactures, the representative value of the income elasticity for all developing countries may have risen—say it is one. If the price elasticities of export demand and supply are both 0.3, then one can calculate that the purchasing power of LDC exports (volume plus price changes) will have an elasticity of about 2.2 with respect to advanced country income (say OECD real GNP). As noted above, econometric estimates usually give numbers of this size.

The next effect is the strength of the dollar. In a simple model a rise in the dollar vis-a-vis currencies of other advanced countries will drive down commodity prices, with the change depending on price elasticities of all three regions (U.S., the rest of OECD, and the developing world). Assume that developing countries remain pegged to the dollar. Then the elasticity of the commodity price change with respect to the dollar exchange rate is the ratio of the non-U.S. industrial countries' demand elasticity to the sum of the demand elasticity and the supply elasticity (treating the United States as the exporter, without loss of generality). Assume a demand elasticity of 0.3 and a supply elasticity of 0.3 from the United States. The result is that the commodity price will have an elasticity of about − 0.5 with respect to the dollar exchange rate. The implication is that dollar depreciation will raise revenues for raw material exporters.

Together with the dollar exchange rate, the interest rate has a major impact on debt burdens. Magnitudes vary across countries, since very poor ones largely obtain foreign aid at fixed, low-interest rates while middle income economies borrow from banks at a spread over the floating London Interbank Offered Rate. For major borrowers, prospects for meeting their debt obligations can be shown to depend at least as much on interest rate changes as on export volumes and prices.

To get a feel for the numbers, we can apply these elasticities to data for the twenty-five largest debtors, taken from the IMF. For the year 1984, their estimated balance of payments figures are, in billions of dollars:

Exports	272	Transfers and direct foreign investment	9
Imports	249	Reserve changes and errors and omissions	− 16
Net Services	− 54	Official loans	15
		Banks and other loans	23
Current Account	− 31	Capital Account	31

Total debt was 640; at an approximate interest rate of 10 percent, interest payments would exhaust net service payments.

Now assume that the capital account items stay constant and postulate the following elasticities:

Real imports with respect to borrowers' GDP	2.0
Value of exports with respect to OECD real income	2.2
Terms of trade with respect to dollar exchange rate	−0.5

The latter two values come from the calculations above, and the elasticity of real imports with respect to real gross domestic product (GDP) in developing countries is consistent with country econometric studies like those summarized in Helleiner (1986).

In a simple trade gap calculation, additional foreign exchange translates into additional capacity to import and permits faster growth. The extra flows of dollars can come from (1) faster OECD growth which generates export revenues at the elasticity 2.2; (2) dollar depreciation which increases the developing countries' terms of trade according to the elasticity 0.5; (3) interest rate reductions which reduce the payments on outstanding debt. Table 2.3 shows two simple calculations based on different hypotheses with respect to changes in these three variables, giving changes in the growth rate of developing countries.

The example is oversimplified but underlines the fact that the borrower LDC's growth rate will be influenced by three forces of roughly equal weight which can move independently of one another in the short to medium run. Reasonable variations in OECD growth, the dollar exchange rate and the interest rate can give rise to a wide range of possibilities for debt burdens and developing country growth. As of mid-1986, the dollar exchange rate and interest rates were moving favorably and OECD growth prospects were not bad. Whether or not these conditions will persist to support an adequate Third World growth rate in the present system into the 1990s is by no means certain. Following Marris (1985), it is easy to imagine scenarios—say continued bankers' revulsion from lending to LDCs coupled with capital flight from the dollar leading to high interest rates and economic stagnation

Table 2.3
Potential Effects of Changes in World Macro Variables on LDC Growth

	"Optimistic"		"Pessimistic"	
	Level	Contribution to LDC Growth (%)	Level	Contribution to LDC Growth (%)
OECD growth rate	0.03	3.6	0.01	1.2
Growth rate of dollar exchange rate	−0.10	2.7	0.05	−1.4
Change in interest rate	−0.01	1.3	0.01	−1.3
		7.6		1.5

worldwide—which would have disastrous effects on developing economies, especially the small and poor ones which are most open to external shocks.

Country Responses

How in fact have individual countries responded to shocks? From the outside, an economy may be forced to reduce its trade deficit or even run a surplus because of adverse shifts in the terms of trade, reduced export volumes, interest rate increases and so on. Within the national system, several responses are possible. Reductions in consumption (both public and private) or investment cut back aggregate demand and draw in a lesser volume of imports. An increased export effort permits external obligations to be met. Import substitution reduces the trade deficit for given levels of capacity utilization and growth.

Several recent studies use a broadly similar methodology of "differentiating the balance of payments" to try to quantify the importance of these different responses. Table 2.4 presents the results of one such decomposition exercise, reported by Helleiner (1986). The numbers are percentage shares of actual GNP; adverse shocks are positive and response which offset the shock are negative. Thus, Chile had an external shock of 16.3 percent of GNP in 1973–78. It further worsened its balance of payments 0.5 percent by increasing investment, improved it 2.9 percent by cutting consumption, and so on. To Helleiner's reported results we have added a further breakdown of countries by whether their overall policy was "inward-oriented" or "outward-oriented." Such classifications are treacherous. Nonetheless, they are widely discussed and for this reason we include one. The policy orientation split is based on Balassa (1985) as supplemented by Balassa and McCarthy (1984) and personal judgment, and is allegedly relevant for the mid-1970s. It also bears noting that the countries in the table are mostly middle-income and fairly large; data were simply not available to do decompositions for the smaller, poorer countries that were probably more severely affected by external events.

The first point that stands out in the numbers is that countries increasingly cut back investment to restrain import demand in 1978–82 as opposed to 1973–78—the potentially unfavorable effects on future growth have already been noted.

Second, most countries in the sample at least partially offset the shocks by improving their trade performance, raising export penetration in world markets and/or cutting import shares in GNP. Very broadly speaking, trade improvements outweighed domestic contraction as the main

Table 2.4
Responses to External Shocks as Shares of GNP

	1973–1978					1978–1982				
		Domestic Contraction		Trade Improvement			Domestic Contraction		Trade Improvement	
	Shock	Inv	Cons	Exps	Imps	Shock	Inv	Cons	Exps	Imps
Outward-Oriented										
Chile	16.3	0.5	-2.9	-9.3	2.1	3.8	-1.3	1.7	-5.0	2.6
Costa Rica	-2.8									
Indonesia	-6.8					-14.1				
Korea	8.2	3.4	-2.6	-19.8	11.4	9.2	-2.2	0.7	-7.2	-0.2
Pakistan	3.1	-0.2	0.2	2.4	0.9	7.6	-0.1	-0.1	-2.9	-2.3
Sri Lanka	-3.0					65.9	5.7	-10.1	-11.4	-42.1
Thailand	10.6	0.8	-1.4	-4.4	-3.2	9.5	-1.7	0.4	-8.8	-3.2
Uruguay	11.3	1.6	-2.4	-6.8	1.0	0.7	0.2	0.1	-2.0	2.3
Inward-Oriented										
Argentina	1.9	0.1	-0.4	-2.5	0.2	-0.9	-0.4	-0.0	-1.7	-1.1
Brazil	1.2	-0.2	0.4	0.5	-1.5	4.4	0.6	0.1	1.8	0.8
Colombia	-0.9					3.7				
Dominican Republic	5.5	0.3	0.2	-0.2	1.2	4.6	-1.0	1.1	-0.8	-4.5
Egypt	14.9	1.8	-4.0	-5.0	2.1	-0.9				
India	1.4	0.1	-0.2	-1.5	-0.1	1.5	0.0	0.1	-0.8	2.4
Ivory Coast	-3.7									
Mexico	0.2	0.1	-0.1	-1.0	0.2	-0.9				
Morocco	4.4	1.6	0.6	4.8	1.3					
Peru	3.2	-1.1	-0.1	-1.7	-6.5	-1.6				
Philippines	7.3	1.7	-0.8	-0.1	1.3	4.8	-0.3	0.2	-2.9	0.2
Sudan	3.8	0.5	1.2	5.0	-2.4	-1.3				
Tanzania	-3.6					8.9	0.4	-2.6	-5.4	-5.2
Turkey	3.0	0.5	-0.4	1.8	-3.7	4.7	-0.5	0.2	-3.6	1.4
Venezuela	-11.7					-13.2				
Zaire	5.8	-2.5	-6.9	11.2	-12.5					
Zambia	29.9	-6.1	2.0	5.0	-12.9	10.0	-6.3	8.7	8.6	-14.2

Source: Decompositions of shocks from Helleiner (1986); country classification based on Balassa (1985) and Balassa and McCarthy (1984).

Table 2.5
Summary of Responses to External Shocks by Policy Orientation

| | | | *1973–1978* | | | | | | *1978–1982* | | | |
| | | | *Domestic Contraction* | | *Trade Improvement* | | | | *Domestic Contraction* | | *Trade Improvement* | |
	Number	*Shock*	*Inv*	*Cons*	*Exps*	*Imps*	*Number*	*Shock*	*Inv*	*Cons*	*Exps*	*Imps*
Outward-Oriented	5						6					
Mean		9.9	1.2	-1.8	-7.6	2.4		16.1	0.1	-1.2	-6.2	-7.1
Median		10.6	0.8	-2.4	-6.8	1.0		9.3	-0.7	0.2	-6.1	-1.1
Inward-Oriented	13						8					
Mean		6.3	-0.0	-1.0	1.3	-2.6		4.7	-0.9	1.0	-0.6	-2.5
Median		3.8	0.1	-0.1	-0.1	0.2		4.7	-0.4	0.2	-0.8	-0.5

Source: Table 2.4.

adjustment mechanism for both groups of countries, especially in the latter period.

Third, adjustment data for the two groups are presented in summary form in Table 2.5. As a share of GNP, shocks were greater in the outward-oriented group, perhaps not surprising insofar as their initial trade shares were higher (presumably this was one of Balassa's criteria for classification). Relative to the magnitudes of their shocks, the outward-oriented countries were *not* substantially more successful in promoting trade improvement. Their record on maintaining investment demand was not better either, when one discounts Sri Lanka's success in keeping the externally financed Mahaveli irrigation project underway during the latter period. Taylor (1986) argues that presence or absence of trade distortions does not influence growth. The results in Table 2.5 further suggest that outward orientation (which is at least highly correlated with absence of distortions in the eyes of the orthodox) is no buffer against external shocks. Relative to GNP, the shocks themselves may be greater; relative to the size of the shock, trade improvement may be no stronger with an outwardly than an inwardly oriented policy stance. This point is developed more fully in terms of the historical experience of specific countries in Singh (1985).

Finally, it bears repeating that the large economies are over- represented in Table 2.4. The only countries with population markedly less than the convenient cutoff point of 20 million are Chile, Costa Rica, Sri Lanka, Uruguay, Dominican Republic, Ivory Coast, Peru, Venezuela, and Zambia. Their external shocks were large relative to GNP, reflecting the difficulties inherent in a small economy's unavoidable vulnerability to external forces when the external environment turns harsh.

Beyond countries' efforts to deal with acute foreign exchange shortages, several other aspects of the adjustment process are worth noting.

First, the major debtors in some ways enjoyed a foreign exchange bonanza in the 1970s. They reacted as common sense might predict, engaging in rapid, debt-led growth associated with exchange rate appreciation. They faced a difficult readjustment process in the 1980s. Before even their versatile economies recovered, major debtors like Korea and Brazil had spells of slow growth.

Second, the adjustment was more difficult for large debtors with open capital markets. They suffered capital flights of billions of dollars—Mexico lost $26.5 billion, Venezuela $22 billion, and Argentina $19.2 billion according to the World Bank's 1985 *World Development Report*. By contrast, exchange losses in Brazil, Colombia and Korea which have traditionally maintained functioning (if imperfect) controls on the capital market were far smaller. For the open countries, the dynamic sequence featured euphoria and capital inflows in the 1970s followed by massive outflows thereafter.

Third, as Singh (1985) points out, the large economies of India and China have traditionally followed conservative foreign borrowing practices. China, indeed, has massive reserves. As a consequence, they rode out the crises well. Southeast Asian countries on the whole borrowed more prudently than the Latin Americans, and this made their position in the 1980s less difficult.

Finally, with regard to inflation, fifteen of twenty-six countries receiving adverse shocks in 1979–82 according to Balassa and McCarthy (1984) saw their inflations accelerate, eight had rates which stayed essentially stable (within two percent per year) and three experienced declines. Though the period was one of inflation worldwide, the accelerations in many cases were large, suggesting that inflation is a common means of dealing with social conflicts arising from the output contraction that an unfavorable external shock entails. Those whose incomes are not fully indexed to price increases—some classes of workers, small farmers, the economically less powerful in general—will cut back consumption as their real purchasing power falls.

Some Conclusions

Economic discourse is lamentably abstract. What exactly do growth rate projections to the 1990s based on debatable hypotheses about global macroeconomic developments and wildly imprecise statistical estimates of the relevant parameters have to do with the health and nutrition of children and adults in the Third World? The answer, no doubt, is a great deal, but it is difficult to add much to that.

What we do know is that given their debt situation and poor external prospects, developing countries will have to undertake massive belt tightening in the foreseeable future. Even on the most Panglossian assumptions, the external situation may allow three or four percent annual output growth, scarcely enough to keep up with expansion of the population. More restrained projections are for substantially slower GDP increases, implying further reductions in national income per capita. Insofar as demand is restrained to fit external constraints by cutting back investment projects (*including* the investment involved in nutrition and education of children), prospects of future recovery become even more bleak.

Of course, things may change. The OECD countries may recover their buoyancy of the 1960s, stimulating imports from the poor countries. The debt obligations of the Third World in one way or another may not be met, which would release resources for domestic uses. Developing economies may learn to resume the growth rates of at least the 1970s even while externally constrained. Or, on the other hand, a run from the dollar may cause a worldwide economic crash unrivalled since the 1930s. We live in interesting times. It is not obvious that the poorer citizens in the poor economies will gain very much economically thereby.

References

Balassa, Bela. "Outward Orientation." Washington, D.C.: Development Research Department, World Bank, 1985.

Balassa, Bela, and F. Desmond McCarthy. "Adjustment Policies in Developing Countries, 1979–1983." Washington, D.C.: World Bank, 1984.

Behrman, Jere. "The Impact of Economic Adjustment Programs." Chapter 5 of this volume.

Blanchard, Olivier, and Lawrence Summers. "Perspectives on High World Real Interest Rates," *Brookings Papers on Economic Activity* 2 (1984): 273–324.

Chu, Ke-Young, and Thomas K. Morrison. "The 1981–82 Recession and Non-Oil Primary Commodity Prices," *International Monetary Fund Staff Papers* 31 (1984): 93–140.

Cline, William R. *International Debt: System Risk and Policy Response*. Washington, D.C.: Institute of International Economics, 1984.

Evans, David. "International Commodity Policy: UNCTAD and NIEO in Search of a Rationale," *World Development* 7 (1979): 259–277.

Fleisig, Heywood, and Sweder van Wijnbergen. "Primary Commodity Prices, the Business Cycle and the Real Exchange Rate of the Dollar." London: Center for Economic Policy Research, 1985.

Helleiner, G. K. "Balance of Payments Experience and Growth Prospects in Developing Countries: A Synthesis," *World Development* 14 (1986): 877–908.

International Monetary Fund. *World Economic Outlook*. Washington, D.C., 1984.

Kaldor, Nicholas. "Inflation and Recession in the World Economy," *Economic Journal* 86 (1976): 703–714.

Kindleberger, Charles P. "Historical Perspectives on Today's Third World Debt Problem," *Economies et Societés* 19 (1985): 109–134.

Kuznets, Simon S. *Modern Economic Growth*. New Haven, CT.: Yale University Press, 1966.

Lewis, W. Arthur. "The Slowing Down of the Engine of Growth." *American Economic Review* 70 (1980): 555–564.

Marquez, Jaime, and Caryl McNeilly. "Can Debtor Countries Sustain their Debts? Income and Price Elasticities for Exports of Developing Countries." Washington, D.C.: Federal Reserve Board, 1986.

Marris, Stephen. *Deficits and the Dollar: The World Economy at Risk*. Washington, D.C.: Institute of International Economics, 1985.

Nurkse, Ragnar. *Patterns of Trade and Development*. Stockholm: Almqvist and Wicksell, 1959.

Prebisch, Raul. "The Economic Development of Latin America and Its Principal Problems," *Economic Bulletin for Latin America* 7 (1950): 1–22.

————. "Commercial Policy in the Underdeveloped Countries," *American Economic Review* 49 (1959): 251–273.

Singh, Ajit. "The World Economy and the Comparative Economic Performance of Large Semi-Industrialized Countries: A Study of Asian and Latin American Economies." Cambridge: Faculty of Economics, University of Cambridge, 1985.

Spraos, John. *Equalizing Trade?* Oxford: Clarendon Press, 1983.

Taylor, Lance. "South-North Trade and Southern Growth: Bleak Prospects from a Structuralist Point of View," *Journal of International Economics* 11 (1981): 589–602.

————. "Trade and Growth," *Review of Black Political Economy* 14:4 (1986): 17–36.

van Wijnbergen, Sweder. "Fiscal Policy and World Interest Rates: An Empirical Analysis." Washington, D.C.: Country Policy Department, World Bank, 1985.

3

Sri Lanka: A Case Study from the Third World

S. W. R. de A. Samarasinghe

In recent years economic adjustment programs have been implemented in many developing countries, often with the help of the International Monetary Fund (IMF) (see, for example, Killick, 1984a and 1984b), with a mixture of short-term and long-term objectives in mind. The short-term objectives are to reduce the balance of payments (BOP) deficit and/or high rates of inflation. The long-term goals are a shift in the economy from state activity and state control to private sector activity and market control and the acceleration of economic growth.

This chapter examines the nature of economic adjustments attempted in Sri Lanka after 1977 and their impact on the country's health and nutrition. Such an impact study can have two related but conceptually distinct dimensions. One is the impact of the adjustment program on "intervening" or "input" variables, such as employment, income, government food subsidies, food output, government expenditure on health, that affect the community's health and nutrition. The other is the ultimate result in health and nutrition as measured by indices of mortality, morbidity, and nutrition and health status.

There have been some studies on certain aspects of these issues in relation to Sri Lanka's experience after 1977. In particular, the changes in the food subsidies and the impact of those changes on nutrition have

*This chapter was prepared while the author was a Takemi Fellow in International Health at the Harvard School of Public Health in 1985–86. The author wishes to thank the Takemi Program and the Ford Foundation for the Fellowship, the University of Peradeniya for giving sabbatical leave of absence, and participants in the Takemi Symposium and seminars for their comments.

been comprehensively reviewed by a number of official and unofficial studies. A few other studies have examined the effects of the 1978 reforms on income distribution. In this chapter we shall refer to the more important findings of some of these and review some other areas that deserve further attention.

Two other points about the focus of this chapter should be noted. Because the outcome variables such as mortality and morbidity are only partly related to the intervening variables that are directly affected by the adjustment program, it is methodologically difficult to distinguish sharply between the effects of the adjustment program and the influence of other factors many of which are structural. Secondly, based on Sri Lanka's experience, we hope to raise certain conceptual issues concerning the management of health and nutrition and, more broadly, social welfare in the face of national and international economic crises. An economic crisis normally has negative implications for social welfare. But it also forces a society to re-examine traditional structures and systems which, having outlived the original purpose for which they were created, can become inefficient. Thus not all sacrifices that a society is called upon to make need be in vain if the system that emerges from the crisis can be made to work better than the one that it replaced.

The chapter is divided into six sections. The first discusses some conceptual perspectives on adjustment programs as they relate to social welfare. The second describes the political and economic conditions that prevailed in Sri Lanka when the adjustment program was initiated. Next I outline the principal elements of the 1977 adjustment program. The fourth section analyzes the impact of the adjustment program on the intervening variables. The fifth section discusses the changes, if any, in nutrition status, morbidity and mortality during the adjustment period and the extent to which they can be attributed to the adjustment program. Finally, the Sri Lankan experience is used to make some generalizations and to draw some implications for stabilization policy.

Conceptual Issues

In the analysis of short-term instability, Keynesian and monetarist models agree on the manifestations of instability but differ on some initial assumptions that each make. Both agree that an excess of aggregate demand over aggregate supply is responsible for the instability and that such instability is manifested in inflation, an over-valued exchange rate, and a BOP deficit. However, the Keynesian model assumes initially unemployed resources and therefore infers that higher demand will produce additional output in non-tradeables while generating inflation and a BOP deficit. The monetarist model assumes "full employ-ment" initially. Thus any additional demand will generate a BOP deficit, higher inflation and (under a fixed exchange rate) shift production from tradeables to non-tradeables.

The usual remedy proposed is a reduction in aggregate demand and/or an exchange rate devaluation. Both aim to reduce the BOP deficit by shifting resources from non-tradeables to tradeables. This poses no difficulty for monetarists who assume flexible prices and nom-inal wages—because deflation and devaluation will shift output from non-tradeables to tradeables, reduce the money income of factors in the non-tradeables sector, eliminate excess demand, remove the BOP deficit and reduce inflation. For monetarists, in principle, the short-term adjustment process entails no serious long-term growth costs. However, Keynesian models in the context of developing economies stress struc-tural rigidities that prevent a quick transfer of resources from non-trade-ables to tradeables (Taylor, 1981). In this view, deflationary policies reduce real incomes, create unemployment, and lower output in the non-tradeables sector.

Based on the above, it is possible to identify three principal types of social costs in a short-term stabilization program:

- Loss of output in the non-tradeables sector and consequent un-employment
- Possible reduction in real wages in the non-tradeables sector due to (1) a fall in demand for labor; (2) an increase in the price of tradeables
- Negative impacts of cuts in government spending and increases in taxes on real wages, reflected in (1) reductions in social welfare programs; (2) increases in direct and indirect taxes

As against the points listed above which reduce incomes and employ-ment, depending on factor mobility, the rate of investment, and the overall growth rate following stabilization, certain income and employ-ment augmenting forces may also quickly come into play. To some degree, these will offset the negative social costs of the stabilization program. However, it may also be necessary to have a special program as a transitional measure to guarantee a minimum level of consumption for the very poor until economic growth improves their position (Tim-mer and Guerrerio, 1980). The net result will depend very much on the particular policy mix in the stabilization package and the time se-quence of the negative and positive forces. The policy mix in turn will primarily depend on two factors. The first is the set of objectives of the program. They could be to control inflation, to change the trade regime to restore equilibrium in the BOP or some combination of the two. The second is the set of conditions that prevail in the economy when the program is undertaken. In this regard, the strength of commitment of the state to the maintenance of a minimum standard of living for the poor is especially important. If it is a strong one, as has been the case in Sri Lanka, an attempt will be made to combine overall reductions in social welfare expenditure with judicious changes in the composition of programs and their targeting so that benefits for the poor can be maintained or even enhanced.

The income and employment augmenting processes essentially relate to the long-term aspects of the adjustment program. Typically, this has involved a shift away from the *dirigisme* policies adopted by a large number of Third World countries following independence from colonial rule after the second world war. There are several reasons for this shift. Firstly, the confidence that these countries placed on the bureaucracy and planning—largely under the influence of the Soviet example—for economic growth has not produced the anticipated results. The recent trend towards liberalization seen in India and China are two prominent examples. Secondly, the success stories of Asian countries such as South Korea, Taiwan and Hong Kong that relied less on *dirigisme* and more on the market have forced other countries to rethink their state-centered development strategies. Thirdly, there have been challenges to the notion embodied in the Kuznets inverted "U" hypothesis and the International Labour Office (ILO) basic needs approach, that suggests that in the absence of active state intervention the fruits of growth fail to trickle down to the poorer sections of the community. It has been pointed out that not only does trickle-down occur under rapid growth (Lal, 1976), but that an elaborate welfare system in a developing country such as the one found in Sri Lanka cannot be viable in the long-term in the absence of sustained growth (Snodgrass, 1974). Those who challenge the "egalitarian development" model argue that a distinction must be made between inequality and absolute poverty. If the choice is between greater inequality and less absolute poverty (higher growth) on the one hand and less inequality and more absolute poverty (lower growth) on the other, the developing countries are better served to choose the former (Lal, 1985: 88–94).

The above discussion suggests the following as guidelines for the empirical analysis to follow.

1. There is no one adjustment program. One important point on which the available body of literature on this subject agrees is that the programs are situation-specific and that any truly meaningful analysis should go beyond generalizations to take into account the specific circumstances of the country and the time in which the adjustment program is implemented (Krueger, 1981; Sutton, 1984: 9).

2. The dynamic nature of the adjustment process is central to a fruitful analysis of the issues. The time sequence of the adjustment process must be taken into account, especially when the social costs and benefits are considered; that in turn influences the political feasibility of the program. Thus, as Dervis (1981: 503–506) points out, methodologically a dynamic model that shows relative speed of adjustment of the important policy and target variables is to be preferred to a comparative static model. Such an approach also implies that the "conventional separation between stabilization and development, or short-term and long-term policies has become increasingly inappropriate to the international economic problems of this decade, in which adjustment policies of individual countries must be assessed over periods of five to ten years. . . ." (Chenery, 1981: 115).

3. The experience with past adjustment programs demonstrates the need to integrate the economic analysis of the economic costs and benefits of such programs with an analysis of the political conditions that constrain or permit such programs. Programs which are abandoned midway due to political unacceptability can result in vain sacrifices and could be worse than no program at all (Killick and Sharpley 1984: 48–50).

Background to the Adjustment Program

The right-of-center United National Party led by J. R. Jayewardene was swept to power in the parliamentary elections held in July 1977 to replace the centrist-left Sri Lanka Freedom Party government led by Mrs. Sirima Bandaranaike. Jayewardene's electoral victory was overwhelming—he secured more than two-thirds of the 168 seats and reduced the opposition to a relatively ineffective rump. In fact, the Tamil United Liberation Front, which had an ethnic focus in policy and returned members exclusively from the Tamil regions in the north and east, had the largest number of MPs for any single opposition party and secured the position of Leader of the Opposition for its leader. The major left parties, the Communist Party (Moscow) and the Trotskyte Lanka Sama Samaja (Equal Society) Party, which traditionally returned a small but highly articulate group of MPs representing mainly urban constituencies, failed to gain a single seat between them. The relative weakness of parliamentary opposition with a national focus and the total absence of left wing MPs weakened any parliamentary opposition that might have arisen to the adjustment program under review. It is particularly useful to note that in 1953 the left, then strongly represented in the parliament, used their powerful trade union base to mobilize the urban working class to stage a general strike ("Hartal") and successfully spearheaded a campaign to prevent a sharp reduction in the consumer rice subsidy which the government had attempted as an adjustment to an increase in the world market price of rice and the post-Korean War economic slump (Wriggins, 1960).

The other important political development relevant to our theme concerns a major constitutional change Sri Lanka made in 1980. The Second Republican Constitution of 1978 replaced the Westminster model of government with a presidential model. Wilson (1980) describes the new system as the "Gaullist System in Asia" in order to highlight the strong executive that it created. Defending the new constitution that undoubtedly weakened the legislature, the administration argued that a strong executive was necessary to make difficult and quick decisions which at times may not be popular with the electorate (*Sri Lanka Hansards*, 1978 Series).

The Dirigisme Regime

In 1977 the Jayewardene administration inherited a highly *dirigisme* economy that had evolved in Sri Lanka since about the mid-1950s. It went beyond the social welfare system that is so well known (Richards and Gooneratne, 1980) and extended to direct state control of major segments of the economy and an elaborate system of price controls, licensing, quotas, foreign exchange control and other such devices to regulate and direct the private sector. Direct state participation in economic activity evolved through a series of nationalizations that started with omnibus transport (1958) and later extended to petroleum (1962), plantations (1972 and 1975), and other areas. The state also took over in stages, especially after 1970, an important slice of the import trade. The *dirigisme* economy also evolved partly through state initiative in developing Sri Lanka's comparatively small manufacturing industrial sector. The system of controls over the private sector grew partly from ideological considerations that believed in a mixed economy where private gain was to be made subordinate to the larger needs of society as expressed in state policy and economic planning. Secondly, it was also the result of a series of essentially *ad hoc* decisions taken in response to short-term economic difficulties such as the foreign exchange shortage that later became institutionalized when the problem became chronic or in response to electoral pressure as in the case of price control.

The extent of state involvement in the economy that finally evolved can be judged by the following. Before 1972, state ownership of plantations was not significant. Land reforms in 1972 and 1975 (Peiris, 1978) gave the state ownership or management of all the large tea and rubber estates, which numbered 530 and covered 66 percent and 33 percent respectively of the total acreage of the two crops (Ministry of Finance and Planning, 1985: 71). State corporations accounted for less than 2 percent of manufacturing value added in 1960, but by 1977 this had risen to 39 percent (World Bank, 1979: 2). By the latter year about two-thirds of the capital stock in Sri Lanka's manufacturing industry in the organized sector was owned by twenty-five state corporations each of which, on average, employed about 2000 workers compared with an average of forty-two in the private manufacturing sector. In the key services the state-owned commercial banks controlled about 80 percent of the banking business, and the state-owned Ceylon Insurance Corporation (1962) had a monopoly of all insurance business. By the end of 1976 about 75 percent of the country's imports were in the hands of government agencies and corporations, many enjoying a monopoly over such imports. In industrial policy official approval was essential to establish a new industry. At a more general level of control the Central Bank noted that in 1976 "all categories of imports were subject to an overall scheme of foreign exchange and licensing of imports." (Central Bank, *Annual Review of the Economy 1976*: 186). The Bank also reported that in 1976 some twenty-six categories of consumer goods were added to the already long list of such goods under price control.

The Economy: 1971–77

Table 3.1 presents some basic macroeconomic data on Sri Lanka. In terms of economic performance the period 1971–1984 clearly divides itself into two sub-periods—the period before the adjustment program (1971–1977) and the period of the adjustment program (1978–1984). Broadly speaking, the first was characterized by relatively slow growth, high unemployment, a low and fluctuating rate of investment, moderate deficits in the current account of the BOP that were financed largely with long-term loans from official sources, and a relatively modest but fluctuating rate of inflation.

The nature of the disequilibrium that the Sri Lankan economy confronted in 1977 is best described as a disequilibrium between actual economic growth and the economic growth warranted to meet the pressure exerted on the labor market by a rapid increase in the country's population, which doubled between 1945 and 1974 from 6.65 million to 13.3 million. It was not a disequilibrium of the traditional type that the IMF normally deals with (Killick, 1984a) that manifests itself in high inflation and/or large BOP deficits caused by large budget deficits that are financed by money creation. To be sure, as Table 3.2 shows, the government did run relatively large budget deficits that showed a grow-

Table 3.1
Sri Lanka: Selected Macroeconomic Indicators, 1971–84

Year	Real GDP Growth Rate (%)	Gross Domestic Investment Ratio	Balance of Payments Balance (SDR m)		Colombo Working Class Cost of Living Index (% Increase)	Rate of Open Unemployment (%)
			Trade	Basic		
1971	0.2	17.8	−35	31	2.7	18.7
1972	3.2	17.3	−29	14	6.3	
1973	3.7	13.7	−21	4	9.7	17.4
						24.9
1974	3.2	15.7	−113	−76	12.3	
1975	2.8	15.6	−91	−25	6.7	19.9
1976	2.4	16.2	−5	58	1.2	
1977	4.2	14.4	117	179	1.2	25.0
1978	8.2	20.0	−75	60	12.1	22.7
1979	6.3	25.8	−177	−13	10.8	14.8
1980	5.8	33.8	−507	−322	26.1	
1981	5.8	27.8	−381	−69	18.0	
1982	5.1	30.6	−516	−45	10.8	18.0
						11.7
1983	5.0	28.8	−441	−57	14.0	15.0
1984	5.0	26.3	−26	327	16.6	14.0

Source: Central Bank of Ceylon, *Annual Reports. Ministry of Finance and Planning (1985).*

ing trend in nominal terms and varied between one-third and one-half of revenue. It was also true that the government was financing a sizable net food subsidy bill that increased by 135.4 percent from Rs 605 million (45.2 percent of the deficit) in 1971 to Rs 1424 million (46.3 percent) in 1977. However, in three of the seven years government budgetary borrowing from the banking system was negative and in the remaining four such funding was kept below one-fifth of the total deficit. The

Table 3.2
Sri Lanka: Budget Deficits and Bank Financing, 1971–77

Year	Budget Deficit (Rs m)		Deficit as a % of Revenue	Net Bank Credit Rs m	Bank Credit as % of Deficit
	Amount	Change			
1971	1336	141	45.6	128	9.5
1972	1366	30	41.6	226	16.5
1973	1425	59	35.3	−116	−8.1
1974	1599	174	33.4	−15	−0.9
1975	2699	1100	53.1	153	5.7
1976	3576	877	62.3	639	17.9
1977	3074	−502	45.9	−224	−7.3

Source: Central Bank of Ceylon, *Annual Review of the Economy.*

government relied mostly on foreign funds and captive savings from the state-run Employees' Provident Fund, Insurance Corporation and savings banks to finance the deficits.

However, this budgetary policy had negative implications for growth. First, the virtually untargeted food subsidy diverted resources to consumption, and some of that could have been saved for capital formation had the scheme been targeted to help only those in genuine need. Second, the captive use of savings collected by the state-run financial institutions and the substantial borrowings made by the public sector including the state corporations and cooperative enterprises from the banking system limited, in effect, the financial resources available to the private sector. In that context, this limitation had negative effects on growth because many of the state-owned enterprises were relatively inefficient. For example, in 1977, in the organized manufacturing sector, the state-owned enterprises as a group had two-thirds of the capital stock but contributed only one-third of the total value-added, whereas private industries as a group had the opposite ratios (World Bank, 1979: 3).

It is also not possible to argue that the disequilibrium in the Sri Lankan economy—and there was a serious BOP disequilibrium—was a monetary phenomena that was attributable to an excessive expansion in the overall money supply (Table 3.3). Between 1971 and 1975 the rate of increase of the money supply (currency and bank demand deposits owned by the public) varied between 4.9 percent and 15.4 percent. Only in 1976 and 1977 did it reach an appreciably higher rate of increase. Of those years, only in 1976 did public sector credit, but more

Table 3.3
Sri Lanka: Factors Affecting Changes in Money Supply, 1971–77 (Rs m)

	1971	*1972*	*1973*	*1974*	*1975*	*1976*	*1977*
External banking assets	201	80	350	−179	−215	471	1943
Private sector	−48	−101	246	21	198	−60	−238
Other liabilities of commercial banks	−82	−97	95	−292	30	−46	−676
Public sector	10	470	−401	544	176	716	166
Central government	(53)	(148)	(−249)	(−261)	(273)	(540)	(−677)
Corporations	(68)	(233)	(−135)	(621)	(−79)	(85)	(320)
Cooperatives	(−15)	(89)	(−17)	(184)	(−18)	(91)	(523)
Adjustments	5	−19	7	75	−47	−3	4
Change in money supply	182	333	297	169	142	1078	1199
Percent change in money supply	9.3	15.4	12.0	6.0	4.9	34.9	28.8

Source: Central Bank of Ceylon, *Annual Review of the Economy.*

particularly the government budget, make a major contribution to the expansion. In 1977, although the public sector was a mildly expansionary force, the government budget was a major contractionary force against the expansion caused by the foreign sector. In 1973 as well, public sector credit operations had a major stabilizing influence on the money supply. In 1974 the government budget had a similar impact. In 1971, 1972 and 1975 the public sector and the foreign sector acted as offsetting influences on the money supply. In sum, the picture that emerges is not one of persistent internal or external disequilibrium directly attributable to fiscal deficits and excessive monetary expansion. On the contrary, even if we allow that shortcomings in computations of the consumer price index probably understate inflation to some extent, it is reasonable to say that price inflation in Sri Lanka in 1971–77 was quite moderate and a part of it was imported inflation. This point must be qualified by noting that the relatively stable but over-valued exchange rate and price controls were partly responsible for the moderation.

The situation was different with respect to the BOP which was in serious disequilibrium. Economists use various criteria to measure disequilibrium in the BOP (Killick and Sharpley, 1984a: 17). By most such criteria Sri Lanka faced a BOP disequilibrium. Thus, as Table 3.4 shows, there was a persistent deficit in the trade balance (Table 3.1 shows deficits in the current account balance). Except in 1977 the external assets of the nation were barely sufficient to finance three or four months of imports even at the severely curtailed levels (see the import volume index) that prevailed during much of 1971–77. In 1972 and again in 1975–77 the external debt increased significantly (with little prospect of significant increases in export earnings) and the debt service ratio averaged about 20 percent. Most important of all, the deficit was contained even at the level it was only with the help of severe import restrictions that cost the economy heavily in terms of productivity and growth. For example, it was estimated that mainly as a consequence of shortages of imported raw materials and spare parts, capacity utilization in manufacturing industry dropped to 40 percent in 1974 and even after imports increased in later years capacity utilization was no higher than 69 percent in 1977 (World Bank, 1979: 10).

More generally, the government responded to the oil shock of 1973 and the consequent adverse movement in the terms of trade by following an essentially deflationary set of policies. Import restrictions would have functioned as a serious disincentive to private investors who could not secure essential imported complementary inputs. The Central Bank took several restrictive monetary measures including two ceilings on bank credit, one effective on May 24, 1974 and the other on October 4,

Table 3.4
Sri Lanka: External Trade and Balance of Payments, 1971–76

	1971	*1972*	*1973*	*1974*	*1975*	*1976*	*1977*
Trade Balance (SDR m)	−47	−38	−39	−158	−168	−73	29
Export volume index (1978=100)	104	102	103	89	107	102	94
Import volume index (1978=100)	68	67	60	42	52	57	73
Terms of trade (1978=100)	98	94	82	72	58	78	102
External assets (SDR m) year end	81	109	112	111	92	137	305
External assets to total goods imports ratio (%)	23.7	33.1	30.8	18.6	16.1	28.6	91.9
External debt (SDR m) year end	293	352	362	360	439	510	541
Debt service ratio	21.9	21.8	23.0	17.8	22.9	20.1	16.0
Nominal exchange rate index (1978=100) year end	38.2	43.2	43.5	43.2	49.7	57.0	100.3

Source: Central Bank of Ceylon, *Annual Review of the Economy.*

1976. In 1973 gross capital formation in the private and the state sector declined by 40 percent and 21.2 percent respectively in nominal terms and probably by higher percentages in real terms. Even with such deflationary adjustment policies the country failed to achieve a surplus in the trade and current account balance of the BOP in 1974 and 1975. Although gross investment showed an upward trend in nominal terms over 1974–77, overall economic growth itself was not impressive during this period, partly due to bad harvests in one or the other of the major crops.

The Sri Lankan BOP disequilibrium was caused largely by structural factors. The principal factor responsible was the sharp deterioration in the terms of trade over 1973–75 (Table 4.4). The first oil shock and the sharp rise in world food prices that were primarily responsible for this were almost entirely beyond Sri Lanka's control. However, a country's terms of trade are also partly determined by its export structure. A country which has some measure of control over its export prices is better able to respond to an increase in import prices. This Sri Lanka was totally incapable of doing. Tea, which accounted for about 50 percent of the country's exports, was the only commodity in which Sri Lanka was an important supplier in the world market. However, tea itself was a weak commodity in the world market—with problems of over-supply and stagnant or falling demand in some major markets such as the UK. More generally, although the combined share of the value of tea, rubber and coconut in total exports had fallen from 90.6 percent in 1966–67 to 71.1 percent in 1976–77, they still were dominant. Moreover, if the export value of petroleum products, which were largely re-exports and were unimportant in 1966–67, is removed from the denominator, the share of the three staples increases to 79.1 percent even in 1976–77.

It is true that, aided by a number of fiscal and exchange rate incentives, manufactured exports (excluding gems and petroleum products) grew continually over 1971–77. Their total value increased from US $9 million in 1972 to US $60 million in 1978 (World Bank 1979: 2). However, since such exports started from a narrow base, even in 1978 they accounted for just 7 percent of total goods exports. In particular the high effective protection given to import substitution industry was a major disincentive to a relative switch of resources to the export sector (Athukorala, 1981).

Finally, the other key question that needs to be raised is the extent to which the exchange rate policy was responsible for the BOP disequilibrium. From 1968 onwards, until the scheme was abandoned in November 1977, all non-traditional exports were entitled to a rupee premium on the official exchange rate (55 percent from 1968–72 and 65 percent thereafter) as an incentive. From 1972 a convertible rupee account scheme operated that gave those who earned foreign exchange from non-traditional exports an exchange entitlement to import goods that were otherwise prohibited. However, the three staples were exported at the official rate which, in effect, was a tax on that sector. This undoubtedly would have been an important factor that discouraged greater supplies of these products. Over the period 1971–77 output in tea, rubber and coconut combined declined at an annual average rate of 1.7 percent. However, this negative growth is also partly the result of several other interrelated factors such as management dislocation caused by the land reform, political uncertainty, under-investment, liquidity shortage, weak prices, high tax rates, the shortage of inputs such as fertilizer, and the disruption caused to labor supply by the repatriation of Indian labor. In the case of coconut products the decline in output was compounded by the steady rise in local consumption that rapidly reduced the export surplus. The net result of this supply constraint has been a trend decline in the volume exported.

By 1977 it was evident that due to a prolonged effort to run the economy with the help of a set of administered or semi-administered prices—prices of tradeables and non-tradeables especially utilities, exchange rate, interest rates, wage rates—relative prices were seriously distorted in relation to domestic resource endowments and the international economy. For example, the World Bank (1983: 57–63) notes that Sri Lanka's wage rates in formal employment were fixed at a level higher than what were justified by productivity gains and changes in terms of trade. An adjustment program had to resolve the price distortion problem while taking into account the potential adverse social welfare consequences of an attempt to establish a set of relative prices that were in harmony with Sri Lanka's medium to long-term growth potential.

To summarize, the disequilibrium in the Sri Lankan economy in 1977 was a structural problem that required simultaneous resolution in two fronts, rapid growth in the domestic economy to remove the disequilibrium in the labor market and strong export growth and independent capital inflows in the external sector to remove the disequilibrium in the BOP. The experience of 1971–1977 demonstrated that it was not possible to achieve the former without the latter.

The Adjustment Program

The adjustment program was prepared by the new government between August and November 1977 in consultation with the IMF and announced in Parliament on November 15, 1977 along with the first budget of the government. The program focused on remedying, in the long term, the persistent deficit in the BOP and on finding an answer to the growing unemployment problem. These two objectives need not be in conflict. However, in programs of this nature, insofar as the IMF is concerned the growth objective is of secondary importance (Killick, 1984a: 185). More importantly, our analysis of the 1971–77 period showed that Sri Lanka's BOP disequilibrium had little to do with excessive monetary expansion, which usually calls for severely deflationary measures through reductions in bank credit and government budget deficits. It was more of a structural problem that required resource augmentation in the export-oriented industries and more efficient use of resources in domestic enterprise, especially in import substitution industry. The need to create more jobs also implied that national savings had to be increased and resources, especially budgetary resources, had to be diverted to productive investment. By implication, this called into question some of the subsidies the government gave consumers. More generally, the strategy called for a more efficient allocation of resources where prices and private economic decision making were to play a larger role than hitherto. However, it appears that the IMF, in agreeing to support a substantial aid package as a part of the program, implicitly recognized the limited scope that existed for resource/expenditure switching in the Sri Lankan economy.

Related to the above, three other factors that influenced the formulation of the program must be noted. First, it has been pointed out that after 1974 the IMF came to realize the importance of the need for a longer time horizon and structural adjustment to make adjustment programs successful (Sutton, 1984: 5). Second, given the Sri Lankan political conditions, especially the need of the government to be responsive to the welfare needs of the people, there were obvious constraints to any expenditure switching strategy. Third, and related to the second point, the speed of the program became crucial to its social acceptability. In other words, in expenditure switching a certain tradeoff had to be expected between welfare losses from cuts in government spending and income gains through new jobs, provided the income gains do not lag far behind the welfare losses. Given all other factors, the reduction of this time lag will depend on the volume of supporting finances available. Thus, the underwriting of the adjustment program by a western aid consortium was an indispensable part of the entire process. In fact, over 1978–83, western official aid commitments to Sri Lanka totalled US $2363 million and private (loan) commitments US $1312 million. The country also used US $1948 million in IMF credit, making up a grand total of US $5623 million, the equivalent of 47.5 percent of total value of imports of goods and services and half of gross domestic investment over the same period (*World Bank*, 1985: 272–275).

The major specific objectives of the adjustment program were the following:

1. The liberalization of the economy to permit a greater role for the market and private sector
2. Rapid economic growth to provide employment for the jobless
3. Strengthening of exports and further development of efficient import-substitution, especially in domestic agriculture (food production), to eliminate the BOP disequilibrium
4. The improvement of productivity in public enterprises

The major reforms of the program are described below with some details of those which have had a direct bearing on health and nutrition.

1. Exchange rate reform. The dual exchange rate that prevailed was replaced with a unified exchange rate that was allowed to float. The new rate at the end of December 1977 was Rs 15.56 = US $1.00. This implied a 46 percent depreciation of the rupee. Since then the rupee has depreciated by another 75 percent against the US dollar and stood at Rs 27.85 = US $1.00 at the end of April 1986.

2. Import liberalization. The trade and payments regime was liberalized by abolishing licensing, exchange control and permits for most imports. With the exception of a few commodities, the state monopoly on imports was removed. The tariff structure was revised and simplified. Certain basic consumer goods such as rice, wheat, full-cream milk, pharmaceuticals and fish were allowed to be imported at zero duty.

3. Price controls were abolished for most commodities.

4. Nominal interest rates were increased and were made more flexible.

5. Fiscal reform. The tax structure was simplified to increase the elasticity of revenue. Personal and corporate tax rates were reduced as incentives for higher productivity and investment.

The major fiscal reform that had direct health and nutrition implications concerned the changes effected in the food subsidy program. When the new administration took office the subsidy scheme was as follows. All non-income tax paying households (about 90 percent of the total) were entitled every week to one pound of rice free of charge and three pounds at Rs 1.00 per pound. Wheat flour, bread, sugar and infant milk powder were sold to everyone at subsidized prices.

Beginning February 1, 1978, the rice ration was restricted to households with five members (or less) with an annual income of Rs 3600 or less. This income ceiling was increased by Rs 720 for each additional member of the household beyond five. However, those households with an annual income exceeding Rs 9000 were totally excluded from the ration scheme.

In September 1979 the ration scheme was replaced by a food stamp scheme. The eligibility criteria were identical to the revised ration scheme of February 1978. The monthly food stamp entitlements were as follows.

Age under 8:   Rs 25
      8–12:   Rs 20
   Over 12:   Rs 15

In addition, each household was given kerosene stamps worth Rs 9.50 which could also be utilized to buy additional food for the household but food stamps could not be used to purchase kerosene. However, both types of stamps were convertible to savings deposits.

At the beginning 7.26 million people joined the scheme. By January 1980 it increased to 7.42 million (50 percent of the population). Since then no new additions have been permitted.

By a series of price increases the government reduced the subsidy on wheat flour to zero by 1982 and that on sugar by 1983.

Impact of the Adjustment Program

The most striking immediate impact of the adjustment program was the sharp increase in the real gross domestic product (GDP) growth rate to 8.2 percent in 1978 and its continuation at an average rate of 5.9 percent over 1978–1984 when compared with 2.9 percent over 1971–1977 (Table 3.5). Initially the high growth rate was helped by the availability of unused installed capacity in industry and highly profitable investment opportunities in areas such as transport, trade, tourism and urban construction that could readily be exploited in the new economic environment.

Table 3.5 shows that all the major sectors except the staple exports recorded relatively high growth rates. The latter, which has been plagued by management difficulties, market uncertainties and other problems mentioned before, has just managed to reverse its declining trend in output. It made practically no net contribution to employment creation during this period.

From the point of view of the adjustment program one of the clear social benefits of rapid growth, especially in services and construction with their high labor absorptive capacity, was the opportunity it provided to create a large number of new jobs. This was particularly important

Table 3.5
Sri Lanka: Changes in GDP, 1971–77 and 1978–84 at 1970 Constant Factor Cost Prices

	Value Rs m. 1970 Factor Cost Prices				Average Growth Rate, %	
	1970	1977	1978	1984	1971–77	1978–84
GDP	13187	16078	17401	24382	2.9	6.1
GDP per capita Ts	1054	1153	1226	1543	1.3	4.3
Value added in agriculture	3732	4299	4532	5615	2.1	3.9
of which tea, rubber and coconut	1191	1052	1111	1072	−1.7	0.3
Paddy and other	2541	3247	3421	4605	3.5	5.1
Manufacturing	1304	1534	1701	2481	2.3	7.1
Construction	744	619	794	1020	−2.6	7.4
Services	6419	8288	8315	13596	3.7	7.3

Source: Ministry of Finance and Planning, *Public Investment 1985–1989*, Colombo, 1985.

because much of this activity was urban-based—Sri Lanka, like most developing countries, reported an urban unemployment rate 31 percent higher than the rural rate in 1973 and 41 percent higher in 1978–79. Moreover, organized opposition to any adverse welfare impact of government policy is typically articulated in urban centers. In such a context it is relevant to note that in the urban sector the rate of open unemployment was only 18 percent higher than in the rural sector in 1981–82.

The Ministry of Finance and Planning (1985: 9) estimated that between 1978 and 1984 the employed population increased by 1.65 million—helping to cut the unemployment rate by almost half from 25 percent to 14 percent. This estimate, however, needs to be qualified in two respects. First, available figures suggest that about 100,000 of these jobs were the result of people emigrating to the Middle East (Women's Bureau, 1985: 85). Second, some doubt has to be cast on the reliability of an official estimate of a net increase of 519,000 of employed persons in 1983. In that year the net increase in employment in the state sector was 9357; in the "organized" private sector it was 158,000. However, the latter is calculated on the basis of the net increase in registrants at the Employees' Provident Fund, which probably overstates the figure to some extent because those who retire are not taken out of the roll immediately. More importantly, in 1978 when gross investment increased by 63 percent in nominal terms and at least by half as much in real terms only 211,000 new jobs were created in the entire economy. In 1983 the increase in gross investment in real terms was only 7.3 percent, which makes the official job estimate look rather improbable. These qualifications notwithstanding, there is no doubt that the adjustment program helped lower the unemployment rate appreciably in Sri Lanka, probably for the first time in three decades of independence. As a parenthetic point it may be noted that the under-employment rate—defined as the number of man-days lost due to non-availability of work as a percentage of total number of man-days for which employed persons were available for work—in the rural and estate sectors declined by 12 percent and 21 percent respectively between 1978–79 and 1981–82.

As one would have expected, expenditure switching induced by the new set of relative prices that came into force following exchange depreciation and import liberalization did create some unemployment in industries that lost their competitive advantage. For example, in agriculture, producer margins were greatly reduced for several subsidiary food crops. One notable example is chillies which were grown largely in the north—a factor believed to have contributed to the alienation of the northern Tamil farmers from the Jayewardene administration—and another was small scale sugar cultivation in the south. Both were adversely affected by liberal imports. In manufacturing industry, according to an official survey (Athukorala, 1985:90), over the period 1977–79 unregistered industries as a group suffered a decline in output (6 percent) and employment (16 percent) due to liberalization. Handloom textile weaving, for which there were 1706 centers in 1976 providing employment mostly to women, is one such industry that suffered badly due to imports. The sugar cane syrup and jaggary (raw sugar) industries also suffered a similar fate; in the organized sector, the light engineering industry also experienced a decline in output. With regard to the social welfare implications of such unemployment three points should be noted. First, many of the activities that were adversely affected were located in the rural areas or in small towns. Some of the industries were restricted to a certain geographical region. Thus those who lost their jobs might also not have had access to new jobs in the towns or in different regions. Second, many who are engaged in cottage industry or small scale farming are at the lower end of the income scale. To that extent pockets of unemployment and poverty could have been created, the overall increase in employment notwithstanding. Third, given the important role that independent female incomes could play in family and especially child welfare, the loss of female employment would have had negative welfare implications. (Between 1973 and 1981–82 the male unemployment rate dropped by 58.7 percent and the female rate by 41.3 percent).

The rapid expansion of the economy combined with the sharp deterioration in the terms of trade following the second oil shock of 1979–80 and the world recession of the early 1980s created a large deficit in the current account of the BOP that equalled 11.9 percent of GDP in 1978 and rose to 15.8 percent by 1983. The sharp increase in tea prices in 1984 that cut the ratio to 3.6 percent proved to be a temporary respite. In making provision for a substantial aid package the authors of the adjustment program were prepared for a large external payments deficit as an unavoidable temporary phase of the adjustment process. However, the IMF was not happy with the serious domestic disequilibrium that emerged in the early 1980s. Consumer prices rose by 26.1 percent in 1980 (Table 3.1). As is the experience in many developing countries, budgetary spending in Sri Lanka proved to be more elastic with respect to rising prices than tax revenue. Thus in 1980 the budget deficit reached a record 116.8 percent of current revenue and 23.1 percent of GDP. No less than 45.8 percent of the deficit was financed with bank credit. The IMF reacted in late 1980 by suspending standby credit. This pressured the government into cutting the 1981 budgeted public spending by a minimum of 10 percent across the board.

The Central Bank imposed a credit squeeze that cut the increase in total domestic credit from 69.6 percent in 1980 to 31.9 percent in 1981 and the increase in the narrow money supply from 22.9 percent to 6.3 percent. Gross bank credit to the private sector increased by 67 percent in 1980 but only by 36 percent in 1981. These budgetary and monetary restraints initiated in 1981 have been continued in the years that followed. (However, beginning 1984 large scale military spending caused by the Sinhalese-Tamil ethnic conflicts has introduced a new destabilizing element to the government budget. See Samarasinghe, 1985.) In particular, budgetary spending on programs which would not yield quick economic returns, including those with a social welfare bias such as new housing development, were discouraged. No new major capital investment projects were permitted over 1981–84, and some tax concessions were withdrawn to increase revenue. In the Sri Lankan case these events did not add up to an abandoning of the adjustment program. However, they highlighted the difficulties of managing such a program in a developing economy with a weak international trading position, especially when one has to balance immediate welfare needs by sustaining growth, employment and real incomes against factors dictated to it by what Timmer and Giuerreiro (1980:3) call the "real" economy. This was vividly illustrated by the July 1980 strike of government employees who demanded a monthly wage increase of Rs 300. The government, faced with adverse international prices and a serious domestic disequi-

Table 3.6
Sri Lanka: Percentage of Total One Month Income Received by Each Ten Percent of Ranked Income Receivers, Selected Years

Decile	1963	1973	1978–79	1981–82
Lowest	1.77	1.80	1.20	1.21
2nd	2.70	3.17	2.56	2.49
3rd	3.56	4.38	3.60	3.47
4th	4.57	5.70	4.76	4.61
5th	5.55	7.10	5.93	5.56
6th	6.82	8.75	7.29	6.93
7th	8.98	10.56	9.11	8.57
8th	11.46	12.65	11.23	10.64
9th	16.01	15.91	15.26	14.82
Highest	39.24	29.98	39.05	41.70
Gini coefficients				
All island	0.49	0.41	0.49	0.52
Urban	0.49	0.40	0.51	0.54
Rural	0.44	0.37	0.49	0.49
Estate	0.27	0.37	0.32	0.32

Source: Central Bank of Ceylon, *Consumer Finance Surveys* (years as above).

librium, not only refused to yield to the demand but also dismissed 40,000 workers who disobeyed a government order to return to work.

Income

One of the most controversial aspects of the adjustment program concerns its impact on incomes. There are two issues. One concerns the impact on the distribution of income and the other on the level of absolute poverty. Related to the absolute poverty level is the question of food availability and nutritional welfare of the poorer sections of the community; we shall discuss this later.

Tables 3.6 and 3.7 present figures on income distribution and the relevant Gini coefficients. They reveal that for the country as a whole the equalizing trend that occurred between 1963–73 had sharply reversed itself between 1973 and 1978–79 and that the trend towards inequality had continued up to 1981–82. An examination of the shares received by each decile of income receivers and spending units reveal that between 1973 and 1978–79 all but the highest decile suffered a decline in the share of income. In terms of income receivers the same trend continued from 1978–79 to 1981–82 except for an insignificant gain made by the lowest decile. However, the gain made by the highest decile was a slight one. In terms of spending units, gains were made by the lowest, seventh, ninth and the highest deciles.

Relative inequality may not be directly relevant to the absolute welfare of the poor unless through its impact on the distribution of factors of

Table 3.7
Sri Lanka: Percentage of Total One Month Income Received by Each Ten Percent of Ranked Spending Units

Decile	1963	1973	1978–7	1981–8
Lowest	1.50	2.79	2.12	2.18
2nd	3.95	4.38	3.61	3.55
3rd	4.00	5.60	4.65	4.35
4th	5.21	6.52	5.68	5.24
5th	6.27	7.45	6.59	6.35
6th	7.54	8.75	7.69	7.02
7th	9.00	9.91	8.57	8.69
8th	11.22	11.65	11.22	10.71
9th	15.54	14.92	14.03	14.52
Highest	36.77	28.03	35.84	37.29
Gini coefficients				
All island	0.45	0.35	0.44	0.45

Source: Central Bank of Ceylon, *Consumer Finance Surveys* (years as above).

production that skews the production structure against wage goods. Nevertheless, the question of extent to which the adjustment program contributed to the trend in inequality from 1973 to 1978–79 is of some importance because income inequalities that can be blamed on the program can make it politically vulnerable (see, for example, Sharpley, 1984, on Jamaica).

In the absence of income distribution data for a period before the adjustment program began (1978) but close to it we have to infer from other available information the extent to which income distribution would have continued on its egalitarian trend between 1973 and 1977. The principal institutional change after 1973 that would have had an egalitarian bias was the land reform. As against this the rapid growth in unemployment which affected all sectors of the economy would probably have exerted a considerable influence in the opposite direction. Moreover, consumer prices as measured by the Colombo Cost of Living Index (COLI) increased by 23 percent over 1974–77. However, given the shortage of goods and extensive price controls—which were used to calculate the index but were not very effective—that were found during much of this time, the above rate probably understates the true rate of inflation. For example, the consumer goods wholesale price index showed an increase of 41 percent over the three years 1975–77. Thus, it is difficult to agree with the observation made, for example, by Lakshman (1986) that 1970–77 would have produced an "equalizing tendency" in income distribution.

In the wake of the 1977 reforms some factors would have come into play that would have worsened income inequality. Removal of price controls, higher interest rates, depreciation of the rupee and the overall increase in productivity would have contributed to a quick increase in income from profits, interests and rents. In contrast, wage incomes would have lagged behind but only to a limited extent. Wage rates of state employees in the clerical and minor grades, plantation workers and most workers who were in trades where government-appointed wages boards fixed wages, got pay rises along with the reforms (Table 3.8) in 1978 and again in 1979. Although there would have been a delay in wage increases in the informal labor market because of the large pool of unemployed labor that was available at the initial stages of the economic boom, as we show below, there is evidence to believe that by the third quarter of 1979 rural and urban informal wage rates were rising quite rapidly under the impact of falling unemployment. The withdrawal of the rice subsidy from the upper 50 percent of income earners in February 1978 would have operated as an income equalizing factor, a point confirmed by Alailima (1984).

Three other observations need to be made about the income distribution implications of the Sri Lankan adjustment program. First, in terms

Table 3.8
Sri Lanka: Real Wage Rates in the Formal Sector, 1973–84
(Index 1978 Dec = 100)

	Private Sector (Daily Rate Rs)			Government Sector (Monthly Salary Rs)		
	Agricultural	Manufacturing and Commerce	Service Industries	Non-Clerical Officer Grades	Minor Grades	Teachers
1973	50.8	75.6	N.A.	100.6	91.0	102.4
1977	76.3	93.7	N.A.	105.1	101.5	106.7
1978	99.0	102.6	N.A.	107.8	105.3	105.3
1979	116.0	105.2	107.8	109.7	112.6	106.6
1980	115.9	105.4	98.9	94.9	99.4	90.5
1981	98.3	96.2	93.2	89.4	96.4	84.9
1982	104.2	92.6	97.7	103.9	112.0	95.7
1983	100.4	82.5	89.7	103.4	114.2	95.1
1984	108.0	72.9	77.8	100.1	112.8	91.4

Source: Central Bank of Ceylon, *Annual Review of the Economy.*

of the Gini coefficients, although inequality increased between 1978–79 and 1981–82 in the urban sector where 20 percent of the population lives, it remained unchanged in the rural and estate sectors (Table 3.7). Second, the trend towards income inequality islandwide from 1978–79 to 1981–82 is less significant in terms of spending units than in terms of income receivers. Third, the Gini coefficient that consistently records a lower value in terms of spending units suggests that in the lower income deciles there are relatively more income earners whose combined income helps to reduce income inequality. This is of considerable relevance to the social welfare implications of the adjustment program because, as we have already seen, it relied heavily on job creation as an antidote to cuts in welfare programs.

With respect to the impact of the adjustment program on absolute incomes and poverty, the first point to be noted is the sharp increase in absolute real incomes overall between 1973 and 1978–79 (Tables 3.9 and 3.10). Even if some allowance is made for underestimating inflation—this was less acute after price controls were removed in 1977—the increases still would be significant. Second, in this regard the higher deciles have done better than the lower deciles. However, it is only the bottom decile that stands out as having fared relatively poorly although even their income had risen by 54 percent in real terms. Third, real income increases between 1978–79 and 1981–82 appear to be very slight. Given the usual statistical deficiencies of income data, these small temporal changes probably mean that nominal incomes

Table 3.9
Sri Lanka: Mean Monthly Income Per Income Receiver by Deciles: Selected Years (Rs)

Decile	Mean Monthly Income at Current Prices			Mean Monthly Income at 1973 Constant Prices			Rate of Growth (%)	
	1973	1978–79	1981–82	1973	1978–79	1981–82	1973 to 1978–79	1978–79 to 1981–82
Lowest	41	74	134	41	51	54	24	6
2nd	72	158	277	72	108	112	50	4
3rd	100	223	385	100	153	156	53	2
4th	130	295	512	130	202	208	55	2
5th	161	367	619	161	252	251	57	—
6th	199	451	770	199	309	313	55	2
7th	240	563	951	240	386	386	61	—
8th	288	695	1182	288	477	480	66	1
9th	362	944	1646	362	647	668	79	3
Highest	682	2414	4632	682	1656	1880	143	14
Mean	228	616	1111	228	422	451	85	7
Median	180	408	612	180	280	248	56	−11

Note: Colombo consumer price index used as deflator.

Source: Central Bank of Ceylon, *Consumer Finance Surveys* (years as above).

barely managed to keep pace with prices and real incomes declined. The behavior of real wage rates in Table 3.8 (and 3.12) lend some support to this argument. However, it is useful to note that over this period the real income increase both in terms of income receivers as well as spending units for the lowest decile is above the mean/median increase for the sample as a whole. In fact the survey data show that the bottom quintile of income receivers in the urban and rural sectors increased their absolute incomes by 26 percent and 10 percent respectively over the three year period but that estate incomes in the same group declined by 6 percent. Fourth, and most important, the evidence discussed here suggests that the Sri Lankan adjustment program had a trickle down mechanism that acted through the job market and reached the weaker sections of the community. For example, Table 3.11 shows that in the first round of job creation almost all the education groups with the exception of GCE General Certificate of Education—Advanced Level (AL) qualified category benefitted but that in the 1978–79 to 1981–82 round the less well educated did better.

The most impressive evidence in favor of the trickle-down theory comes from the behavior of wage rates in the informal labor market. Data in Table 3.12 show that between the last quarters of 1978 and

Table 3.10
Sri Lanka: Mean Monthly Income Per Spending Unit by Deciles: 1973, 1978–79, 1981–82 (Rs)

Decile	Mean Monthly Income at Current Prices			Mean Monthly Income at Constant 1973 Prices			Rate of Increase (%)	
	1973	1978–79	1981–82	1973	1978–79	1981–82	1973–79	1979–82
Lowest	87	195	356	87	134	145	54	8
2nd	136	333	580	136	228	235	68	3
3rd	174	428	711	174	294	288	69	−2
4th	203	523	857	203	359	347	77	−3
5th	232	607	1038	232	416	421	79	1
6th	272	709	1148	272	486	466	79	−6
7th	308	790	1421	308	542	577	43	6
8th	362	1034	1751	362	709	711	96	—
9th	464	1293	2390	464	887	970	91	9
Highest	871	3225	6096	871	2212	2474	154	12
Mean	311	921	1635	311	632	664	103	5
Median	250	658	1159	250	451	470	80	4

Note: Colombo consumer price index used as deflator.
Source: Central Bank of Ceylon, *Consumer Finance Surveys* (years as above).

1979 there have been substantial increases in real wages in certain representative categories of workers in rural and urban employment. Furthermore, such increases have continued, albeit at a reduced rate, in 1980 and 1981. The Agrarian Research and Training Institute (ARTI), in in-depth micro studies in the principal paddy growing areas,

Table 3.11
Sri Lanka: Percentage Reduction in Unemployment Rate by Educational Status, 1973 to 1981–82 (percent)

	1973 to 1978–79	1978–79 to 1981–82
No schooling, illiterate	58.7	31.4
No schooling, literate	59.4	32.1
Primary	53.1	27.3
Secondary	74.5	31.5
GCE (OL)	41.8	11.2
GCE (AL)	17.9	4.3
Graduates	67.5	+83.0
All	38.5	20.9

Note: Graduate unemployment increased between 1978–79 and 1981–82.
Source: Central Bank of Ceylon, *Consumer Finance Surveys* (years as above).

Table 3.12
Sri Lanka: Real Wage Rates in the Informal Sector, 1978–84
(Daily Rate Rs)

| | Rural Male Paddy Worker* | | Urban Construction (Masonry) | | | |
| | | | Skilled Male Helper | | Unskilled Male Helper | |
	Rs	Per-centage Increase	Rs	Per centage Increase	Rs	Per-centage Increase
1978 Sept–Oct	13.63	—	13.73	—	10.45	—
1979 October	15.35	12.6	17.64	28.5	12.16	16.4
1979 annual avg.	16.41	—	19.07	—	12.55	—
1980 annual avg.	17.30	5.4	19.82	3.9	14.91	18.8
1981 annual avg.	17.96	3.8	21.19	6.9	16.01	7.4
1982 annual avg.	18.39	2.4	21.62	2.0	15.97	−0.2
1983 annual avg.	18.29	−0.5	21.27	−1.6	16.02	0.3
1984 annual avg.	16.29	−10.9	19.99	−6.0	15.10	−5.7

*Ploughing with hoe. The value of meals provided to paddy workers is excluded. Nominal wage rates deflated by the Colombo Consumer Price Index. 1979 October figures are at 1978 Sept-Oct prices. 1980 to 1984 figures are at 1979 prices.

Source: Nominal wage rates from Central Bank of Ceylon, *Social and Economic Statistics*, 1979, 1980 and 1984.

also reported increases in nominal wage rates in the neighborhood of 50 percent between 1978 and 1979. (ARTI, 1980a, 1980b, 1981). Thus, given the increases in consumer prices in 1978 and 1979—12.1 percent and 10.8 percent in terms of the Colombo Consumer Price Index (CCPI) and 9.1 percent and 19 percent in terms of Central Bank Cost of Living Index (COLI)—there is little doubt that there was an improvement in real wage rates in informal employment—where the poorest generally find employment—in 1978–79, the first two years of the adjustment program. However, in 1980, the third year of the adjustment program, inflationary pressures increased sharply, with consumer prices rising by 26.1 percent in terms of the CCPI and by 37.8 percent in terms of the Central Bank COLI. The rise in domestic spending, especially on projects such as the Accelerated Mahaweli Multi-Purpose River Diversion Project that had long gestation periods was one major reason for the higher rate of inflation. The sharp increase in import prices—by 52 percent in 1979 and by 43 percent in 1980—following the second oil shock also contributed. About one-third of the increase in import prices in 1980 can be attributed to the depreciation of the Sri Lanka rupee by 16.5 percent in that year after maintaining a steady value in 1978–79. The rupee came under pressure because of the large current account deficit—12 percent of the GDP in 1979 and 22.6 percent in 1980—that resulted from the growing volume of imports, but particularly from rising import prices. The acceleration in inflation—which was partly if not largely exogenous to the adjustment program and stemmed from structural weaknesses in the economy that the program was designed to correct in the long term—eroded real earnings. Nevertheless what is striking is that workers in the informal sector continued to make modest to considerable gains over 1980–81 and even in 1982, whereas many categories of workers in the formal sector suffered considerable drops in real earnings in 1980–81 (Table 3.8). However, in 1983–84—with the exception of plantation agriculture workers in 1984 (Table 3.8), no group in our sample managed to keep pace with inflation. Given the modest absolute earnings of the low income groups, the drop in real wages reduced the degrees of freedom that the government had to further adjust relative prices in line with resource availability and to cut direct subsidies to households—a principal objective of the adjustment program. Thus, the welfare consequences of fiscal policy—taxes, government spending on social welfare and especially on food subsidies—in the adjustment program had a major bearing on the welfare of the poor.

Taxes

Table 3.13 presents data on Sri Lankan government taxes. What is most striking is that the tax revenue structure has practically remained unchanged between 1977 and 1983. Personal income taxes and corporate income taxes yielded almost identical percentages of total tax revenue despite faster income growth after 1977 and the higher income gains made by the upper income groups. Even if one were to consider the total of export duty revenue as a substitute income tax, not more than 25 percent of total tax revenue would have come from direct taxes in each of the years. The rest came mainly from sales taxes and import duties.

Tax revenue has been only mildly elastic with respect to overall income growth, showing an income elasticity of 1.28 with respect to GNP. Personal and corporate tax revenues have shown an income elasticity of 1.2. Given the rapid income growth enjoyed by the higher income deciles noted earlier in the context of reductions in income and corporate tax rates effected in 1977, these tax yields suggest that tax incidence of the rich would have declined significantly, a fact confirmed by Alailima (1984). However, the rate structure itself remained highly progressive so that the incidence of direct taxes also remained progressive.

As for the incidence of indirect taxes, many of the selective sales taxes and import duties are designed to reduce the regressivity associated with

Table 3.13
Sri Lanka: Revenue of the Central Government, 1977 and 1983

	1977		1983	
	Rs m	*Percent*	*Rs m*	*Percent*
Personal income tax	275	5.0	891	4.3
Corporate tax	662	12.0	2475	11.9
General sales tax	711	12.9	6224	30.1
Selective sales tax	1407	23.5	3230	15.6
Import duties	518	9.4	4836	23.4
Receipts from FEECS (net)	1158	21.0	—	—
Export duties	620	11.3	2459	11.9
License taxes	54	0.9	188	0.9
Property transfer taxes	37	0.6	336	1.6
Estate duty	18	0.3	17	0.1
Wealth tax	25	0.4	33	0.2
Other capital taxes	25	0.4	33	0.2
Profits from food sales	—	—	—	—
Total tax revenue	5510	100.0	20700	100.0
Other revenue	1178	17.7	4508	17.9
Total revenue (TR)	6688		25208	
TR as percentage of GNP		19.4		23.2

Note: FEECS = Foreign Exchange Entitlement Certificates.
Source: Central Bank of Ceylon, *Annual Review of the Economy.*

such taxes. For example, basic foods and drugs continue to be imported duty free. Thus Alailima (1984) found that the tax incidence for the poorest 24 percent of income earners had fallen marginally between 1973 and 1980 from 7.2 percent to 6.9 percent. The overall tax structure had also retained its progressive character while the 1978 tax rate changes had not made an appreciable difference to income concentration. Thus, overall, although the 1977 tax changes have helped the rich to raise their after-tax incomes substantially, they have remained more or less neutral with respect to the absolute incomes of the lower income groups.

Government Expenditure

One of the most politically controversial aspects of the adjustment program was the attempt to restructure government expenditure. The overall thrust of this restructuring was to de-emphasize public consumption spending, especially transfers to consumers, and emphasize spending on economic infrastructure development that would directly enhance the productive capacity of the economy.

Table 3.14 shows that the government has had considerable success in achieving its objective. Current spending had been sharply reduced from 75.5 percent of total spending in 1977 to 57 percent in 1983, with a corresponding increase in capital spending. Recurrent spending on social services and transfers to households have been cut by a third each in proportionate terms. However, the percentage devoted to capital development in the social services sector had been increased relative to total government spending.

Table 3.15 shows the total welfare expenditure and its composition. One should note that the share of social welfare expenditure in the total budget had been halved from 38 percent in 1977 to 18.7 percent in 1983. Second, when the total of Rs 7834 million is deflated by the Gross Domestic Product (GDP) deflator it is found that in real terms 1983 expenditure is Rs 3348 million, which is almost the same as the 1977 figure. Given a population growth rate of 10.6 during the intervening seven year period, this implies a reduction of about one-tenth in per capita real expenditure on social welfare. Third, Table 3.15 also shows that the structure of welfare expenditure itself underwent some significant changes. The most important of these is the sharp reduction in transfer payments to households in the form of food subsidies which accounted for almost half of the total welfare budget in 1977 but which

Table 3.14
Sri Lanka: Central Government Expenditure, 1977 and 1983

	1977		1983	
	Rs m	*Percent*	*Rs m*	*Percent*
Current expenditure	(6554)	(75.50)	(23837)	(57.0)
Administration	999	11.3	4273	10.2
Social services	1637	18.6	3756	9.0
Economic services	212	2.4	680	1.6
Gross payments to trading enterprises	500	5.7	1447	3.5
Intra-government payments	10	0.1	17	—
Transfer payments to private accounts	3174	36.0	11098	24.1
Other transfers	279	3.2	2567	6.1
Capital expenditure	(2194)	(24.8)	(17078)	(40.8)
Civil administration	90	1.0	717	1.7
Social services	239	2.7	1437	3.4
Economic services	784	8.9	3313	7.9
Domestic transfers	936	10.6	10739	25.7
Transfers abroad	1	—	11	—
Loans	135	1.5	801	1.9
Other payments	66	0.7	923	2.2
Total	8813	100.0	41839	100.0

Source: Central Bank of Ceylon, *Annual Review of the Economy.*

Table 3.15
Sri Lanka: Central Government Expenditure on Social Welfare,
1977 and 1983

	1977		1983	
	Rs m	*Percent*	*Rs m*	*Percent*
Current Account	(3114)	(92.9)	(6397)	(81.2)
A. *Social Services*	(1637)	(40.8)	(3756)	(47.9)
Education	860	25.6	2324	29.7
Health	455	13.6	1268	16.2
Housing	5	0.1	11	0.1
Special Welfare Services	28	0.8	75	1.0
Community Services	20	0.6	78	1.0
A. *Subtotal Social Services*	1637	40.8	3756	47.9
B. *Transfers*	(1747)	(52.1)	(2641)	(33.7)
Food Subsidies	1424	42.5	81	1.0
Food Stamps	—	—	1427	18.2
Kerosene Stamps	—	—	287	3.7
Other Transfers to Households	323	9.6	846	10.8
B. *Subtotal Transfers*	1747	52.1	2641	33.7
Subtotal Current Account (A + B)	3384	92.9	6397	81.6
Capital Account	(239)	(7.1)	(1437)	(18.3)
C. *Social Services*	239	7.1	1437	18.3
Education	116	3.5	507	6.5
Health	43	1.3	777	10.0
Housing	43	1.3	69	0.9
Special Welfare Services	15	0.5	10	0.1
Community Services	239	7.1	1437	18.3
C. *Subtotal Social Services*	239	7.1	1437	18.3
Grand Total (A + B + C)	3353	100.0	7834	100.0

Source: Central Bank of Ceylon, *Annual Review of the Economy.*

now took about one-fifth, in the form of food stamps. It is useful to recall that in 1977 the food subsidies absorbed 16.4 percent of total government spending whereas in 1983 it was only 4.3 percent (including kerosene stamps which were largely used to buy food).

Alailima (1984) investigated the incidence of government expenditure on different income classes in 1973 and 1980. She concluded that the incidence of such benefits was highly progressive in both years and remained "pro-poor." It was also noted that the subsidies had a much greater impact in 1980 than in 1973 in reducing income concentration (Alailima, 1984: 82). This happened principally because of the withdrawal of the consumer food subsidies from the higher income groups. However, there was also a major reduction in the food subsidies to the lower income groups. As we show later in this chapter, that, in combination with a decline in real incomes caused by inflation, has had a negative impact on family food intake and nutrition standards.

Health and Allied Welfare Expenditure

The adjustment program, especially its market bias, affected health policy in one significant respect. The market orientation principle was applied to the health sector in a limited fashion by encouraging the scope for the provision of fee levying services in patient care.

Sri Lanka always had a private patient care system that co-existed with the state system. This included private clinics and hospitals (both western and Ayurveda) as well as a limited number of fee-levying beds in a few major government hospitals. However, after 1977 four important qualitative changes took place. Firstly, government doctors were allowed to do "private practice" (for a fee service) outside their normal duty hours. This was meant to augment their income (and thereby reduce the demand for higher salaries that can be a burden on the budget) and also increase the supply of doctor services. Second, the government increased the number of pay beds in the state sector hospitals by constructing an ultra-modern 1001-bed hospital in Colombo. Third, the government used tax breaks and other incentives to encourage the establishment of private for-profit hospitals, an enterprise which has already attracted a sizable amount of capital. Fourth, the import of pharmaceutical products was liberalized. This reversed the then existing policy that prevented the import of brand names when cheaper generics of comparable quality were available. Fifth, the government abolished the monopoly held by the state-run university system to train medical doctors, and allowed a private fee-levying medical school to be established in 1981.

It is yet too early to assess the impact of these different measures. Moreover, a systematic study requires considerable data gathering from field surveys. However, taken together they spell out a new orientation in health care with the following implications. First, it is a clear attempt to shift a significant share of responsibility for patient care to the private sector and individuals. Second, given the relatively large proportion—around 75 percent—of the state health budget that is taken by patient care (Table 3.16), any steps that will help reduce that will, *ceteris paribus*, release resources for community health ("preventive") programs. Third, and this is perhaps the most important implication, the distributional consequences of the new orientation need to be examined. In principle, it may well augment resources overall and hence may not harm the relatively poor section of the community by draining resources from

Table 3.16
Sri Lanka: Composition of Health Expenditure (%), 1976–83

Year	General Administration	Patient Care	Community Health
1976	5.2	68.8	26.0
1977	6.2	69.3	24.5
1978	6.3	66.2	27.5
1979	6.6	64.2	29.2
1980	7.2	73.3	19.5
1981	7.8	71.1	21.2
1982	5.8	74.8	19.5
1983	3.7	80.7	15.6

Source: Ministry of Health.

the state sector. For example, the new beds in the private hospitals may relieve the pressure on hospitals in the state sector. Similarly, the private medical school may augment the total supply of doctors. On the other hand, the private sector can simply attract resources away from the state sector and make the health care system less equitable with means rather than need becoming the important factor in distribution. Moreover, urban-based and sophisticated curative facilities—often financed with foreign aid—may begin to claim an increasingly large share of the health budget. Another danger to equity is that the government could reduce the resources that are allocated to the state health care system, creating a sharp dichotomy between rich and poor in the delivery system.

With respect to the several points that were raised above, the data that are available yield a picture that has both negative and positive features. First, the cyclical variations in state health expenditure seen in Table 3.17 were partly precipitated by exogenous shocks that the economy felt. For example, the cut in expenditure seen in 1974–75 was associated with the first oil shock; and the cut in 1981 was connected with the mid-stream adjustment made in the 1977 program which was also precipitated, at least in part, by the second oil shock.

Second, Table 3.17 also shows that there has been no substantial trend growth in state health expenditure. (The sharp increase in 1983 is entirely due to provision being made to finance the large hospital referred to earlier with Japanese aid.) This is not sufficient proof of gradual "privatization" of health care under the liberalized economy. Computations based on data in the 1963, 1973, 1978–79 and 1981–82 *Consumer Finance Surveys* (Part II of Report) of the Central Bank of Ceylon reveal that households spent Rs 130 million, Rs 273 million, Rs 639 million and Rs 1068 million respectively on health care during the

Table 3.17
Sri Lanka: Government Health Expenditure, 1973–84

Year	Recurrent		Capital		Total				Total Real Expenditure (1970 Prices)	Per Capita Total Real Expenditure (Rs)	Per Capita Real Expenditure on Community Health (Rs)
	Rs m	Percent	Rs m	Percent	Rs m	Percent of Government Expenditure	Percent of GDP				
1973	268	98	5	2	273	5.1	1.53		216	16.50	N.A.
1974	297	98	6	2	303	4.8	1.30		190	14.30	N.A.
1975	334	95	18	5	352	4.6	1.37		205	15.19	N.A.
1976	407	94	25	6	432	4.8	1.54		238	17.35	4.51
1977	463	95	22	5	485	5.2	1.40		225	16.14	3.95
1978	524	85	80	15	604	3.4	1.49		260	18.32	5.04
1979	648	84	105	16	753	3.6	1.51		280	19.35	5.65
1980	762	84	122	16	884	3.2	1.42		278	18.86	3.68
1981	853	88	100	12	953	3.3	1.20		249	16.61	3.52
1982	999	82	183	18	1182	2.8	1.29		281	18.50	3.61
1983	1368	66	716	34	2084	4.0	1.83		425	27.58	4.30
1984	1621	92	129	7	1750	3.1	1.27		—	—	—

Note: Real expenditure figures have been calculated by deflating the nominal values using the Central Bank of Ceylon GDP deflator. Per capita expenditure on community health has been computed using the community health expenditure ratio in Table 14.6.

Source: Ministry of Health.

Table 3.18
Sri Lanka: Selected Indicators of Government Health Services,
1977 and 1983

	1977	1983	Change (%)
Doctors (western)	2168	2245	3.6
Nurses	6266	7112	13.5
Midwives	1995	2812	40.9
Assistant Medical Practitioners	1050	933	−11.1
No. of hospital beds	36281	37716	4.0

Source: Ministry of Health, *Administration Reports.*

years in question—as ratios of the government health budget these amounts were 82 percent, 54 percent, 80 percent and 85 percent respectively. In view of the relatively high ratio of private to government expenditure in 1963, it is difficult to judge, without more information, the significance of the increase in the ratio between 1973 and the later years. However, the data in Table 3.18 suggest that there has been no attempt to scale down the overall operations of the state health care system.

Third, the proportion of the state health budget taken by patient care has increased from less than 70 percent in the late 1970s to over 75 percent in the early 1980s (Table 3.16). The share devoted to community health has shown a corresponding decrease. A matter for some concern is the fact that per capita real expenditure on community health has been lower in the early 1980s than in the late 1970s.

Fourth, during the adjustment program period, up to 1981–82, there has been no significant change from the pattern that existed earlier in the distribution of medical expenses incurred by households in the different income groups. Calculations based on data in the *Consumer Finance Surveys* (Part II of the Reports) of the Central Bank of Ceylon reveal that in the three survey periods 1973, 1978–79 and 1981–82, the top one-fifth of the households in terms of income accounted for about half of total household expenditure on western health care—and also on health care of all types—and that the remaining four-fifths accounted for the other half. Table 3.19 shows that between 1978–79 and 1981–82 urban households as a group have increased their share of the total spent on western health care—in 1981–82 they spent almost double the share warranted by their population ratio. This in itself is not sufficient proof of a growing urban bias in the provision of health care facilities, or inaccessibility of such facilities to the rural population. On the one hand, given the higher incomes enjoyed by the urban population—in 1981–82 the median income of the rural household

Table 3.19

Sri Lanka: Sectoral Distribution of Household Expenditure on Western Health Care, 1973, 1978–79 and 1981–82

	Urban			Rural			Estate		
	Popu-lation Share (%) 1	Share of Total Health Care Expend-iture (%) 2	2/1 3	Popu-lation Share (%) 1	Share of Total Health Care Expend-iture (%) 2	2/1 3	Popu-lation Share (%) 1	Share of Total Health Care Expend-iture (%) 2	2/1 3
1973	22.3	34.3	1.54	68.5	60.1	0.88	9.2	5.6	0.61
1978–79	21.5	28.6	1.33	72.2	67.9	0.94	6.3	3.5	0.55
1981–82	21.5	40.3	1.87	72.2	56.8	0.79	6.3	2.8	0.44

Note: The 1973 population shares refer to the 1971 population census and those for 1978–79 and 1981–82 to the 1981 census.

Source: Calculated from data in Central Bank of Ceylon, *Consumer Finance Surveys* (years as above).

was 80 percent of that of the urban (Central Bank of Ceylon, 1984: 205)—higher private expenditure on health care in the urban sector is to be expected. On the other, this may release more state health care facilities for the rural and estate populations. However, no definite answer to this question can be given without further investigation.

Fifth, an attempt is being made to improve the managerial efficiency of the health sector and to prioritize activity with a focus on primary health care. This is being done with a rolling national health development plan, which is a new concept introduced in 1984 to Sri Lanka's health sector administration. The underlying economic reasoning behind this plan is the need to be cost-effective in utilizing the limited resources that are available under rather difficult economic conditions.

Sixth, several programs described below which are of considerable importance from the perspective of an integrated approach to health care have been undertaken, especially after 1980.

1. Beginning in 1981 the government supplies textbooks free of charge to all school children. The main purpose is to discourage the poor from dropping out of school due to lack of textbooks. Nevertheless, there is some evidence to suggest that the rate of school dropouts and illiteracy have risen since the late 1970s. (The crunch in real incomes of the poor and/or increased employment opportunities in the informal sector may explain the increase in the dropout rate.)

2. It was estimated that at the end of 1982 Sri Lanka had a housing backlog of 400,000 units. The current annual incremental demand is

around 50,000 units in the urban sector and 150,000 in the rural sector. Between 1978–84, 115,000 new housing units were constructed by the state sector. This has been one of the major social development programs of the government. The target for 1985–90 is to construct or upgrade 1 million housing units (one-fourth of national housing stock). Unlike in the 1978–85 program the state will not normally construct houses but will assist private individuals and firms in the construction by financing loans, etc. Obviously the housing program will have major long-term effects on public health.

3. In 1981, 27 percent of the people were supplied with pipe-borne water. By 1983 this had risen to 38 percent. The government has initiated a major program to raise this ratio, especially in the rural areas where it is still below 30 percent. Where pipe-borne water is not feasible, protected wells are being constructed to supply potable water. The water supply schemes that are planned envisage a total capital outlay of Rs 9 billion over 1985–1995 and a further Rs 2.4 billion will be spent on urban sewerage development. Here too there has been a major departure in pricing policy: beginning in 1981 the government has charged water users a fee to recover cost.

4. A special effort is being made to improve the educational and health status of the plantation community that suffers from comparatively high rates of illiteracy, morbidity and mortality. For instance, approximately 15 percent of the US $212 million invested under the Medium Term Investment Program (MTIP) in the state-owned estates have been earmarked for health, education and housing facilities (Ministry of Finance and Planning, 1985: 78–80). This may be considered as a good example of targeting of social welfare expenditure under the adjustment program.

Changes in Food Supply, Nutrition Status, Morbidity and Mortality

Food Supply and Nutrition Status

One of the key elements in the post-1977 food policy was to maintain an adequate overall supply of food through domestic production supplemented by imports. For example, the domestic production of rice—rice supplies about two-fifths of the calorie intake of Sri Lankans—increased by 71 percent from an average of 952,000 metric tons in 1975–77 to 1,629,000 metric tons in 1982–84. Inclusive of imports, domestic per capita annual gross rice availability over the two periods was 104.0 kg and 113.7 kg respectively. Wheat—which is a close substitute for rice in the Sri Lankan diet—was freely imported to maintain supplies. In the case of milk foods and sugar overall availability was considerably higher after 1977 compared to the mid-1970s when there was strict rationing. In general, the overall supply situation of almost every major food item improved after 1977. Moreover, in addition to rice, the home output of several other principal foodstuffs, notably potatoes, fish and fresh milk, increased over 1978–84. These were tradeables whose prices rose, when price controls were relaxed and the rupee was depreciated, giving an incentive to the producer. Thus, insofar as the poor were concerned the problem was not one of absolute scarcity of food but one of inadequate purchasing power to buy it in the open market.

The food stamp scheme that replaced the subsidized rice ration scheme was the principal income transfer scheme that operated in Sri Lanka after 1979 to help the low-income households. According to available estimates, in nominal terms, the food stamps were worth about Rs 95 to the average recipient family (Ministry of Plan Implementation (MOPI), 1981: 9; Edirisinghe, 1986: 32). Edirisinghe notes that this represented 112 percent of the value of the rice ration subsidy that was abolished. However, food stamps were fixed in money terms. In 1983 the kerosene stamp value was increased twice from Rs 9.50 to Rs 15.50 in March and to Rs 21.72 in August. Except for this marginal increase the food stamp cash values remained unchanged. Consequently, in terms of the price of rice—on which about three-quarters of the stamps were spent in 1984—the stamps of the average recipient family were worth only a little over 40 percent of the 1979 value. In view of the fact that for the poorest 20 percent the stamps accounted for at least 20 percent of household income (Edirisinghe, 1986: 32) and possibly more—according to one survey (MOPI, 1981: 9) it could have been as high as 55 percent—this represented a serious erosion of real purchasing power. Consequently, according to one official study (MOPI, 1982: 9–15), for a hypothetical family of five, food stamps supplied 36 percent of energy requirements and 34 percent of protein requirements in 1979, but the corresponding ratios for 1981 were only 18 percent and 17 percent respectively.

More generally, inflation and the reduction in food subsidies have affected the poorer sections of the community. First, both official (MOPI, 1984: 14) as well as unofficial (Edirisinghe, 1986: 63) analysts note that the three lowest income deciles have suffered a decline in their caloric intake between 1978–79 and 1981–82. Indeed, Lipton's "ultra-poor" (Lipton, 1983), defined as those who devote at least 80 percent of their expenditure to food but fail to achieve 80 percent of the recommended calorie allowance—2200 per day in Sri Lanka—had risen from 19.5 percent to 25 percent of households in the bottom quintile (Edirisinghe, 1986: 68). Finally, again both official (MOPI, 1984: 18–19) and unofficial (Sahn, 1985) sources note that in 1981–82 around one-third of pre-school children were chronically under-nourished (stunted) and about one-eighth were acutely undernourished (wasted). More disturbing from the point of view of the adjustment strategy is the fact that wasting appears to have worsened between 1975–76 and 1981–82 which indicates a deteriorating nutritional status (Sahn, 1985: 10). It should also be noted that in general the nutritional status was the lowest among the estate population.

Morbidity and Mortality

The infant mortality rate (IMR) has declined by almost 50 percent from 42.4 per 1000 in 1977 to 23.1 per 1000 in 1984 (Table 3.20). IMR is generally acknowledged to be a highly sensitive index of social wellbeing of the poor. For example, in Sri Lanka IMR increased from 46.3 per 1000 in 1973 to 51.2 per 1000 in 1974 when the domestic food situation deteriorated following the first oil shock. Therefore, the decline in IMR after 1977 taken in conjunction with the drop in morbidity rates as-sociated with nutrition deficiencies (Table 3.21) is difficult to be recon-ciled with the apparent deterioration of nutrition status of the bottom one-fifth of the population discussed earlier. One explanation for this apparent contradiction is that it would be possible for the overall mor-bidity and mortality rates to decline while those that apply to some population subsection deteriorate. It may also reflect the efficiency of the health care system in protecting the most vulnerable. The immuni-zation program is a case in point. It was accelerated in 1985 in collabo-

Table 3.20
Sri Lanka: Mortality Rates, 1976–84

Year	Crude Death Rate	Infant Mortality Rate	Neo-Natal-Mortality Rate	Maternal Mortality Rate
1976	7.8	43.7	26.1	0.9
1977	7.4	42.4	25.9	1.0
1978	6.6	37.1	25.0	0.8
1979	6.5	37.7	24.2	0.8
1980	6.1	34.4	22.7	0.6
1981	6.0	29.5	19.1	0.6
1982	6.1	30.5	18.1	0.6
1983	6.1	27.4	N.A.	N.A.
1984	6.5	23.1	N.A.	N.A.

Note: 1983 and 1984 figures are provisional.
Source: Ministry of Health, *Annual Health Bulletin 1983*. Registrar General's Department.

Table 3.21
Sri Lanka: Morbidity and Mortality per 100,000 Population in Selected Subgroups of Government Hospital Patients, 1970–83

	1970		1975		1980		1983	
	A	B	A	B	A	B	A	B
Intestinal infections	949	19.3	942	18.2	965	0.4	1186	13.15
Tuberculosis (all forms)	103	6.6	114	8.3	43	1.3	86	3.6
Helminthiasis	517	3.5	231	1.6	210	0.5	144	0.4
Malignancies	137	9.3	156	8.8	130	6.4	134	7.8
Nutritional deficiencies	151	1.7	198	10.4	136	1.3	120	1.7
Anaemias	508	5.7	431	9.4	338	3.3	292	2.5
Hypertension & ischaemic heart diseases	167	9.3	198	13.6	303	17.6	337	19.8
Injury and poisoning	2055	17.8	1751	21.2	1743	27.5	1257	22.5

Note: A = Cases per 100,000 population.
   B = Deaths per 100,000 population.
   Excludes admissions to the Peradeniya Teaching Hospital.
Source: Ministry of Health, *Annual Health Bulletin 1983.*

ration with UNICEF to immunize all children against tetanus, diptheria, whooping cough, polio, tuberculosis and measles and pregnant women against tetanus. The Health Ministry has targeted the less advantaged for special attention under this scheme and figures in Table 3.22 suggest considerable success. This means that the government's free medicine and hospital care provides a life support system to a section of the population who may not necessarily be healthy in the true sense of the term.

Conclusion

Based on the foregoing analysis, we consider some general questions concerning the relationship between stabilization measures and health and nutrition status. Here it is useful to note certain conditions whose

Table 3.22
Sri Lanka: Infant (one year old) and Pregnant Women Immunization Coverage Rate, 1981–85

	1980–Percent	1984–85 Percent
TB	61	71
DPT	46	70
Polio	48	71
Measles	nil	02
Tetanus (pregnant women)	72	41

Source: Grant, 1986.

combination is special, if not unique, to Sri Lanka—conditions that may affect the outcome in unexpected ways. One is the high literacy rate of 87 percent. Another is the politically conscious and highly competitive plural political system found in the country. It has a long reputation for sensitivity to voter needs, especially in relation to other countries. Sri Lanka held its first national election with universal suffrage for men and women over twenty-one in 1931, just three years after British women won suffrage and twenty-one years before India held such an election. Third, although Sri Lanka has no superhighways, it has a dense road network that permits even the more remote villages access to a town. Fourth, Sri Lanka has had a long established history of institutionalized health care. The Vaccination Ordinance, requiring the provision of immunization against disease, was passed in 1886. These and other similar factors may help to soften the adverse impact, if any, of economic policy on mass welfare.

However, the Sri Lankan experience after 1977 also highlights important dimensions of economic stabilization and adjustment that might have more general validity. First, Sri Lanka is a good example of adjustment with growth. We have argued here that it was that factor (growth) operating via employment that made the adjustment program socially bearable and even desirable for at least a majority of the population if one were to take the election victory of President Jayewardene in October 1982 as an endorsement of policy.

Second, the Sri Lankan experience showed the important role of international factors in third world adjustment programs. The large aid package helped to combine adjustment with growth. The adverse impact of the terms of trade showed that countries such as Sri Lanka will find it extremely difficult to cope with the adjustment demands made by the international economy without some sort of international support.

Third, it showed that the orientation of domestic investment towards domestic agriculture, food production in particular, was helpful to soften the social impact of the adjustment program.

Fourth, the Sri Lankan experience highlighted the importance of properly targeted social welfare programs to make adjustment programs humane and socially and politically acceptable and, at the same time, economically successful. Even with the same level of budgetary resources the food stamps scheme could have improved its actual benefits to the poor if the considerable leakage to higher income groups had been prevented. More generally, the adjustment experience forced the authorities to seek out the more vulnerable groups, especially in matters of health and nutrition, for state assistance and programs.

Fifth, it is important to go beyond national averages in health and nutrition matters and to identify the relatively less fortunate in terms of their regional, occupational, ethnic and other characteristics. This is needed if health and nutrition programs are to be made more cost-effective and socially beneficial.

Sixth, the crisis has opened new ways of thinking on and management of issues vital to health and nutrition. For example, nutrition policy is no longer considered in isolation as a matter only for the health officials. Now there is a serious attempt to integrate nutrition policy with food and agriculture policy. However, it is also useful to note that progress in such matters, which often are major departures from established bureaucratic procedures, is slow.

Seventh, given Sri Lanka's past record as a provider of free or subsidized food, free health care and publicly financed education to the mass of people, the adjustment program forced the country to rethink fundamental economic questions that any society must face in providing such services—namely who pays, how much, and who benefits. Though put simply, these are questions for which there are no easy answers. Sri Lanka made a decision, for example, that some who hitherto did not pay the market price for rice should do so. Health services are still free; however, after the adjustment program the government has encouraged those who can afford to pay for such services to do so. We have pointed out that such policies can have major equity implications that need to be studied.

Finally, we would like to note that the economic crisis and the adjustment program in particular forced the country to reexamine long-standing institutions, policies, and the assumptions that underlay them in public policy. This is useful; they should not be regarded as permanent fixations in the polity that simply require minor adjustments from time to time until conditions return to normal. The one matter of which we can be reasonably certain is that the present economic difficulties will be with us for quite some time to come.

References

Abyeratne, Seneka, and Thomas T. Poleman. *Socioeconomic Determinants of Child Malnutrition in Sri Lanka: The Evidence from Galle and Kalutara Districts.* Ithaca: Cornell University, 1983.

Agrarian Research and Training Institute (ARTI), Sri Lanka. *Hired Labourers in Peasant Agriculture in Sri Lanka.* Colombo: ARTI, 1980a.

———. *A Study of Five Settlement Schemes Prior to Irrigation Modernization, Vol. V Padaviya.* Colombo: ARTI, 1980b.

———. *The Economics of Seasonal Labour Migration in Sri Lanka.* Colombo: ARTI, 1981.

Alailima, P. *Fiscal Incidence in Sri Lanka.* Geneva: International Labour Office, 1984.

Athukorala, Premachandra. "The Impact of the 1977 Policy Reforms on Domestic Industry," *Upanathi* 1:1 (1986).

———. "Import Substitution, Structural Transformation and Trade Dependence: A Case Study of Sri Lanka," *The Developing Economies* 24:2 (1981).

Central Bank of Ceylon. *Report on Consumer Finances and Socio-Economic Survey 1981/82 Sri Lanka*, Part I. Colombo: Central Bank of Ceylon, 1984.

Chenery, Hollis. "Comments" on Anne O. Krueger's Paper in Cline and Weintraub, 1981.

Cline, William R. and Sidney Weintraub, eds. *Economic Stabilization in Developing Countries*. Washington, D.C.: The Brookings Institute, 1981.

Dervis, Kemal. "Comments" on the paper by Lance Taylor in Cline and Weintraub, 1981, pp. 503–506.

Edirisinghe, Neville. *The Food Stamp Program in Sri Lanka: Costs, Benefits and Policy Options*, Washington, D.C.: International Food Policy Research Institute, 1986.

Grant, James P. *The State of the World's Children 1987*. New York: Oxford University Press for UNICEF, 1986.

Killick, Tony. *The Quest for Economic Stabilization*. New York: St. Martin's Press, 1984a. See especially Killick, "The IMF Stabilization Programs," pp. 183–226.

———. *The IMF and Stabilization*, New York: St. Martin's Press, 1984b.

——— and Jennifer Sharpley. "Extent, Causes and Consequences of Disequilibrium" in Killick, 1984a, pp. 15–54.

Krueger, Anne O. "Interactions Between Inflation and Trade Regime: Objectives of Stabilization Programs," in Cline and Weintraub, 1981, pp. 83–118.

Lakshman, W. D. "State Policy in Sri Lanka and Its Economic Impact 1970–85: Selected Themes with Special Reference to Distributive Implication of Policy," *Upanathi* 1:1 (1986): 5–36.

Lal, D. "Supply Price and Surplus Labour: Some Indian Evidence," *World Development* 4 (1976): 10–11.

———. *The Poverty of Development Economics*. Cambridge: Harvard University Press, 1985.

Lipton, M. *Poverty, Undernutrition and Hunger*. World Bank Staff Paper No. 597, Washington, D.C.: World Bank, 1983.

Ministry of Finance and Planning, Sri Lanka. *Public Investment 1985–1989*. Colombo, Sri Lanka, 1985.

Ministry of Plan Implementation (MOPI), Sri Lanka. *Nutritional Status: Survey in the Mahaweli H. Area*. Colombo: 1981.

———. *Survey Report of the Food Stamp Scheme*. Colombo: 1982.

———. *Evaluation Report on the Food Stamp Scheme*. Colombo: 1982.

———. *National Agricultural, Food and Nutrition Strategy*. Colombo: mimeo, 1983.

———. *A Preliminary Analysis of the Determinants of Nutrition Welfare in Sri Lanka*. Colombo: 1984a.

———. *Nutrition Strategy*. Colombo: 1984b.

———. *Nutritional Status and Its Determinants and Intervention Programmes* (Final report). Colombo: 1984.

Ministry of Plan Implementation and the International Food Policy Research Institute. *Sri Lanka Nutritional Surveillance Programme*. Colombo, 1985.

Peiris, G. H. "Land Reform and Agrarian Change in Sri Lanka," *Modern Asian Studies* 12:4 (1978).

Richards, Peter, and Wilbert Gooneratne. *Basic Needs, Poverty and Government Policies in Sri Lanka*. Geneva: International Labour Office, 1980.

Sahn, David E. *Food Consumption Patterns and Parameters in Sri Lanka: Causes and Control of Malnutrition*. Washington, D.C.: International Food Policy Research Institute, 1985.

Samarasinghe, S. W. R. de A. *Ethnic Conflict and Economic Development in Sri Lanka*. Kandy, Sri Lanka: International Centre for Ethnic Studies, mimeo, 1985.

Sharpley, Jennifer. "Jamaica, 1972–80," in Killick, 1984b, pp. 115–163.

Snodgrass, D. R. "Sri Lanka's Economic Development During Twenty-five Years Since Independence," *The Ceylon Journal of Historical and Social Studies* 4:1–2 (1974).

Sutton, Mary. "Introduction and Summary of Companion Volume" in Killick, 1984b, pp. 1–18.

Taylor, Lance. "IS/LM in the Tropics: Diagrammatics of the New Structuralist Macro Critique," in Cline and Weintraub, 1981, pp. 465–506.

Timmer, C. Peter, and Mathew Giurreiro. *Food Aid and Development Policy*. Colombo: ADC/RTN Conference, mimeo, 1980.

Wilson, A. J. *The Gaullist System in Asia: The Constitution of Sri Lanka 1978*. London: Macmillan, 1980.

Women's Bureau, Sri Lanka. *Impact of the U.N. Decade for Women in Sri Lanka*. Colombo: Ministry of Women's Affairs, 1985.

World Bank. *Sri Lanka: Issues and Prospects for Industrial Development*. Washington, D.C.: 1979.

———. *World Development Report 1983*. New York: Oxford University Press, 1984.

———. *World Debt Tables*. 1984–85 ed. Washington, D.C.: 1985.

Wriggins, W. H. *Ceylon: Dilemmas of a New Nation*. Princeton: Princeton University Press, 1960.

4

A UNICEF Perspective on the Effects of Economic Crises and What Can Be Done

Richard Jolly

The 1980s will almost certainly be recorded by future development historians as a decade of rising poverty and malnutrition in many if not most countries of the world. Certainly this is true for the vast majority of countries in Africa and Latin America. It is probably true also for many of the better-off countries in the Middle East. Even the US, Britain and some of the other industrialized countries have experienced increases in poverty—and possibly in malnutrition among the poorest as well. Only in the economically dynamic Asian countries can one be reasonably sure that malnutrition and poverty are declining rather than increasing—in both the proportion of the population affected and the depth of poverty and malnutrition they experience.

What has been happening in the majority of countries is a widespread and marked *deterioration* in the human condition.[1] Poverty and malnutrition are worsening, not merely persisting as for so long before. Nor, as often before, is it a matter of worsening poverty in some countries with improvements in others. The early 1980s have produced a strong, sustained, and systematic set of downward international pressures on the majority of developing countries, with the consequence that living standards have very seriously deteriorated. There is still time for change, but without it, the second half of the 1980s will be little better.

*A version of this paper was originally prepared for a conference in honor of Prof. H. W. Singer and will be published in *Poverty, Development and Food: Revisited*, edited by Edward Clay and D. John Shaw.

81

This chapter will focus on the situation and the need for offsetting action in that majority of countries whose economies are open to global influences, especially the economic repercussions of world recession. In most cases, it is extremely difficult to disentangle the effects of global influences from national influences and to distinguish causes from the effects of policy actions they often engender. Such disentangling, while not without interest, is not essential for deciding that remedial action needs to be taken both nationally and internationally. Action is the concern here, just as action for development has been the focus of most of Hans Singer's life work. For this reason, this chapter shows what a broader approach to adjustment policy would involve and how this content relates directly to earlier development concerns with basic needs and redistribution with growth. This is done in five parts:

- The context—rising malnutrition and economic decline in the 1980s
- The impact of adjustment policy
- Adjustment with a human face
- Links with basic needs and redistribution with growth
- Monitoring of the human dimension of adjustment

The Context—Rising Malnutrition and Economic Decline in the 1980s

The increase in the levels of severe and moderate malnutrition of children under age five in six African countries is shown in Figures 4.1 through 4.6. These figures are of double interest. In the first place, they show the seasonal fluctuations in the levels of child malnutrition—a typical situation in predominantly rural countries where for poor families food shortages become increasingly common in the pre-harvest period. For young children, the period of food shortages is often compounded by seasonal patterns in the incidence of diseases like measles or diarrhea, with their own downward pressures on growth and weight gain.

In the second place, the figures highlight the increasing pressures on child nutrition in all parts of Africa in recent years—the starting point of this discussion. Ghana showed the most serious increase of those recorded. The proportion of children moderately or severely malnourished almost doubled from 1980 to 1983. Fortunately, the situation improved somewhat during 1984, though malnutrition levels remained well above those for 1980–81. Botswana and Burundi also record clear increases in the proportion of children malnourished.

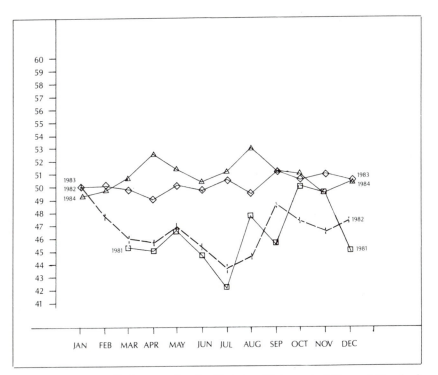

Figure 4.1. *Burundi: Percent of under 5's below 80 percent of Harvard Standard Weight for Age.*

Although the changes in Lesotho, Madagascar and Rwanda are relatively small, one should note that in every case the changes are upward and from unacceptably high base levels—20 percent or so in Lesotho, 30 percent in Rwanda, and 45 percent in Madagascar.

These figures also show the possibility of regularly monitoring nutrition, one of the most basic indicators of the human conditions. But for the moment, let us return to the economic pressures creating or contributing to much of the human deterioration observed.

The forces at work can be illustrated in graphs and references. Figure 4.7 shows schematically the movement over time of per capita consumption (the C curve) in a hypothetical developing country—one highly dependent on primary commodities with an economy open and highly sensitive to changes in the world economy. With deteriorating terms of trade for primary commodities, sluggish world demand for manufactures, rises in interest rates and debt servicing, stagnation in private capital flows, often compounded by other influences, it is not surprising that per capita income has fallen and with it per capita consumption.

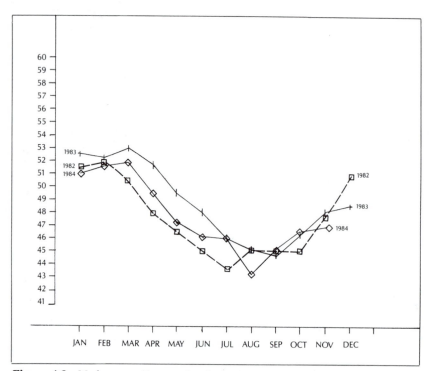

Figure 4.2. *Madagascar: Percent of under 5's below 80 percent of Harvard Standard Weight for Age.*

There are, of course, many possible variations in the decline in income (GNP) and consumption per capita. In Figure 4.7, C^0v shows a sharp fall followed by unmitigated long-term decline. If we assume that "adjustment policy measures" are taken nationally or internationally, and that domestic policies are severely inadequate, without major corrections the downward path of production and per capita consumption seems likely to continue. In other cases, as C^iv, there may be hope of some future upturn if external conditions improve.

A 1983 UNICEF study explored the impact of world recession on children, especially the poor and vulnerable, using data from a dozen country case studies. It showed that the impact was usually magnified rather than diminished in the process of transmission from rich to poor countries and from rich to poor within countries. In general, and in the absence of special offsetting action, world recession took its greatest toll on children. Two major reasons account for this result.

The mechanisms of international transmission usually magnify the economic effects of global recession on the poorer countries. These countries in turn have a greater proportion of their populations poor,

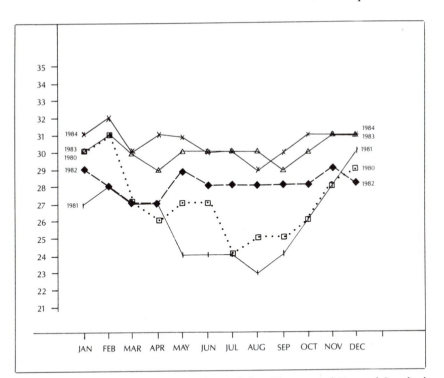

Figure 4.3. *Botswana: Percent of under 5's below 80 percent of Harvard Standard Weight for Age.*

young and in the vulnerable groups. The extent of this multiplied impact is often disguised by referring to *average annual* growth rates for the main regions of the world rather than rates per capita of total *decline since peak year* for individual countries. Table 4.1 summarizes the number of developing countries recording declines in per capita income each year since 1980.

In addition, another six or so countries (twelve in 1985) recorded per capita growth of less than 1 percent per year. Over the period shown, almost two-thirds of the developing countries recorded negative or negligible per capita growth. The lowest income countries of Africa were affected the worst.

The net effect was cumulative decline of a substantial magnitude (over 20 percent, 1980–85) in eighteen of the seventy-nine countries for which we have data and of 10–20 percent in another seventeen. Altogether fifty countries experienced negative growth from 1980–85. These economic setbacks, because of their size and sustained effect, stand in sharp contrast to the slow but mostly positive growth of the industrial countries over the same period.

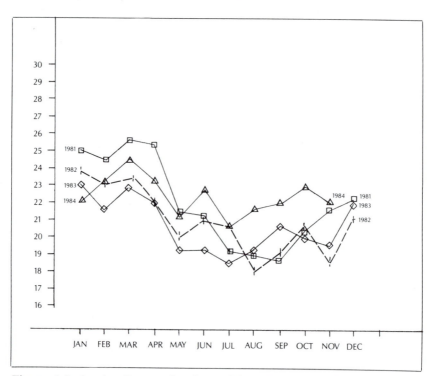

Figure 4.4. *Lesotho: Percent of under 5's below 80 percent of Harvard Standard Weight for Age.*

Within countries, this decline in average per capita income has a magnified impact on the poor and on children. There are three main factors at work:

1. the tendency for cutbacks in employment and wages to hit the poor more severely than the better-off

2. the tendency for health education and other social sectors to be cut back more than the so-called productive sectors of government spending

3. the tendency for poorer families to have larger numbers of children and others who are vulnerable

The effects of declining income are offset for some of the rural population because the more remote rural areas are comparatively insulated from government and the urban and international economy. Just as this part of the rural population commonly received only limited benefits from the expansion of government services, so also it has suffered relatively less from the cutbacks and withdrawal of these services.

Table 4.1

Number of Developing Market Economies with Growth Rates of Real GDP At or Below the Rate of Growth of Population,* 1979–85

	Total Number of Countries	Number of Affected Countries						
		1979	*1980*	*1981*	*1982*	*1983*	*1984*	*1985*
All developing market economies	83	26	32	38	55	51	45	49
Africa	32	14	15	21	25	21	25	21
Latin America	23	6	8	12	21	19	11	18
West Asia	14	4	5	5	7	8	8	7
South and East Asia	14	2	4	0	2	3	1	3

*Excluding India.

In Brief, GDP per capita has been declining or stagnating for between half and two-thirds of the eighty-two developing market economies included in the sample, while in 1985, 718 million people, or 42 percent of the population of the developing market economies (excluding India) were affected by negative growth rates of GDP per capita. In Africa 84 percent of the population experienced a negative growth rate in GDP per capita in the same year.

The cumulative decline in GDP per capita experienced by many developing market economies over the 1980–1985 period has been very large in many cases. In about one-fifth of the eighty-two countries the cumulative decline was extremely large (greater than 20 percent). In the next fifth it was also quite severe (between 10 and 20 percent). Only in a little more than a quarter of the countries has there been sustained growth from 1980 to 1985.

Source: United Nations Department of International Economic and Social Affairs, Table II-2. New York: UN-DIESA, 1986.

However, too much should not be made of this insulation. The truly subsistence economy is rare, and subsistence economies have always left much to be desired in the area of basic health and nutrition—especially when land is limited and population has grown. Nevertheless, the change in per capita consumption conveyed in Figure 4.7 may overstate the extent of decline in the subsistence sector where consumption will probably have fluctuated less but around a lower level. The major setbacks in this sector will be more the result of drought and much less the result of national and international factors.

But for major parts of the population, national and international forces will have had a marked effect on household incomes—especially on the incomes of the poor and vulnerable groups, shown as Cv in Figure 4.7. This figure also shows consumption in relation to a minimum level of basic needs (BN) consumption, defined in reference to the minimum requirements for nutrition, clothing, shelter, health and education. The declines of income and consumption soon reduce consumption to levels below minimum requirements, as Figure 4.7 illustrates.

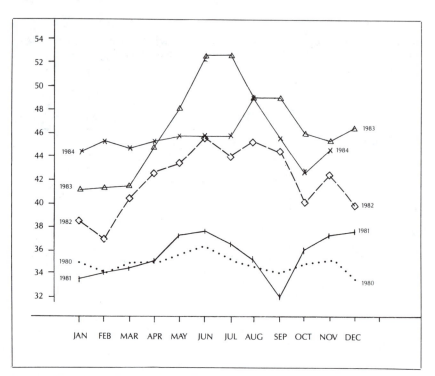

Figure 4.5. *Ghana: Percent of under 5's below 80 percent of Harvard Standard Weight for Age.*

Note that because there is a certain arbitrariness about the precise line, numbers below it may be imprecise—but there is less doubt about changes.

There are, of course, many possible trends in Cv. Figure 4.7 shows perhaps the most favorable of the likely options, in the absence of special action. In this scenario, the consumption pattern of the vulnerable changes pro-rata with per capita income—implying unchanged factor shares and unchanged income shares by income group. However, if all the tendencies listed earlier were operating, Cv would decline even more than shown.

The Impact of Adjustment Policy

So far—at least conceptually—the argument has tried to portray the direct impact of world recession against some background of broadly unchanged domestic and international policy. In practice, there will almost always be some immediate policy adaptations to the worsening

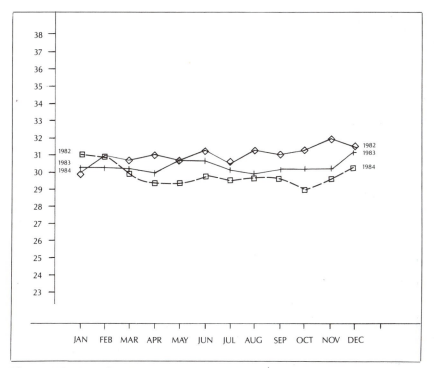

Figure 4.6. *Rwanda: Percent of under 5's below 80 percent of Harvard Standard Weight for Age.*

international situation, but as a frame of reference it will be convenient to ignore them.

What now of national "adjustment policies," that set of domestic policy changes and international pressures and support consciously designed to curb the macro deficits in the balance of payments and the government budget and to restore a pattern of non-inflationary economic growth over the medium term?[2]

These measures of domestic adjustment policy may be adopted independently of any international *quid pro quo* or as part of some formal or informal international agreement, whereby the domestic measures are part of a total package of reform and international financial support. Either way they will further affect the level of consumption and living standards of the population. Usually these measures involve some conscious reduction of consumption in the short run in the hopes of restoring balance, investment, and growth of the economy in the medium to longer run.

This is shown in Figure 4.8 as the curve $C^i v$—a reduction of the consumption curve in the short run and, after a period, some return

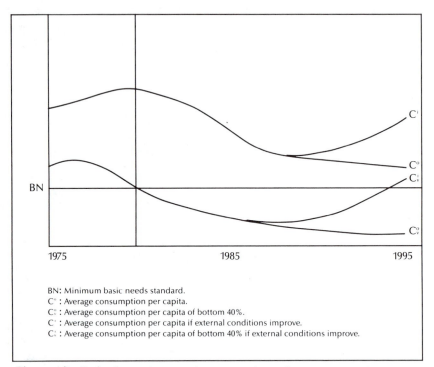

BN

1975   1985   1995

BN: Minimum basic needs standard.
C" : Average consumption per capita.
C⁰ᵥ : Average consumption per capita of bottom 40%.
Cⁱ : Average consumption per capita if external conditions improve.
Cᵢᵥ : Average consumption per capita of bottom 40% if external conditions improve.

Figure 4.7. *Paths of average per capita consumption and average per capita consumption of bottom 40 percent when no adjustment measures are taken.*

to growth of income and consumption. This addition to growth will result, in principle, both from restructuring the economy and from an extra inflow of funds from abroad. In practice, as the controversy over orthodox adjustment policy shows, neither in theory nor in actual achievement is it clear that the orthodox policies generally have led to such an acceleration or "restoration" of growth.

Recently there have been calls for more growth-oriented adjustment, giving more conscious attention to policies and measures to stimulate growth during and as an objective of the process of adjustment. Figure 4.8 illustrates a more growth-oriented adjustment path as Cⁱⁱv, corresponding to the emerging orthodoxy of a more conscious concern with accelerating growth in the adjustment process. Note that if the adjustment process is accompanied by a marked increase of net foreign exchange inflow from abroad, both Cⁱv and Cⁱⁱv could be somewhat shifted upwards.

But for the present the purpose of the diagram is to illustrate a separate and simpler point. How are the consumption and the living standards of the poor and vulnerable affected by the process of adjust-

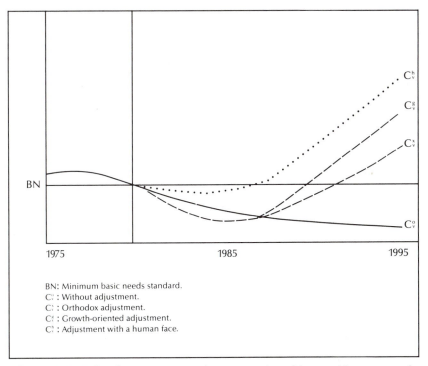

Figure 4.8. *Paths of average per capita consumption of bottom 40 percent under different adjustment policies.*

ment? There are three basic possibilities, corresponding to whether the income distribution effects of the adjustment policies followed are positive, neutral or negative.[3] If neutral, the consumption levels of the poorest will fall by the same proportion as the consumption levels of other groups; if positive, by not so much; if negative, by more.

However, I argue that the critical issue is not whether income distribution as such is worsened or unchanged, but where the consumption and living standards of the population are left in relation to their basic needs. If the proportion of the rural or urban population whose basic minimum needs for nutrition, food, or health are unmet is increased, and if the deficiency between their needs and their actual levels of consumption is also growing, there will be growing numbers in the country who are less and less able to support the process of economic revival and participate in its achievement. In economic parlance, there will be a disinvestment of human capital, affecting both the short and the longer run. In the short run, low levels of nutritional intake and probably increased levels of illness will take direct tolls on productivity and economic production, especially in the small scale agricultural sector and the informal urban sector. Even in the small scale agricultural sector, where most farmers will have access to their own production, there are likely to be some repercussions as the result of cutbacks in agricultural equipment and materials, essential drugs such as antimalarials, and other things needed for basic services.

The longer-run effects may be even more serious, especially for children under five years old. This is the age group most vulnerable to short-term health and nutritional deficiencies and the period of life over which critical needs cannot be postponed without considerable risk. If the purpose of adjustment policy is to lay the foundations for sustained growth in the economy over the longer term, it is senseless to ignore the most basic needs of the population in the process. Yet if nutrition standards fall or basic health and basic education services are cut back, this is precisely what is being done.

Adjustment with a Human Face

We have now provided the frame within which a broader policy of adjustment with a human face can be illustrated. Such an approach would combine the basic economic elements of adjustment policy with conscious efforts to ensure that the basic nutrition and health and education needs of the entire population are satisfied. This is shown in Figure 4.8 as the curve $C^{iii}v$, which includes special measures to raise the consumption levels of the most vulnerable to the basic needs minimum during the periods of adjustment when consumption levels in general are most constrained. In this respect, the consumption path of the most vulnerable would be kept as near as possible along the horizontal BN line until point BN', after which it would rise along the curve $C^{iii}v$ as shown.

As I have explained elsewhere (Jolly, 1985), this would involve three types of policy action:

First, a clear acknowledgment in the goals of adjustment policy of concern for basic human welfare and a commitment to protect the minimum nutrition levels of children and other specially vulnerable groups of a country's population.

Second, the implementation of a broader approach to the adjustment process itself, comprising four components:

1. Actions to maintain a minimum floor for nutrition and other basic human needs, related to what the country can in the long term sustain.

2. Restructuring within the productive sectors—agriculture, services, industry—to rely more upon the small-scale, informal sector pro-

ducers and to ensure their greater access to credit, internal markets and other measures which will stimulate growth in their incomes.

3. Restructuring within health, education and other social sectors, to restore momentum and ensure maximum coverage and benefits from constrained and usually reduced resources. Already, there are important examples of what can be done to reach all of a country's population, but still at relatively low cost.

4. More international support for these aspects of adjustment, including more finance, flexibly provided and with longer term commitments. The extremes of the present situation will often require a ceiling on outflows of interest and debt amortization if the protection of human needs is to be feasible in the short run.

Third, a system for monitoring nutrition levels and the human situation during the process of adjustment. We should be concerned not only with inflation, balance of payments, and GNP growth—but also with nutrition, food balances and human growth. The proportion of a nation's households falling below some basic poverty line should be monitored and treated as one of the most relevant statistics for assessing adjustment.

There is one point about adjustment with a human face which is frequently misunderstood. Because the focus is on human need, there is a common tendency, almost a reflex of the economic mind, to think of the program as a welfare program. I would stress that it is primarily a program of enhancing production and investment—in an area of production and investment often overlooked and downplayed in spite of clear economic evidence of the positive and often high economic returns accruing to these activities.

This is not the place to summarize the literature, but it may help to remind readers of the basic points and evidence in the key areas concerned.

Economic Efficiency of the Small-Scale Producer

Many studies have documented the relative efficiency of the small-scale producer, rural or urban. In terms of productivity per acre, use of resources and equipment, and returns to capital, the small-scale farmer usually achieves much better economic efficiency than the large-scale farmer. The same is frequently true of the small-scale urban producer in both the formal and informal sectors, though here the evidence is more limited. A strong case can be made, therefore, for expecting that a shift of emphasis in production to the small-scale producer will increase, not reduce, productivity and growth. There is overwhelming evidence that increasing production by the small-scale producer is the most effective way to increase incomes in the producer's household.

Labor intensive investment generally is both efficient and employment creating. This was the basis of the East Asian success. It is not, therefore, just a question of *adding* some small-scale production to the existing industrial structure but of changing the industrial structure radically and also shifting to rural industrialization by:

1. promoting small-scale production throughout the economy
2. fostering linkages between the agricultural sector and rural industry and processing

Productivity

Alan Berg (1981) writes:

> Overcoming deficiencies in nutrition produces stronger, more energetic workers, reduces the number of work days lost because of illness, lengthens the working lifespan, and increases cognitive skills. The flow of earnings is thereby increased above what it would have been in the absence of improved nutrition and health. (Berg, 1981: 14).[4]

The same publication summarizes the links between improved nutrition and increases in the benefits to children and society from education, family planning programs, anti-poverty programs and, in general, human well-being and the capacity "to enjoy whatever sources of human satisfaction are available."

It is important also to recognize that these nutritional benefits accrue to workers in the recognized (or formal sector) part of the labor force but also to others, especially but not only women, who are engaged in household activities which may not be counted in national income but which greatly influence economic production and household living standards.

Investment

Investment, the long-run contribution to enhancing productivity, may be even more important, especially in the case of children. The failure to provide adequate nutrition during the first five years of life may lead to lifelong impairment of all the human and productive capacities mentioned above. The economic evidence of positive returns to basic levels of human investment has been frequently documented. For instance, the World Bank's *World Development Report 1980* gives estimates from sixty developing countries showing that the social returns to primary education averaged 22 to 27 percent higher than the typical returns to physical investment. Moreover, the rates of return to primary education were significantly higher than the returns to secondary and higher education and showed only a mild tendency to decline over time as education expanded. In addition, investment in primary education also tends to be redistributive towards the poor, thus enhancing income distribution *and* poverty alleviation. These direct estimates are supported by the evidence of education's long-run, qualitative benefits to worker productivity: for instance, the effects of primary education of women in improving child care, reducing infant and child mortality rates, and reducing fertility and thus population growth rates.

Evidence of the economic return from basic health services and expenditure is more limited. But there are impressive examples of the high cost-effectiveness of preventive health services over curative, precisely the sorts of health actions to which a basic needs approach would give priority.

The Impact of Adjustment with a Human Face on Economic Growth

With these reminders of the positive contributions to productivity and investment of expenditures on basic needs, it is time to return to the effects of an adjustment strategy protecting human needs on the subsequent path of economic growth and consumption. Figure 4.8 showed this as $C^{iii}v$, in which the upturn took place sooner and the rate of consumption growth was higher than for any of the strategies which omitted direct attention to the human factor.

This, however, is only one of several possible growth paths. It corresponds to a case in which basic needs expenditures strongly and immediately enhance productivity—as, for instance, when the initial deficiencies in health, nutrition and incentives of the active labor force are very considerable. To redress these deficiencies will then have an immediate effect on production.

At the other extreme, if the basic needs expenditures have a weak immediate effect on productivity but the long-run investment effects are strong, the total adjustment package will still help to accelerate economic growth, but only after an interval. In this case, the upward shift of consumption will occur later, as shown in $C^{iii}v$ (b), Figure 4.9.

The relationship of the various C^{iii} paths to the conventional or more growth-oriented adjustment paths (C^i or C^{ii}) will also depend on the sources of support for the basic needs measures. If they are taken from consumption of higher income groups, from "unproductive" uses of government expenditure, or from additional foreign aid, the adjustment with a human face path will at every point do as well as the growth-

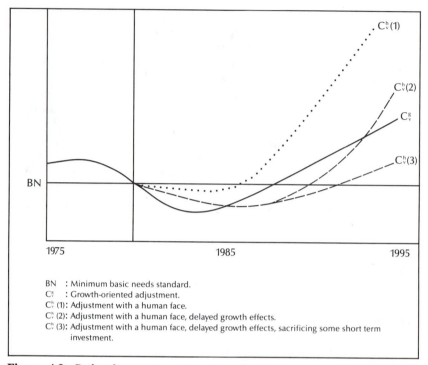

Figure 4.9. *Paths of average per capita consumption of bottom 40 percent under growth-oriented adjustment and alternative options of adjustment with a human face.*

oriented path, and at some point it will accelerate and do better—following some path like $C^{iii(a)}$ or $C^{iii(b)}$. If, however, the sources of support for the basic needs measures are taken from resources which would otherwise have supported the conventional adjustment program, long-run growth may be accelerated, assuming the rates of return on the human investment are higher than those on the foregone investment in physical investment—but it may take longer for the higher returns to materialize. In this case, the curve $C^{iii(c)}$ might start its upward acceleration later than C^{i} or C^{ii} but after a point cross over to produce the greater long-run growth which it promises.

Obviously these are only the polar cases of possible combinations. And it must be emphasized that they are analytical abstractions from a real world in which many other factors, economic, political, social, inevitably enter. But with appropriate attention to the right conditions, it should be possible to aim for a $C^{iii(a)}$ path with as much probability of success as any of the other paths sketched out.

In the short run, this is likely to be the significant tradeoff, relievable only to the extent that additional outside support is provided to ease it. In the long run, by making more rapid growth possible, this tradeoff can be greatly eased if not made to disappear.

And this is the parallel with the arguments for redistribution with growth or for a basic needs growth strategy. Within a considerable margin of options, one can show that over the long run a country can pursue a positive-sum growth strategy in which all groups can be better off than they would otherwise be, especially but not only the poor. One can identify a number of countries which have in fact achieved just such a combination of growth and increasing basic needs satisfaction, sometimes with considerable redistribution, over the post-war period.

I have stressed the need for restructuring *within* the social sectors, in addition to the continued concern with restructuring the economic sectors. Here I must make another general point of fundamental importance. Adjustment policy with a human face will remain a sham—an attempt to paint a smile on a face with tears—if it is seen only as a matter of a change in the macroeconomic policy of government. Instead it must involve a move to a more people-focused process of adjustment, a more fundamental restructuring—a shift to much greater self-reliance, to decentralization, small-scale production and community action, empowerment of people and households. These are the groups and approaches which in fact provide the goods and services and generate the incomes for the low-income sections of most populations. These are also the sectors which more often than not are squeezed by adjustment approaches as conventionally implemented. Yet for sheer cost-effectiveness, as well as protection for the poor, these are the approaches that matter.

Antecedents

Precisely because this broader approach to adjustment differs from much current thinking, it may be helpful to set it within the context of earlier development thinking. The obvious links, as explained, are with strategies of redistribution with growth and of meeting basic needs. Both were part of the rethinking of development strategy in the early 1970s and both are closely associated with the work of Hans Singer.

Singer himself played an important part in the evolution of redistribution from growth thinking, initially in his contributions to the ILO Kenya Mission report, *Employment, Incomes and Equality*. Later these ideas were generalized and developed more formally in the IDS/World Bank study, *Redistribution with Growth*, which explored both the economic rationale and the approaches for such strategy.

As Paul Streeten has aptly summed up in the World Bank Study, *First Things First*, the emergence of basic needs thinking in the 1970s was in one sense a

> homecoming. For when the world embarked on development thirty years ago, it was primarily with the needs of the poor in mind. Third World leaders wanted economic as well as political independence, but independence was to be used for man's self-fulfillment. The process got sidetracked. . . . (Streeten, 1981).

Streeten points out the compelling logic of basic needs. It is not only a strategy for efficiently meeting the needs of the poorest 40 percent of the population but of increasing their productivity and thereby enabling them to contribute efficiently to their own development and the alleviation of their own poverty.

In the same book, Mahbub ul-Haq sums up the core of the argument (Streeten, 1981).

> It is true that the only way absolute poverty can be eliminated on a permanent and sustainable basis, is to increase the productivity of the poor. But direct methods to increase the productivity of the poor need to be supplemented with efforts to provide their unmet basic needs, for at least the following four reasons:
>
> - First, education and health are required—in addition to machines, land, and credit—to increase productivity. Sufficient empirical evidence is now available to suggest that education and health services often make a greater contribution to improving labor productivity than do most alternative investments.
>
> - Second, many poor people have no physical assets—neither a small farm nor a small industry. They are the landless or urban poor. The only asset they possess is their own two hands and their willingness to work. In such a situation the best investment is in human resource development.
>
> - Third, it is not enough to enable the poor to earn a reasonable income. They also need goods and services on which to spend their income. Markets do not always supply wage goods, particularly public services. Greater production of wage goods and the expansion and redistribution of public services become essential if basic needs of the majority of the population are to be met.
>
> - Finally, it may take a long time to increase the productivity of the absolute poor to a level at which they can afford at least the minimum bundle of basic needs for a productive life. In the interim, some income groups—particularly the bottom 10 to 20 percent—may need short-term subsidy programmes.

This quotation underlines again the basic argument for making the protection of basic needs the highest priority in the adjustment process.

With this priority, the living standard of the poor will not only be protected, but their productivity will be considerably enhanced. Indeed, without concern for the human dimension, not only will productivity be set back, but investment in the next generation will also decline.

Monitoring the Human Dimensions of Adjustment

If human concerns are to be given proper attention during the process of adjustment, it will be essential to develop some monitoring system to ensure that some indicators of the extent to which human needs are met or unmet are regularly and rapidly collected, analyzed and published in a form which policymakers can take into account in devising remedial action. Experience suggests this is less momentous a task than might at first appear, even in data-weak, low-income countries. Many of the indicators required are already being collected in the course of day-to-day operations by the government departments or private organizations working at the grassroots level and in touch with poor and vulnerable communities. The statistical reliability of this information may not be perfect—but, almost by definition, it matches the administrative capacity and outreach of the services available to play some role in remedial action. The challenge is therefore to develop ways to ensure that this data is used for monitoring and policymaking at the regional and national level, not only at the level at which the data are originally collected.

The data on nutritional status given earlier in Figures 4.1 through 4.6 provide an excellent example. In the case of Botswana the data are collected as part of regular and largely routine nationwide child health activities, whereby each child is weighed monthly at a health clinic, the weight recorded on weight charts and the clinic takes remedial action as necessary including the distribution of food supplements. In Ghana and the other four countries presented, the data on nutritional status are obtained directly from the food distribution services run by the Catho- lic Relief Services. In these cases, because only a fraction of the country's children are covered by the services and because child weighing is used to determine eligibility for free food, the sample of children covered by the data is undoubtedly biased. But for purposes of monitoring *changes* in the nutritional status of the poorest, including the adequacy of remedial action, the data are both highly relevant and well focused. Some 250,000 children in Ghana are covered by the data, and tabulations are available separately for all ten provinces. Even if coverage is partial, the picture presented of the month-by-month and year-by-year changes in nutritional status is highly indicative and probably much less biased statistically as an indicator of the position of the poorer sections of the population than most of the other statistical indicators available.

In addition to these data, the need for two other classes of information can be identified. First, there is the range of more conventional social indicators already widely collected, analyzed and used—such as school enrollment data, basic health care service data, consumer price and income data, production data from farms and small-scale producers, urban and rural. Here the issue is timeliness and focus. Unlike most of the economic data used for adjustment policy, where collection, processing and often publication is expected and achieved in two or three months, the statistical lag between collection and publication for the human indicators is usually two or three years—if that. The result is that even when willing, economic policymakers seeking to include human concerns into their adjustment deliberations are starved of the data which they need to do so. A priority in every country should be to develop a system for producing a core of human indicators with the same urgency and priority as is routinely accorded to some of the core economic statistics.

The second class of data required relates to the functioning of the key parts of government administration which support the poor and vulnerable. One needs indicators of the adequacy and effectiveness of these services in reaching out to the poor and in responding to their needs. Sample surveys and the routine statistical services have an important part to play in all this.

Even with increased timeliness and a sharper focusing on a critical core of indicators, there will still be a lag between data availability and the indicators needed for policymaking. It is here that the world of social concerns needs to borrow from the world of economic concerns. Some short set of leading social indicators is needed, akin to the leading economic indicators regularly compiled and considered in many of the industrial countries. These should be available some six to nine months ahead to indicate likely trends in the human situation, based on such statistics as:

household foodstocks at end of last harvest

forecast rainfall

planned government expenditures in key areas such as primary health care

vaccines and essential drugs

maintenance of village water supplies

credit for small farmer inputs and small-scale industrial producers

As before, the issue is not the lack of data or the intrinsic difficulty of devising appropriate weights for an effective system of leading indicators. The essential issue is one of perceptions and priorities. To recognize that the human dimension is central to the formulation of all economic policy and, especially at times of severe economic constraint and adjustment, cannot be assumed to follow as an inevitable by-product of general economic policy. There is a need for conscious attention to the human dimensions and for indicators to guide this.

Interestingly, this was the Keynesian lesson of the 1930s out of which grew direct concern with the level of unemployment in the formulation of macroeconomic policy and from which, in turn, grew the present system of national accounts which provides a focus and priority of much of the economic statistical work in most countries. Ironically, it was this original *social* and *human* concern underlying GNP which is now being lost in the over-preoccupation with GNP and the neglect of the human dimensions of the people involved in its creation and use.

Notes

1. Paradoxically, the sheer size of China and India, accounting for almost 40 percent of the world's population, makes it difficult to be sure whether (in terms of the total number of persons affected) worldwide *poverty and malnutrition* is growing, constant or declining. The economies of China and India by their size and structure are relatively insulated from world economic repercussions, their populations therefore being more affected by domestic changes of policy, the results of which in terms of poverty and malnutrition are not yet clear.
2. This is an orthodox and optimistic view of the *goals* of adjustment policy. Critics would point out that the actual measures of adjustment adopted often fail to achieve these goals—as some of the IMF's own evaluations have made clear. There is also the matter of *international* adjustment policy, international action (or inaction) to correct major imbalances in the pattern of trade or income flows between countries, or of deficiencies in the total level of global economic activity. We return to this point later.
3. The measurement of income distribution is complex. Here I refer to the effects of income distribution on consumption levels of the poor and vulnerable, that is, on Cv.
4. See also World Bank, *Poverty and Hunger*, 1986.

References

Barker, R. and R. Herdt, with B. Rose. "Who benefits from the new technology?" in *The Rice Economy of Asia*. Washington, D.C.: Resources for the Future, Johns Hopkins University Press, 1984.

Berg, Alan. *Malnourished People—A Policy View*. World Bank, Poverty and Basic Needs Series, 1981.

Chambers, R., R. Longhurst and A. Pacey, eds. *Seasonal Dimensions to Rural Poverty*. London: Frances Pinter, 1981.

Collis, W. "On the Ecology of Child Health and Nutrition in Nigerian Villages," *Trop. Geog. Med.* 14 (1962): 140–163, 201–228.

Dey, J. "Development Planning in the Gambia: The Gap between and Farmers' Perceptions, Expectations and Objectives," *World Development* 10 (1982): 377–396.

Food and Agriculture Organization. *Integrating Nutrition into Agricultural and Rural Development: Six Case Studies*, Nutrition in Agriculture no. 2. Rome, 1984.

Ghai, D. and S. Radwan, eds. *Agrarian Policies and Rural Poverty in Africa*. Geneva: International Labour Office, 1983.

.Hanger, J. and R. J. Moris. "Women in the Household Economy," in Chambers, R. and J. Moris, *Mwea: An Irrigated Rice Settlement Scheme in Kenya*. Munich: Afrika Studien, 1973.

Hayami, Y. "Induced Innovation, Green Revolution and iIcome Distribution: Comment," *Economic Development and Cultural Change* 30:1 (1982): 23–44.

Jolly, Richard. "Adjustment with a Human Face," Barbara Ward Lecture, *Development*. Rome: SID, 1985.

Levinson, F. J. "Towards Success in Combatting Malnutrition: An Assessment of What Works," *UNU Food and Nutrition Bulletin* 4:3 (1982): 23–44.

Lipton, M., with R. Longhurst. "Modern Varieties, International Agricultural Research, and the Poor," *CGIAR Study Paper* no. 2. Washington, D.C., 1985.

Lipton, M. "Land Assets and Rural Poverty," *World Bank Staff Working Paper* no. 744. Washington, D.C., 1985.

Longhurst, R. "Farm Level Decision Making, Social Structure and an Agricultural Development Project in a Northern Nigerian Village," *Samaru Miscellaneous Paper 109*. Zaria: Ahmadu Bello University, 1982.

Norman, D., J. Haywood and H. Hallam. "An Assessment of Cotton Growing Recommendations as Grown by Nigerian Farmers," *Cotton Growing Review* 51 (1974): 266–280.

Popkin, B. "Time allocation of the mother and child and nutrition," *Ecology of Food & Nutrition* 9 (1978): 1–14.

Streeten, Paul, and associates. *First Things First: Meeting Basic Human Needs in Developing Countries*. World Bank, Oxford University Press, 1981.

Tripp, R. "Farmers and Traders: Some Economic Determinants of Nutritional Status in Northern Ghana," *Journal of Tropical Pediatrics* 27 (1981): 15–21.

UNICEF. *State of the World's Children*. New York, 1985.

Wolfe, B. and J. Behrman. "Determinants of Child Mortality, Health and Nutrition in a Developing Country," *Journal of Development Economics* 11 (1982): 165–193.

World Bank. *Poverty and Hunger*. Washington, D.C., 1986.

5

The Impact of Economic Adjustment Programs

Jere R. Behrman

Most developing economies face periodic macroeconomic problems of imbalance between aggregate demand and supply, inflation, unemployment, and foreign exchange shortages. Such problems may originate in the international economic environment (e.g., declines in demand for exports, increased interest charges for foreign debt, and increased costs for critical imports such as petroleum); in the domestic economic environment (e.g., policies that discriminate against traditional products and exports); or, more generally, in both. Whatever the sources, the affected developing countries in such circumstances often undertake macroeconomic adjustment programs to attempt to resolve the problems. These adjustment programs may be developed and undertaken by the countries themselves or, particularly if foreign exchange shortages are severe, in collaboration with the IMF and (at least implicitly) with important international lenders. Such programs typically have involved currency devaluations, governmental budget reductions, monetary restrictions, freeing of previously controlled prices, and wage restraints. This paper focuses on the impact of the economic adjustment programs undertaken by the developing countries on health and nutrition in those countries.[1]

Some observers, such as Jolly (1985), Jolly and Cornia (1984), UNICEF (1984), the Inter-American Development Bank (1985), and the

*I thank David Bell and Sam Preston for useful comments on the first draft of this study; participants at the Takemi symposium—particularly Alan Berg, Frances Stewart, Lincoln Chen, William McGreevey, Andrea Cornia, and Per Pinstrup-Andersen —for useful comments on the revised draft at the symposium; and NIH for research support. The standard disclaimer applies.

103

World Food Council (1985), have concluded that recent economic recessions and associated macro adjustment programs in developing economies have had significant deleterious effects on health and nutrition in these societies. Jolly (1985) summarizes the results of these studies as follows:

> As it mostly operates at the moment, adjustment policy . . . transmits and usually multiplies the impact on the poor and vulnerable. The result, as shown in many countries, is rising malnutrition in the short run—and in the long run, reinforcement of a style of development which will primarily rely on accelerated growth and trickle down, if it works at all, to reduce malnutrition in the future.

Based on this kind of generalization, UNICEF (1984), Jolly and Cornia (1984), and Jolly (1985) call for what Jolly (1985) calls adjustment with a human face:

> First, *a clear acknowledgment in the goals of adjustment policy of concern for basic human welfare and a commitment to protect the minimum nutrition levels of children and other specially vulnerable groups of a country's population.*
>
> Second, *the implementation of a broader approach to the adjustment process itself, comprising four components:*
>
> (a) actions to maintain a minimum floor for nutrition and other basic human needs, related to what the country can in the long term sustain;
>
> (b) restructuring within the productive sectors—agriculture, services, industry—to rely more upon the small-scale, informal sector producers and to ensure their greater access to credit, internal markets and other measures which will stimulate growth in their incomes;
>
> (c) restructuring within health, education and other social sectors, to restore momentum and ensure maximum coverage and benefits from constrained and usually reduced resources. Already, there are important examples of what can be done to reach all of a country's population, but still at relatively low cost;
>
> (d) more international support for these aspects of adjustment, including the provision of more finance, flexibly provided and with longer term commitments. The extremes of the present situation will often require a ceiling on outflows of interest and debt amortization if the protection of human needs is to be feasible in the short run.
>
> Thirdly, *a system is needed for monitoring nutrition levels and the human situation during the process of adjustment.* We should be concerned not only with inflation, balance of payments and GNP growth—but also with nutrition, food balances and human growth. The proportion of a nation's households falling below some basic poverty line should be monitored—and treated as one of the relevant statistics for assessing adjustment.

Despite the confident assertions in such studies, however, considerable uncertainty remains about the impact of economic adjustment programs on health and nutrition in developing countries. Because of this, related studies currently are underway at the International Food Policy Research Institute (IFPRI), the World Bank, UNICEF, the United Nations University, and the IMF, among others. The purpose of this chapter is to access what we currently know about the impact of economic adjustment in the developing economies on health and nutrition.

Difficulties in Analyzing the Impact of Economic Adjustment Policies on Health and Nutrition

The analysis of the impact of economic adjustment policies on health and nutrition is very difficult for a number of reasons:

1. There is considerable disagreement about the impact of standard economic adjustment policies on macroeconomic outcomes such as aggregate demand and supply, imports, exports, international financial flows, inflation, and employment.

·2. Whatever the impact on such basic aggregate macroeconomic indicators, the effects on health and nutrition depend critically on changes in composition at various levels, including the nature of income and asset distributions, the breakdown of governmental expenditures and revenues, and relative prices. The health and nutrition effects are likely to be most deleterious if the real resources available to the poorest members of society are reduced by adjustment policies. The poorest groups typically include landless rural laborers, subsistence and small farmers, informal sector urban workers, and disabled or elderly individuals and children. Real output reductions or cuts in social services due to adjustment policies may hit some of these groups hard, but others—such as subsistence farmers—may be unaffected. Moreover, relative price movements may benefit some of these groups at the same time they disadvantage others—e.g., increases in relative food prices may harm poor urban dwellers and at the same time give poor rural producers and agricultural laborers increased purchasing power.

3. The proximate determinants of health and nutrition are the decisions of individuals and households, given their assets and the prices (broadly defined) that they face. But individuals and households have considerable capacities for substitution among products and activities given changes in relative prices. Well documented examples include short-run and longer-run migration in response to employment options, substitution of lower cost sources of nutrients in response to adverse relative price or income shifts, substitution over time by dissaving, sub-

stitution of informal for formal sector activities, and even human energy expenditure adaptations to nutrient intakes.

4. The effects of the components of stereotypical adjustment programs on health and nutrition may partially offset each other and may appear with differential lags. The so-called J-curve response in the balance of payments to devaluation, in which there is observed an initial deterioration and then an improvement, is but one of many possible examples.

5. The empirical basis for monitoring and assessing health and nutrition outcomes and the many complicated links in the overall process is very weak or almost nonexistent in many cases. Therefore deductions often are made on the basis of very imperfect information such as indices of inputs rather than of outputs.

6. The phenomena under examination are complex and are embedded in a complicated, dynamically evolving context. This makes it difficult to maintain *ceteris paribus* assumptions. But without such assumptions, it is almost impossible to identify the health and nutrition impact of economic adjustment policies or to ask the appropriate hypothetical questions, i.e., what would have been health and nutrition without the adjustment policies or with a different economic adjustment policy package?

Implications of Economic Theory in Analyzing the Effects of Adjustment Policies

Economic theory provides frameworks for analyzing many of the possible links between economic adjustment policies and health and nutrition. Such structures are essential for gaining understanding of these complex phenomena given the very imperfect state of relevant information and the difficulty, if not impossibility, of conducting relevant *ceteris paribus* experiments. But before sketching out the implications of economic theory for this topic, I should point out the limitations of economic theory in this regard. First, for some links in the process there is considerable controversy about which of several competing theories is most relevant. Second, economic theory leads to clearcut predictions regarding the direction of changes in many contexts only by abstracting from some possibly relevant characteristics of the situation. Often the net effect depends on which of several counteracting responses is most important, which is an empirical—not a theoretical—question. Third, even if the direction of an effect is predicted clearly by economic theory, the magnitude still is an empirical matter. Fourth, economic theory is most useful regarding comparative statics between equilibrium outcomes, but has very little to say concerning the nature or the lag in adjustments between equilibria. For all of these reasons economic theory often leads more to raising useful questions about responses to the income and price changes induced by economic adjustment policies rather than to precise answers.

With such caveats in mind, I attempt the somewhat heroic task of summarizing the implications of economic theory for assessing the impact of economic adjustment on health and nutrition in terms accessible to a fairly broad audience. Since those who are most vulnerable are the poorest members of society, I begin with a discussion of the impact of the major components of standard stabilization programs on resources under the control of lower-income people. Since many of the proximate determinants of health and nutrition are decisions made by individuals and households and since intrahousehold inequalities are thought by many to be important, I then turn to such decisions given the individual's or household's assets and the prices (broadly defined) that households face.

Impact of Major Adjustment Policies on those in Lower End of Income Distribution

The macroeconomy determines the aggregate supply and demand of goods and services, the overall price and employment levels, and the aggregate balance of trade in goods and services and international financial flows with the rest of the world.[2] In the simplest form, the short-run equilibrium income level and price level are determined by the intersection of short-run aggregate demand and aggregate supply, as at point a for the solid curves in Figure 5.1

Aggregate demand depends on private and governmental consumption and investment and net foreign investment (i.e., exports minus imports). These major demand components, in turn, depend primarily on real permanent income and wealth (and probably the distribution of each among members of society), governmental expenditure minus revenue, prices of international goods and services relative to prices of domestic goods and services, and credit availability and/or interest rates. Expectations also may affect aggregate demand and may cause behavioral responses to offset anticipated policy changes.

The impact of expectations is illustrated in the so-called Phillips curve tradeoff between inflation and unemployment of Figure 5.2. For given inflationary expectations, the economy can be moved along the solid line in this curve, say from a to b, by contractionary policy. However such policy may change (reduce) inflationary expectations with the result that the Phillips curve shifts downward to the dashed line so that the

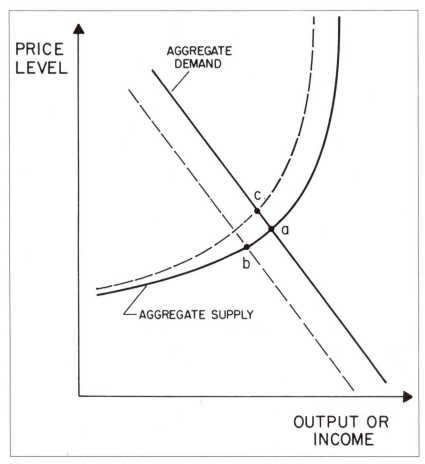

Figure 5.1. *Short-run macroeconomic equilibrium.*

actual movement of the economy is from a to c, with little impact on output and employment. There are those who argue that in fact the impact of privately held expectations offsets any anticipated policy change, thus rendering economic adjustment policies mostly ineffective. I do not think the available evidence warrants such an extreme position, but it does seem to be the case that expectations can affect significantly policy outcomes.

Returning to the aggregate demand curve per se, if interest rates or inflationary expectations rise or any of the other factors mentioned above fall, aggregate demand is likely to shift to the left. This would result in a decrease in equilibrium real output and the aggregate price level, with the balance between price and output changes depending

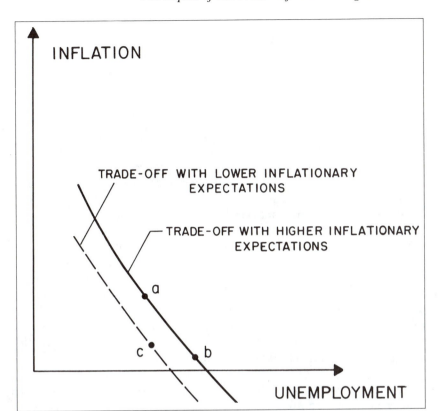

Figure 5.2. *Phillips curve tradeoff between inflation and unemployment conditional on inflationary expectations.*

on whether the initial equilibrium is on a more vertical or more horizontal segment of the aggregate supply curve). The dashed demand curve in Figure 5.1 gives an example, with the new equilibrium at point b.

Short-run aggregate supply reflects the conditions in short-run variable input markets, primarily for labor, intermediate inputs, and financing, given capacity production levels. The short-run supply curve is likely to shift to the left, resulting in a higher price level and lower output (income) level if prices of labor (wages), intermediate inputs, or credit (interest rates) rise, if rationed credit becomes less available (assuming that any parallel or "curb" financial market is not well developed), or if production becomes less efficient. The dashed supply curve in Figure 5.1 is an example, with the associated equilibrium at point c. In the longer run, aggregate supply tends to shift to the right with increased physical (e.g., machinery and equipment) and human capital, improved technology, and improved institutions.

To model all of these processes and the impact of policy changes, the relevant product, factor (i.e., labor, capital, land), and financial markets must be represented. Some of the major components of such a model and the inherent complexities therein are illustrated in Figure 5.3.

Different approaches to modeling macroeconomies for lesser developed countries (LDCs) hinge upon: (1) the importance of rigidities, particularly in wages and prices, that preclude short-run clearing of all markets (which, if it occurred, would obviate the need for short-run economic adjustment policies); (2) the importance of expectations and their relation to policies (e.g., if policies are correctly anticipated, the private sector may adjust to them in ways that make them ineffective); (3) the representation of market fragmentation—widely considered a critical feature of developing economies—at the macro level and the related issue of the extent of detail regarding agriculture and services (with the agriculture vs. manufacturing two-sector model being the most common representation); and (4) which closure rule is adopted (i.e., whether variables such as prices, factor returns and investment are exogenous or endogenous). For the purpose of this review, I assume that considerable rigidities exist (including ones in formal sector nominal wages); that expectations are sufficiently dispersed in a constantly changing environment so that governmental policies have some impact; that disaggregation of distribution, at least among subsistence agriculture, commercial farming, the informal urban sector and the formal urban sector, is required to capture the critical segments of income distribution for the purpose of investigating health and nutrition impacts and the different institutional arrangements in these sectors; and that the closure issue need not be addressed in detail for this level of generality.[3]

With this background, I now turn to consideration of the distributional effects of the major components of stereotypic economic adjustment programs.

Currency devaluation is frequently (though not invariably; see Killick, 1984a: 191–95), a key component of economic adjustment policies—particularly those associated with IMF stabilization programs. Devaluation, however, has been the subject of much heated debate because of controversy over its effectiveness in eliminating supply-demand imbalances, because of its inflationary effects and because of the distributional and related political consequences of devaluation.

Devaluation increases the costs of imports and the prices of exports in terms of the domestic currency. The impact of devaluation on the balance of payments (which presumably is of major concern from the point of view of economic adjustment programs) and on distribution

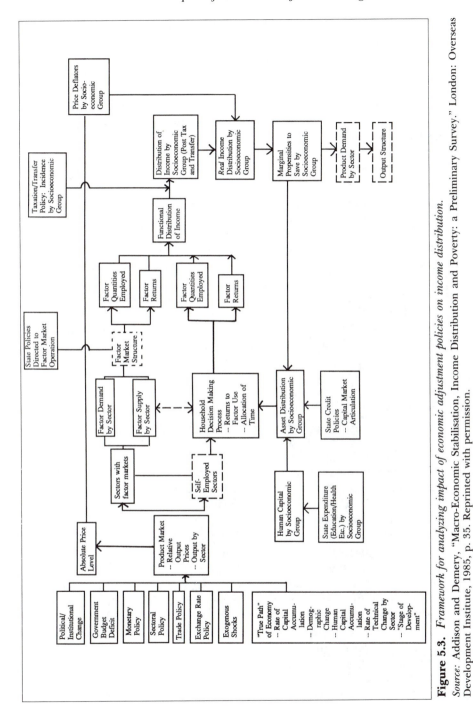

Figure 5.3. *Framework for analyzing impact of economic adjustment policies on income distribution.*

Source: Addison and Demery, "Macro-Economic Stabilisation, Income Distribution and Poverty: a Preliminary Survey." London: Overseas Development Institute, 1985, p. 35. Reprinted with permission.

(of major concern here) depends upon the extent of expenditure switching and the extent of expenditure changes.[4]

Expenditure switching occurs due to the increase in the prices of internationally traded goods (whether imports or exports) relative to nontraded goods. Under strong simplifying assumptions (i.e., perfect competition, profit maximization, no externalities, well-behaved production functions), such shifts benefit the inputs used relatively intensively in traded-goods production and the consumers (relatively) of nontraded goods. The implications within a particular context thus depend on the factor intensity of production and the nature of consumption patterns.

If export production is largely from small farmers, for example, devaluation might increase the incomes of at least some of the poorer members of society from the factor intensity side. If importable production largely is in capital intensive industries, on the other hand, the factor-intensity effect tends to favor profits and increase income inequality. Likewise, the consumption effect depends on the nature of the traded goods and who consumes them. If the exportables are primarily staple foods that loom large in the consumption basket of poorer members of society (e.g., rice in Thailand), for example, the consumption effect in itself is likely to worsen the position of the poor (though poor farmers and landless rural laborers producing this staple may be net gainers if for them the factor-intensity effect outweighs the consumption effect). But if tradeable goods are primarily manufactured products and the basic staples nontraded (e.g., yams, cassava), the opposite result may obtain. Such considerations lead to questions in any particular case about relative factor intensities and relative marginal consumption propensities.

The more one moves away from the simplifying assumptions noted above, the less strong are any predictions about the way expenditure switching due to devaluation affects distribution. If the formal-informal sector distinction is made, for example, the above results hold if and only if factors are mobile. But if, as seems more appropriate for short-run analysis, factors are not completely mobile between the formal and informal sectors, there are no unambiguous predictions (Knight, 1976). Returns to the factor used relatively intensely in the production of traded goods and services increase in response to devaluation, but both the formal and the informal sectors may generate such products with very different factor intensities (i.e., capital intensive in the formal sector and labor intensive in the informal sector as, perhaps, in tourism or textile production).

Devaluation also may induce aggregate real expenditure changes, with feedback on distribution. The conventional result is that *eventually* exports will expand and imports will decline in response to the change in relative prices induced by devaluation under the assumption that these relative price changes persist. This eventually leads to an improved balance of payments in international terms and probably an increase in aggregate demand and (assuming some unused capacity and/or efficiency inducements of devaluation) in output and income. However, such a process may be quite slow, particularly if exports are goods for which gestation periods are long (e.g., tree crops, minerals) and for which initial capacity is more or less fully utilized. There may be offsetting factors, emphasized by the "New Structuralists" such as Buffie (1984), Diaz-Alejandro (1965, 1981), Krugman and Taylor (1978), Ahluwalia and Lysy (1981), Taylor (1979, 1983), Van Wijnbergen (1982), and others, that may lead to devaluation being contractionary. On the aggregate supply side, these offsetting factors include the importance of noncompetitive, imported intermediate inputs in production and wage indexation in the formal sector. Both of these shift the aggregate supply curve to the left with devaluation. Such features are likely to differ greatly among countries with indexed wages—common, at least until recently, in many inflation-prone Latin American countries but relatively unimportant in Africa and Asia. On the demand side, the net trade component of aggregate demand *in domestic currency* may be reduced if there is an initial large deficit, particularly before exports respond. Consumption and investment may decline if wealth falls with devaluation (due to an increase in net foreign debt in terms of domestic currency) or if income falls (due to more rapid induced inflation than changes in factor payments). Finally, investment may be reduced because of higher prices for tradeable investment goods. Once again, such factors vary substantially across countries. For example, the real wealth effects are relatively important in Latin American countries with large private foreign debt but not so important for much of Asia or Africa.

These contractionary demand and supply factors are widely thought to dominate in the short-run response to devaluation. If they do, the resulting reduction in real expenditure is likely to reduce the real purchasing power of many poorer people. This would happen as a result of reduced demand for the services and products of the informal sector. In addition, workers who otherwise might have been employed in the formal sector would move into the informal sector—along with people who enter the labor force because other household members have lost work. This labor surplus, along with reduced demand, would increase unemployment and reduce input returns in the informal sector.

Contractionary monetary and fiscal policies almost invariably are part of economic adjustment programs since excess demand is perceived (particularly, but not exclusively, in orthodox analysis) to be at the heart of the problem.[5] Supply expansion presumably requires some time, so demand restraint is viewed as essential in the short run and contractionary fiscal and monetary policies are widely thought to be the major set of tools for restraining aggregate demand. As suggested above with regard to Figure 5.1, such policies are likely to shift aggregate demand and aggregate supply to the left initially, resulting in a fall in equilibrium output and income and an ambiguous change in the price level.[6] The extent of such an impact, however, may depend critically upon how firms' and individuals' expectations respond to such fiscal and monetary policy changes. Assuming that these policies are likely to have some negative impact on output, the balance of payments is likely to be improved due to the decreased real purchasing power of the economy (thus reducing imports and increasing exports). This trend would be reinforced—if prices are sufficiently flexible—by a decline in the relative price of nontraded goods and services. For reasons discussed above, such output reductions—and the related declines in labor demand—will probably lessen the real income of most of the poorer groups in society, except pure subsistence groups, with respect to the impact of expenditure reduction induced by devaluation. However, there are possible exceptions once again. For example, if prices fall but nominal wages in the formal sector do not fall, workers who receive such wages may experience an increase in real income.

The extent and duration of the negative impact on the income of such groups depends on several considerations beyond the extent of the initial leftward shifts in the aggregate demand and supply curves. One important consideration, of course, is the extent of and gestation required for a longer run positive supply shift. The larger and the quicker such a response, the less the likely toll on the real income of poorer members of society. A second consideration is how the government cuts expenses and increases revenue and how such changes affect the poorer members of society. Reductions in purchases of armaments from abroad, lowered credit subsidies to capital-intensive manufacturers, or increases in income taxes are not likely to have much negative impact on poorer households, but reductions in public health expenditures, food stamps, school lunches or subsidization of inferior foods may have significant negative income and price effects on many of the poorer households. To the extent that the main asset of the poorer members of society is their human capital, cuts in health, nutrition and educational programs from which they benefit are likely to have negative long term effects on their future command over real resources.

Direct wage and/or price controls often are part of stabilization packages. Since wage increases could offset substantially the impact of economic adjustment policies such as currency devaluation by shifting the aggregate supply curve in Figure 5.1 to the left, adjustment policy packages often include some limitation on wage increases for governmental and formal sector employees. If effective, such policies reduce the real income of individuals who would have been employed in the affected occupations without the wage controls. This may increase overall income inequality but is not likely to have a strong negative effect on most of the poorest members of society. This is the case because the poorest members of society are not likely to have been in such occupations if there were no wage policy. In fact, to the extent that the limitation on wages is effective, these relatively high-wage occupations are likely to be more accessible to the otherwise relatively poor members of society than they would be if there were no effective wage controls.

Price interventions as part of an economic adjustment policy package are likely to involve increases in or freeing of previously controlled prices—such as transport, fuel, food staples—to induce supply expansion, reduce government subsidies, and discourage demand. If such price controls had been effective prior to the economic adjustment program, such a policy shift means increased nominal prices for consumers of these items. This is likely to reduce their real incomes, particularly if there is an effective "asymmetrical" price policy, in Foxley's terms (1981: 206), of restraining their wages at the same time that prices are increasing.[7] However, questions immediately arise about how effective price controls have been—in most societies, parallel markets with higher prices readily develop when there are price controls. To the extent that the price controls were not effective to begin with, removing the price controls or increasing price ceilings obviously has little impact on distribution except for reducing the legal and extra-legal incomes of the members of the price control and monitoring organizations (who are not likely to be among the poorer members of society).

Policies to limit foreign exchange uses and to encourage foreign exchange generation are also often part of economic adjustment packages. Countries with balance of payments problems sometimes initiate such policies instead of the others discussed above. Beyond devaluation, imports (and their domestically-produced substitutes) may be made more expensive to discourage their use by increased import tariffs and by a wide range of nontariff barriers (e.g., licensing, quantitative restrictions, prior deposits). Outflows of financial capital likewise can be taxed, limited or prohibited. On the other side of the balance of payments, exports can be subsidized, given special tax breaks, or given special access to foreign exchange for use in imports. Financial inflows can be encouraged by favorable exchange rates and guarantees (if credible) regarding the nature of subsequent reconversion to foreign exchange. While the whole range of such policies has been used by developing economies with cyclical macro problems, adjustment packages developed in conjunction with the IMF generally include prohibitions against introducing or increasing restrictions on imports.

Increased tariffs on imports have at least three types of effects on income distribution. First, such tariffs are a major source of governmental revenues in most developing economies. If increased tariff rates do not discourage imports too much, such revenues increase and thereby reduce the government deficit (or add to its surplus), thus being part of the contractionary fiscal policy discussed above. Second, increased import tariffs change the relative price structure to favor production of importables. Within the simplest trade model, a country exports goods which make the most use of resources which are relatively abundant in the country (presumably labor for a developing country trading with a developed economy). The imposition of an import tariff in this framework favors the relatively scarce factor of production used in importables, which presumably is capital in most developing countries, thus shifting income away from labor. However, this strong prediction is weakened considerably once more realistic complications are introduced into the analysis. Moreover, empirically such a relation is not strongly verified (e.g., Bhagwati, 1978). Third, once again there is an impact on the relative prices that consumers face, and it depends upon the marginal propensities to consume importables relative to alternatives. If the importables are luxuries or other goods consumed relatively by the better off, then the consumption price effect in itself does not worsen the relative position of the poorer—but it does tend to do so if importables are basic goods such as staple foods.

Increasing nontariff import barriers such as quantitative restrictions has the second and third effects noted in the previous paragraph, but not the first. Instead, the gains from having access to such quotas are likely to go to the administrators and recipients of such quotas. Neither of these groups is likely to include much representation of the poor.

Impact on Health and Nutrition Given Changes in Prices and Household Income

The economic adjustment policies described above ultimately affect individuals or households through altering their incomes or the prices that they face. Prices are broadly defined to include the total costs to an individual or household to obtain goods or services, whether from a private vendor or a governmental agency. If, for example, health clinic services are reduced as part of economic adjustment policies so that patients have to wait longer for free (in monetary terms) services, the total price for those services has increased.

Households (including single-individual households) make decisions about time-use and consumption, given their assets and prices that they face for the use of these assets, consumption items, etc. For the poorer households of interest here, the primary asset is labor, with varying degrees of skills. That means that wages and the nature of employment options are particularly important in determining household income. But many such households also have land (e.g., subsistence households and small farmers) and capital (e.g., many households in the manufacturing or maintenance parts of the informal sector as well as farming households), so returns to other assets also may be important in determining their income. The prices of obvious importance, given the interest in health and nutrition, are for the items that help determine health and nutrition—food, potable water, preventive health measures, curative health care, housing, sewage, and clothing. But since the actual use of such items depends on relative prices and real income (which depends on all prices for goods and services important in the consumption basket of the poor), other prices may be important as well.

Economic models of the household assume that individuals in the household have preferences which they express in choices about their own and others' time use, current consumption of goods and services, health, and investments in future command over resources. Investments in future command of resources include human capital investments in health, nutrition and education as well as savings in the form of financial and physical asset acquisition. Household members maximize these preferences within the constraints of budget and production functions. Budget constraints depend on current assets such as time, their returns, and prices for relevant goods and services. Among the production functions are one for health and nutrients. Health is determined by consumption of nutrients, consumption of other items like tobacco and alcohol, the nature of water and waste disposal, preventive and curative health care, the nature of time use, the general environment, genetic endowments, previous health status, and knowledge about how to use such factors. Nutrient intakes are determined by the foods consumed, given preparation procedures, and current health and time use.

Constrained maximization of preferences, whether or not there is bargaining among household members,[8] leads us to suppose a relationship between an individual's health and nutrient intakes and the variables (assets and prices, both broadly defined) mentioned above. These variables can be exogenous (to the household) or predetermined. The impact of economic adjustment policies depends on (a) how the exogenous and predetermined variables in those relations are altered (particularly the relevant returns on assets and prices broadly defined, but possibly also the environment) and (b) how the impact of such changes are filtered through the household. With regard to the latter, there are a number of critical questions. How responsive are individuals or households to relative price differentials? If the price of nutrients from one source increases due to an economic adjustment program, for example, is there little or considerable shifting to cheaper nutrient sources? How much fungibility is there in the use of returns from assets among individuals? To what extent, for instance, is the loss of a formal-sector job due to an economic adjustment program by one member of the household offset by increased activities of other members of the household in the informal sector or elsewhere? To the extent that this occurs, is it at the cost of longer-run human capital investments (e.g., by keeping children out of schooling)? Does it make a difference whose returns to assets are affected (e.g., women versus men)? If women are induced to participate more in the labor force by changes in the economic environment, what are the tradeoffs between their increased command over market resources and any concomitant reduced time in household activities pertaining to health and nutrition? To what extent can the household draw down existing assets in order to tide its members over a transitory bad period? At what point are changes in the economic environment likely to lead to substantially increased probabilities of disintegration of the household, probably to the disadvantage of some of the more vulnerable members?

Empirical Evidence on the Impact of Economic Adjustment Programs on Health and Nutrition in Developing Countries

No empirical studies currently available examine all of the links between economic adjustment programs and health and nutrition in developing countries with theoretical frameworks such as those outlined in the previous section and careful empirical control for all relevant factors. But some studies have considered systematically some of the critical links in the process, and a few others have considered relations in which intervening links have been collapsed to simplify the analysis. I review a number of these studies now, roughly following the order in the previous section by starting with studies on the effectiveness of macroeconomic policy in developing countries, then the nature of governmental cuts at the time of fiscal and monetary contraction, then the nature of household responses to changed income and prices, and finally country studies focusing on "collapsed" relations between economic recessions or adjustments and more direct measures of health and nutrition.

The Effectiveness of Macro Adjustment Policies on Macro Outcomes in the Developing Countries

As is noted earlier, this is a controversial topic. The simple aggregate supply and demand curves in Figure 5.1 suggest to some that macro adjustment policies that shift aggregate demand can be fairly effective in altering equilibrium output if the initial equilibrium is on the more horizontal part of the aggregate supply curve and that they can be fairly effective in altering the equilibrium price level if the initial equilibrium is on the more vertical part of the aggregate supply curve. But some analysts (e.g., Taylor, 1974) have questioned whether well-intentioned policy makers in developing economies have enough policy tools to pursue their multiple macro objectives given realities such as inadequate capital markets and resulting ineffective monetary policy. Others (e.g., Rao, 1952) doubt that the initial equilibrium could be on the more horizontal part of the aggregate supply curve at least in many South and Southeast Asian and African developing economies, because of the severe supply shortages and the critical role of a large traditional semi-subsistence sector. If so, macro adjustment policies primarily affect the price level, but not output nor employment. Still others (e.g., Lucas, 1973; Fernandez, 1979; Barro, 1979) have queried whether expectations may make macro policies ineffective in developing economies as many claim is the case in developed market economies; an example is the Phillips curve tradeoff between inflation and unemployment conditional on expectations that is illustrated in Figure 5.2 and discussed above.

If, for a particular developing country, any of these arguments are correct, economic adjustment policies would not have much impact on output and employment, and therefore probably not much impact on health and nutrition—though conceivably there still could be some composition effects. Therefore, empirical evidence on the effectiveness of macro policies in developing countries is germane to understanding the topic of this paper.

There are a great number of empirical studies that are related to this issue. Unfortunately they do not settle the issue definitively because of the institutional differences among developing countries (such studies tend to focus on the more developed and less agricultural Latin American economies); the difficulties in capturing the macro complexities of any economy in a tractable empirical framework (particularly such features as adjustment lags and expectations formulation); and the problem that some of the results of macro models reflect the initial theoretical model specifications (the "closure" problem alluded to earlier). Nevertheless, a selective review of some of these studies is suggestive.

The tests of the Phillips' curve tradeoff between employment or output and inflation include Lucas's (1973) seminal paper in which he presents tests for eighteen countries, including five in Latin America plus Puerto Rico (the rest are in Europe or North America). His tests suggest that the "apparent short-term tradeoff is favorable, as long as it remains unused" (p. 333), but in countries with a volatile price history in the sample and with relatively high variance in demand (namely Argentina and Paraguay) the inflation-output tradeoff is very unstable. Brodersohn (1979), Fernandez (1979) and Barro (1979) report results that they interpret as basically consistent with Lucas's conclusion for five Latin American countries. Both Barro and Fernandez report that unexpected money supply changes are relatively ineffective in changing output (rather than prices), though Barro does report a significant effect for Mexico. Hanson (1980) reports "a small though significant relation between output or growth and 'unexpected' inflation" for "moderately inflationary" Latin American countries that is substantially stronger than that obtained by Barro and between the Lucas values for the 16 relatively price-stable countries on one hand and the two price-volatile countries on the other hand. Nugent and Glezakos (1982) report estimates for sixteen Latin American countries. They find no significance of unanticipated inflation for the least agricultural countries and a negative (not positive as in the standard Phillips curve) output impact for the more agricultural countries. They interpret the negative association to reflect the lack of supply price rigidities (which the Lucas formulation emphasizes) in agricultural societies in the spirit, in a sense, of Rao (1952).[9]

A second group of studies that attempt to evaluate the impact of macroeconomic policies on aggregate economic output in developing economies involve the construction of models of these economies. For the purpose of the evaluation of short-run impacts of economic adjustment policies, a major long standing tradition is composed of macroeconometric models in the Keynes-Tinbergen-Klein tradition.[10] There exist literally hundreds of macro models in this tradition, with a higher representation of Latin American and a lower representation of African than of Asian economics (Lau, 1975; Beltran del Rio and Schwartz, 1986). Such models initially tended to be specified along Keynesian aggregate-demand oriented lines (i.e., as if the initial equilibrium were along the horizontal supply curve in Figure 5.1), with the implications including fairly substantial impact of economic adjustment policies. However, many subsequent efforts have tried to incorporate supply constraints, devaluation impacts on costs of intermediate inputs and of investment goods, adjustment lags and other more realistic features of developing economies. Such studies usually report some, but much more limited impact of economic adjustment policies, often with substantial lags that make successful detailed predictions and policy formulation extremely difficult (e.g., Behrman 1977).

More recently emphasis has increased on the use of social-accounting matrix (SAM) based and computable-general equilibrium (CGE) models for empirical analysis of economic adjustment impacts in developing economies (e.g., Adelman and Robinson, 1978; de Melo and Robinson, 1982; Dervis, de Melo and Robinson, 1982; Pyatt and Round, 1979; Pyatt and Thorbecke, 1976; Taylor, 1979, 1983). An interesting example of the use of CGE models is provided by the simulation studies of the impact of devaluation on distribution within three archetype economies (i.e., a primary product exporter, a manufacturing exporter, and a relatively closed economy) with CGE models by de Melo and Robinson (1980), which also are summarized in Dervis, de Melo and Robinson (1982). Some of the results of these simulations are that much greater devaluation is required to eliminate an initial balance of payments deficit in the closed economy than in the others because of the greater dependence on imported intermediate inputs in that economy, that devaluation leads to an improvement in the income share for small holders for all three archetype economies, but mixed income distribution effects for other low-income groups depending on the structure of the economy, and that price shifts play a major role in changes in real income. Such approaches tend to have the advantages over traditional macroeconometric models of specifications that are better based in economic theory and more complete, including more attention to income distribution, than those used in most models in the macroeconometric tradition. On the other hand at times the estimation of these models is quite cavalier, and the focus on market equilibria often is accompanied by inattention to adjustment lags and expectations that may vitiate the value of such models for analysis of short run economic adjustment programs. Also, like the macroeconometric models and other models, such models are limited by some of their a priori assumptions (e.g., unitary elasticities of substitution in production in de Melo and Robinson 1980).

A third group of studies are country studies that tend to use less systematic modeling approaches and empirical tests to evaluate the economic impact of stabilization. Probably the best known of these are the volumes edited by Cline and Weintraub (1981) and Killick (1984a,b). The lesser emphasis on formal frameworks in these studies leads to a richer, but also looser, range of interpretations. With regard to income distribution, for example, Cline and Weintraub (1981:35) note: "The contrast between the 30 to 40 percent real wage reductions in the Southern Cone [of Latin America] and nominal wage increases to maintain real wages in Pakistan is striking, and success at reversing inflation was at least as great in Pakistan, although from a lower base." Such results suggest the possibility in practice, and not only in theory, of cushioning at least some of the poorer members of society from negative consequences of economic adjustment programs by appropriate selection of the components of those programs. But since some members of society have their incomes reduced in the short run if the economic adjustment program is successful in its effort to reduce a demand-supply imbalance by contracting demand, the question remains what determines if there is political will and power to protect the poorer members of society.

The empirical studies on the economic impact of macroeconomic adjustment problems have their problems, in part because of the complexities of such economies, the limitations of macroeconomic theories, and data inadequacies. Often there are questions about simultaneity, structural changes, unobserved variables such as price expectations, the time period for observations—almost always a year which may be long for the questions of concern, lag patterns, and a priori restrictions on the implicit or explicit models. Nevertheless, I think that studies do support the conclusions that economic adjustment policies often have some significant impact on macro outcomes such as output and employment which feed back through the income distribution and relative prices potentially to alter health and nutrition and that there have been a range of varied experiences with regard to the income distribution effects of such policies, which suggests that choices may exist to buffer many of the poor if there is sufficient political will to do so.

Changed Composition of Governmental Expenditure in Economic Adjustment Programs

As discussed above, changes in the composition of governmental expenditures as part of economic adjustment programs may affect health and nutrition. The conventional wisdom regarding such changes is that they probably discriminate against social sectors of health, education and rural development. Hicks and Kubisch (1983:2–3) provide some quotations about the alleged vulnerability of these social sectors in various writings of the World Bank:

> In the difficult past few years, budgetary crises have often meant that social services were cut back, in the process unraveling carefully designed programs.
> —*IDA in Retrospect*, p. 52.

> Since many human development programs are publicly funded they are especially vulnerable when growth is threatened and budgets are under pressure . . . The recurrent costs of social programs, especially salary costs, tended to make them a prominent and therefore vulnerable part of government budgets. —*1981 World Development Report*, pp. 97–98

> Quick-fix relief through disproportionate cutbacks—in for example, education or rural development—may well have lasting negative consequences for the entire economy.
> —*Focus on Poverty*, 1983, Introduction by A. W. Clausen

Many member countries have had to reduce and reorient investment programs to curtail recurrent expenditures, and to delay the completion of high priority development projects. Programs in health, education and other social sectors have been particularly vulnerable.
—*World Bank Program of Special Assistance to Member Countries, 1983–84*, p. 1.

In the crisis situations confronting African governments, education, training and health programs are continuously in danger of becoming the residual legates of both resources and of attention by policy-makers.
—*Sub-Saharan Africa: Progress Report on Development Prospects and Programs*, p. 30.

Other examples can be found in other sources, e.g., UNICEF (1984: 161):

Cuts in social services are often the first to take place so that the *share of social expenditures out of the total . . . shrink[s] . . .*

Despite such strong claims about the vulnerability of social service sectors to governmental cut backs, very little empirical work has been undertaken on this topic, particularly prior to the study of Hicks and Kubisch (1983, 1984).

Hicks and Kubisch examine the patterns in such cuts by considering all thirty-seven cases for which there were reported cuts in real governmental annual expenditures in developing countries during 1972–80. For each case they asked whether cuts in governmental expenditures in each of five categories (social, defense and administration, production, infrastructure and miscellaneous—the last largely transfers to local governments) were larger or smaller than the average overall expenditure cut. Table 5.1 summarizes their results with reference to an index of vulnerability defined to be one if the percentage cut in a category is equal to the average overall percentage expenditure cut and less than (greater than) one if a category is relatively protected from (vulnerable to) such cuts. These results suggest that, contrary to the above quotations, on the average social expenditures are the *most* protected of the five categories (somewhat more so in low-income countries than in middle-income countries), with infrastructure and production the least protected (with some differences, again, between low- and middle-income countries). Hicks and Kubisch caution about drawing too firm conclusions from these numbers because of the small number of cases and because the expenditure data are for the consolidated central governmental accounts—they do not include expenditures of publicly owned corporations and enterprises, nor the expenditures of state and local governments.[11] Nevertheless, such results suggest strongly that the frequent assumption that social sectors are particularly vulnerable to cuts in governmental expenditures is wrong—perhaps the social sectors are even favored. On the other hand, cuts in the apparently

Table 5.1

Reduction of Government Expenditures: Capital and Recurrent Expenditures for 32 Developing Countries for Various Periods During 1972–80

	Social	Defense/ Adminis- tration	Produc- tion	Infra- structure	Miscel- laneous[a]
Average percent change in real expenditures	−5	−8	−11	−22	−7
Index of vulnerability[b]	0.4	0.6	1.2	1.7	0.8
Low income (17 observations)	0.2	0.9	0.6	1.2	0.5
Middle income (20 observations)	0.5	0.4	1.7	1.9	1.1

[a] Largely transfers to local governments.

[b] Calculated as e_j/E where e_j is the percentage change in expenditures on the jth sector and E is the percentage change in total expenditures.

more vulnerable production and infrastructure categories may have indirect impact on health and income through associated reductions in labor demands such as construction.

Cheap food policies, including food subsidies, are one form of social expenditure that is particularly relevant for the present concern about health and nutrition and that has been studied in some detail for several countries, perhaps in part because of the urban demonstrations (if not riots[12]) that have accompanied efforts to reduce or remove such subsidies in countries such as Peru, the Dominican Republic, Haiti, Jamaica, Morocco, Sudan and Turkey. What is likely to be the health and nutritional impact of lessening or eliminating cheap food policies, as the IMF has been advocating as part of some recent actual and proposed adjustment programs?

This question is less easy to answer than it might seem to be prima facie. It depends upon the incidence of such subsidies across income classes, whether there would be supply changes associated with the removal of such subsidies (e.g., due to increased prices for agricultural producers), how the affected poor respond to the increased prices for some foods and the reduction in their real income due to such a policy change, and whether there are any compensatory policy measures for those affected.

Pinstrup-Anderson (1985a, 1986a, b) surveys many of the existing studies of the impact of the removal of cheap food policies on the poor. Since food expenditures are such a large proportion of the expenditures of low-income consumers (typically 60–80 percent of their income), increases in food prices considerably decreased the real income of low-income groups and generally have much greater impact on the poor than on the well off, as is reflected in Table 5.2. These estimates are

Table 5.2
Impact of a 10 Percent Increase in the Price of Food on Real Incomes of Low- and High-Income Population Groups

Country	Percent Decrease in Real Income		Source[a]
	Lowest Decile	Highest Decile	
Sri Lanka	8.5	4.1	Sahn
Thailand	6.0	2.0	Trairatvorakul
Egypt	5.6	1.0	Alderman and von Braun
India	7.3	2.9	Murty
Funtua, Nigeria	7.7	6.5	Pinstrup-Andersen and Uy
Gusau, Nigeria	9.0	5.7	Pinstrup-Andersen and Uy
India[b]	5.5[c]	1.2[d]	Mellor

[a] Source of data used for calculations, except for Mellor who reports the estimates shown.
[b] Foodgrains only.
[c] For the lowest 20 percent.
[d] For the highest 5 percent.
Source: Pinstrup-Andersen (1985a: 71). Reprinted with permission of Mouton de Gruyter.

for a 10 percent increase in all food prices, while typically cheap food policies are in effect or are effective for a subset of foods (though often including some basic staples), so these estimates probably overstate the negative impact on real income of adjustment policies that increased currently subsidized food prices by 10 percent.

On the other side of the market, the elimination of cheap food policies is likely to result in increased production prices for food producers.[13] Pinstrup-Andersen argues that recent research (e.g., Mellor, 1978; Sahn, 1984; Trairatvorakul, 1985) indicates that the short-run impact of food prices on the rural poor is much less favorable than might have been anticipated because many of the rural poor do not derive a large share of their income from food production–related activities. He cautions against assuming too high food supply elasticities even with a longer time horizon because of other changes required to alter food production significantly, with concomitant gains to the rural poor.

Based on such considerations and additional studies that have looked at other dimensions of the food subsidy programs (e.g., Gavan and Chandrasekera, 1979; George, 1979; Keenan, 1979; Ahmed, 1979; Alderman and von Braun, 1984), Pinstrup-Andersen (1985) concludes that "food subsidies have increased incomes and improved nutritional status among the poor, particularly, but not exclusively among the urban poor." He also observes, as have many others, that the cost of general food subsidy programs may be quite high, particularly if there is a tendency (as often seems to be the case) to attempt to keep the nominal price of subsidized foods relatively constant in the presence of overall increasing prices. For instance, Alderman, von Braun and Sakr (1982) report that the fiscal costs of Egyptian wheat subsidies increased from 0.05 to 3.5 percent of GDP in the 1970s, and Alderman and von Braun (1985) simulate that by 1986–7 the Egyptian food subsidy will increase by 44 percent in real terms from the 1981–2 level to account for 12 percent of the total governmental budget or one-third of the fiscal deficit if there is no change in the food subsidy program. For other examples, Gavan and Chandraskera (1979) report that Sri Lankan food ration shop scheme fiscal costs increased rapidly in the early 1970s to 15 percent of total government expenditures in 1975 and Mateus et al. (1986) estimate that Moroccan food subsidies reached 2.6 percent of gross domestic product (GDP) and 11.6 percent of current government expenditures in 1985. These orders of magnitudes make it not surprising that curtailment of food subsidies come to the minds of many who are contemplating the nature of economic adjustment programs for such economies.

Reducing the costs of these programs without severely affecting the real income of most of the poor would seem possible in many cases given the broad incidence of many existing cheap food programs. For the Moroccan program, for instance, Mateus et al. (1986) estimate that the *upper* 30 percent of the income distribution receives 47 percent of the subsidies and the lower 30 percent receives only 16 percent of the subsidies. Ahmed (1979) reports that in Bangladesh two-thirds of the subsidized grain was distributed to urban areas even though most of the poor people reside in rural areas. Alderman and von Braun (1984) estimate that the absolute value of the subsidy is almost constant among income groups, including those in the middle and upper parts of the distribution.

For such cases, if targeting (i.e., limiting the beneficiaries of such programs to the poor and nutritionally vulnerable) is administratively and politically feasible at a reasonable cost, it may be very attractive from the point of view of economic adjustment programs. Such costs eventually tend to rise substantially as efforts to limit leakages to other groups increase, but Mateus (1985), Mateus et al. (1986) and a number of others argue that substantial reductions in the governmental budget and distribution costs of existing general cheap food policies can be achieved by greater targeting. Examples of targeting include subsidization of inferior foods (i.e., those that are consumed less as income increases) and direct distribution of food to those thought to be most vulnerable (e.g., infants and pregnant women).[14,15] For Morocco, Mateus et al. (1986) estimate that expanded targeted programs could compensate most of the poor who benefit from current food subsidies at a budgetary cost of 11 percent of current food subsidies. Even if this is a substantial underestimate due to overoptimism about the marginal costs of expanding existing targeted programs and about the extent of leakages, it suggests considerable possible budgetary gains from targeting. Likewise, Gavan and Chandrasekera (1979) claim that a shift in the second half of the 1970s to a more targeted program (including a shift to food stamps and the exclusion of about half of the population from the program) cut by more than half the fiscal costs of Sri Lankan food subsidies to the poor as a share of government expenditure. Alderman and von Braun (1985) have conducted careful simulations of different options for the Egyptian food subsidy system; they conclude that "major fiscal savings may be obtained only by substantial modifications [i.e., reductions] of the bread and flour price subsidy and the subsidies paid to consumers of the cooperative shops (e.g., for meat and poultry, macaroni) or by targeting."[16] From such examples, it would seem that governments in a number of cases could cut budgetary expenditures on cheap food programs without directly worsening the income of most of the poor.

Of course, cheap food policies are not the only social policies related to health and nutrition that may be cut as part of economic adjustment programs. Direct cuts on health services may have both an immediate and a longer run impact, and those on education may have a longer run impact given the evidence regarding the relations between better education and improved health and nutrition (e.g., Isenman, 1980; Behrman and Wolfe, 1984; Rosenzweig and Schultz, 1982a; Wolfe and Behrman, 1982). Jimenez (1984) provides a recent survey of pricing policy for health and education in developing countries which has some important implications for the present paper. He concludes that the efficiency gains from user charges for *selected* types of health and education (i.e., those for which the benefits accrue primarily to the individuals concerned, such as hospital care and university education)[17] could be substantial. He adds that the impact of increased user charges need not be inequitable, since

> the present distribution of subsidies tends to be highly skewed towards higher income groups, who obtain greater access to more costly social services . . . even if they are uniformly free for all. Under these circumstances, the expansionary effect of fee increases for selected services (and if possible, for selected individuals) may actually improve equity in the distribution of public resources.

Such a characterization suggests that as part of economic adjustment programs, social programs in health or education *could* be altered through selected user charges so that the poor were not adversely affected. Politically this may be very difficult, perhaps even more difficult than food targeting—and if it were done, there would seem to be no good reason to reverse the process at the end of the economic adjustment program (in which case there would not be the same option in the *next* economic adjustment program).

Household and Individual Responses to Income and Price Changes

As is discussed in an earlier section, the most important effects of economic adjustment programs on households or individuals are to change their real income and the prices, broadly defined, that they face. This section summarizes some evidence that reducing or eliminating governmental programs such as those providing general cheap food may considerably reduce the short-run income of many of the poor—not infrequently by 10–20 percent, and in some cases by much more. At the same time, relative prices may change substantially, and for cuts of the sort discussed in the last section the relative price changes are likely to be ones that discourage the consumption of goods that are presumably positively associated with nutrition and health.

What is the probable impact of these income and relative price changes? Perhaps the most information on these responses pertains to food consumption. Innumerable studies report large income responsiveness for food expenditures, with reductions in total food expenditures often of eight to nine percent for every ten percent drop in income among poorer populations.[18] Considerable evidence also exists that the poor are very responsive to relative prices in deciding what food items to consume. Table 5.3 summarizes evidence from a number of countries regarding the combined real income and own-price response to rice price increases. The poor tend to cut back on their consumption considerably—and more than the rich—in response to such price changes. The income and price responses of the poor are probably also large with respect to nonfood health inputs, though I am aware of many fewer studies of these than of the food-related responses.

However, such large responses in expenditures on food (or in aggregate quantities of food) do *not* necessarily imply large changes in nutrients. Households also may respond substantially by changing the composition of their food expenditures when relative prices change. Several studies document, for example, that the price per calorie (or other nutrient) paid by households in the same society often varies strongly with income (Murty and Radhakrishna, 1981; Pitt, 1983; Radhakrishna, 1984). At least in cross-section data, households with different income levels may have quite different expenditures on food without much difference in nutrients consumed because the wealthier households

Table 5.3
Price Elasticity of Demand for Rice Among Low- and High-Income Population Groups in Selected Countries

Country	Low Income		High Income		Source
	Percentile	Price Elasticity	Percentile	Price Elasticity	
Colombia (Cali)	1	−0.43	93	−0.19	Pinstrup-Andersen, et al.
Indonesia	8	−1.92	55	−0.72	Timmer and Alderman
Bangladesh (rural)	10	−1.30	90	−0.83	Ahmed
Thailand	12	−0.74	87	−0.46	Trairatvorakul
Philippines	12	−0.73	87	−0.40	Bouis
Brazil	15	−4.31	90	−1.15	Williamson-Gray
Sierra Leone (rural)	16	−2.16	84	−0.45	Strauss
India (rural)	3	−1.39	96	−0.39	Murty
India (urban)	1	−1.23	92	−0.21	Murty

Source: Pinstrup-Andersen (1985a: 72). Reprinted with permission of Mouton de Gruyter.

purchase better tasting, more processed, better appearing, and higher status food (or just prefer greater variety)—but not necessarily much more nutritious food (Shah, 1983). If this is the case, many studies of the nutrient response to income changes that indicate substantial responses may be overstated because they use expenditure or quantity data for fairly aggregate food groups[19] and thereby ignore possible responses to differential prices for calories (e.g., Pitt, 1983; Strauss, 1984).

Behrman and Deolalikar (1987b) provide a recent test of this possibility for a rural south Indian sample. First, they estimate fairly standard relations for the food quantity response to income for major food groups and find elasticities of the order of magnitude of 0.8 to 0.9, suggesting that food quantities are adjusted almost as much as income when the latter changes. Then they estimate direct nutrient elasticities with respect to income for the same sample and find elasticities at most of 0.1, suggesting almost no change in nutrient intakes with income. Even in this relatively poor society in which the variety of food is relatively limited, thus, such results suggest that income decreases cause substantial decreases in food expenditures, but mainly by shifting to less costly sources of nutrients rather than by consuming fewer nutrients. Of course some members of society may be so poor that shifting to cheaper sources of nutrients may not be possible because no cheaper sources are available. But these results suggest that shifting cyclically to cheaper nutrient sources may occur for much poorer individuals than is often assumed.

Behrman and Deolalikar (1986b) undertook a subsequent study using aggregate data from thirty countries. In this study they find that the average food expenditures decrease 8 percent for every 10 percent decline in income, but caloric intakes decrease only 3 percent.[20] They conjecture that households value food variety increasingly as their income rises and therefore diversify their food purchases without great emphasis on nutrient qualities of food. They present empirical estimates that support this conjecture. The implications of these estimates is that, with declines in income, households reduce their food expenditures substantially. However, they do so primarily by purchasing less food variety and reduce purchases of nutrients much less than would be proportional to their lessened food expenditures.

The results from these studies are consistent with the relatively low nutrient responses to income reported in a number of other studies which use nutrients directly as the dependent variable[21] (e.g., Behrman and Wolfe, 1984; Levinson, 1974; Pitt and Rosenzweig, 1985; Wolfe and Behrman, 1983), though there are some such studies that report higher nutrient elasticities (e.g., Mateus et al., 1986). If indeed the nutrient responses to income even among the poor are very limited, as many of these studies suggest, then the impact of economic adjustment policies on nutrients consumed by the poor probably is much less than often assumed. Note that this means that many cheap food policies are mainly means of transferring income, not of affecting nutrition much directly.[22] Therefore if one is concerned with the income or the welfare of the poor, one should be concerned that reductions in food subsidies would decrease income. But one should not too easily assume that these reductions would greatly impair nutrition. Whether such results carry over to other factors affecting health is not obvious. They may if there are a number of differentially priced close substitutes, but it is not clear that this is the case.

A further question pertains to the impact of nutrient changes, if they occur, on health status. This is a somewhat murky area. However, a number of recent studies suggest that the impact of small changes in nutrients may be much more in terms of body heat and perhaps energy expenditure than in terms of somewhat longer run anthropometric or clinical measures of health status (e.g., Behrman and Deolalikar, 1985; Payne, 1985; Srinivasan 1985; Sukhatme, 1982). To the extent that this is the case, the commonly assumed negative impact on health of economic adjustment may be overstated. But again there are some counterexamples. For instance, Isenman (1980) presents time series evidence for Sri Lanka that mortality has responded positively and significantly to the price of paddy, presumably in part through a link between price, nutrient intake, and health.

Country Studies Directed to the Evaluation of the Impact of Economic Adjustment Policies on Health and Nutrition

The most visible of these studies probably are those associated with UNICEF (Jolly and Cornia, 1984; UNICEF, 1984). These studies do not formalize explicitly the links between recession and/or economic adjustment and the health and nutrition of children. But they do attempt to use secondary data to characterize some of the links relating to factors such as unemployment, the composition of governmental expenditures, and direct indicators of health and nutrition.

The individual chapters in Jolly and Cornia (1984) provide a useful catalogue of trends, but relatively little information on changes due to recessions and economic adjustment programs. Given the project focus on finding possible negative recessionary and economic adjustment impact on children, the authors appear to have pressed hard to find examples of deterioration in children's conditions. But they provide relatively little direct evidence of such deterioration. To the contrary, in Preston's (1986) words:

> . . . What is remarkable is that the best data on children's status in most of the countries reviewed—that on infant and child mortality—shows continued declines nearly everywhere. Nutritional status indicators also typically show improvement and so do school enrollment figures, despite downturns in governmental expenditure on health and education in some countries.

Preston therefore suggests, and I concur, that the appropriate conclusion from surveying these studies would seem to be—subject to conceptual and data difficulties—that the available evidence from these studies indicates "how much can be achieved even in the face of unusual economic adversity—surely good news for social policy . . ." Instead of such emphasis, however, the editors have a "penchant for stressing the negative trends . . . (a distinct minority) [which] receive the lion's share of the editors' attention in the introduction and summary." Thus, a set of studies that seem to lead to the conclusion of little, or at least unproven, systematic impact of recession and economic adjustment on health and nutrition, is summarized as finding that adjustment policy usually multiplies negative recessionary impact on the poor and vulnerable—see the quotation from Jolly (1985) in the introduction to this paper and the statements by the other editor in the summary to Jolly and Cornia (1984) that "the present crisis . . . has severely aggravated the situation of several social groups," ". . . child welfare indicators . . . are unambiguous in pointing to a deterioration in child status . . . ," and "In most countries one observes . . . a serious deterioration in indicators of nutrition, health status and school achievements . . ."[23]

Certainly I share the judgments expressed in the UNICEF studies that the situation of millions of poor (including children) is appalling, that substantial deterioration *may* have occurred due to recession and economic adjustment that is not very visible because of the poor quality of data monitoring health and nutrition outcomes, that the effects of such deterioration *may* be lagged and may appear only much later—particularly for children (e.g., Selowsky and Taylor, 1973), and that better data are desirable to understand the impact on nutrition and health outcomes. But I do not see these studies as having demonstrated that economic adjustment policies have had deleterious effects on health and nutrition in developing countries or that health and nutrition would have been substantially better without the economic adjustment policies or with different economic adjustment policies.

Summary and Conclusions

Health and nutrition in developing countries *may* be adversely affected by economic adjustment policies, either concurrently or with substantial lags. Macro and microeconomic theories indicate possible channels for such effects, primarily through altering income and prices broadly defined for the poorest and the most vulnerable. Such theories also consider that such channels are complex and that the effects *may* be small because of the limited effectiveness of macroeconomic policies, the lack of impact of policies on some of the poorest, and the adjustment and substitution capabilities of those of the poor whose real income and prices broadly defined are altered negatively.

Systematic empirical studies illustrate some of these links and suggest that the impact of economic adjustment policies on health and nutrition in developing economies often may be slight. Macroeconomic adjustment policies certainly have some negative impact, particularly on those at the lower end of the formal sector income distribution, with some spillover on those in the informal sector. But those in the formal sector usually are not the poorest and most vulnerable members of society. If anything cuts in governmental expenditures as part of economic adjustment programs apparently have been on the average proportionately less extensive in the health and nutrition areas than for overall governmental expenditures. Staple food prices have been increased in a number of cases with declines in the real income of the poor (as well as of those much better off). But recent evidence suggests that many of the poor adjust the composition of their food consumption in response to price and income changes so that nutrient intakes are affected proportionately much less than are their incomes, though such adjustment possibilities may be limited for the poorest due to the absence of still cheaper nutrient alternatives. The most reliable data on health status, that on infant and child mortality, generally shows continued declines despite economic adjustment programs.

Certainly any conclusion about the impact of economic adjustment in developing countries on health and nutrition must be tentative at this time because of the conceptual and empirical problems in assessing such effects. Subject to such qualifications, the appropriate conclusion seems to be that the coping capacities of societies, households and individuals apparently often have been substantial so that the demonstrable impact on health and nutrition has been surprisingly limited. This assessment contrasts sharply with the view of those summarized in the introduction that the pervasiveness of multiplied negative effects of economic adjustment policies on health and nutrition in developing countries has been demonstrated systematically. The available systematic evidence simply does not support such an assertion. Theoretical and empirical studies raise many questions that would have to be answered before such a conclusion legitimately could be reached. For example, in a particular economy exactly what are the effects of economic adjustment policies on aggregate economic indicators, how do these translate through product and input markets into changes in the real income and prices broadly defined faced by poor individuals and households, to what extent do such individuals and households change their behavior in response to the real income and relative price changes in ways that affect their health and nutrition, and what are the time lags and adjustments periods throughout this complicated system? My tentative conclusion is that, if anything, the available evidence indicates on the average an ameliorated rather than a multiplied impact of recession and adjustment policies on health and nutrition because of substitution possibilities throughout the system. Of course some countries have ameliorated such effects better than others, so there is potential for useful learning from the more successful experiences if the political concern about the welfare of the poorer members of society is strong enough. There also are some fairly widespread possible efficiency and budgetary gains from better targeting of food and health programs. Economic recessions may be catalytic in improving such targeting, but it should be realized that any gains realized should be viewed as once and for all, not cyclical gains to be reversed with the economic cycle.

But there is much that we do not know about such complex events. Better data and more systematic analysis are desirable, may prove enlightening, and may support the multiplied impact assertion of Jolly and Cornia, et al. or may support my tentative more ameliorative conclusion. Likewise, greater consciousness regarding "adjustment policies with a human face" and the initiation of information systems to monitor the impact of adjustment programs on distribution and the welfare of the poor are desirable. It is important that such programs encompass a broad view of income and asset distribution, not just health and nutrition indicators, since the evidence is much more persuasive regarding the impact of economic adjustment on income of the poor per se than on health and nutrition. However, resources devoted to research and to anticyclical social policies have an opportunity cost. At this point, given the inherent complexities of the processes of interest and the limited systematic evidence to date of any impact, I am not at all sure that the expected payoff is high to investment of a lot of resources in research or in policies related primarily to the relation between *cyclical* economic adjustment programs and health and nutrition in developing countries. I well can believe that the expected payoffs are higher to research and policies—including those related to economic growth as well as distribution—that focus on *secular* improvements in health and nutrition, though perhaps with some emphasis on flexibility to accommodate cyclical changes and their impact.[24]

Notes

1. Economic adjustment programs in the developed economies also may affect health and nutrition in the developing economies, primarily by affecting the international markets of importance to the developing countries through, for example, the prices they receive for their exports or the interest rates they pay on their foreign debts. I do not consider such policies in this chapter but treat their impact on international markets as given from the point of view of developing economies. Taylor (1986) considers prospects for these external factors in his useful contribution to the symposium. With respect to the relative importance of these external factors in comparison with ones internal to developing countries in the 1970s, Black (1981: 70–71) concludes:

   Thus, although external factors have generated many of the disturbances to which developing countries have had to respond in the 1970's, it appears to have been largely country characteristics and the internal response to those disturbances and other internally generated disturbances that have spelled success or failure for stabilization policy.

   The present chapter also focuses on short-term economic adjustment programs, not on long-term structural adjustments.

2. I draw extensively in this section on the recent excellent survey on macroeconomic stabilization and income distribution by Addison and Demery (1985), to which the interested reader is referred for a much more extensive discussion. The interesting related paper by Kanbur (1985) came to my attention so late that my chapter has not benefited from it.

3. But the closure issue may be troublesome indeed for actual explicit applications. Addison and Demery (1985: 22) state in this regard: "Clearly, the paradigm will to a large extent pre-determine the results of the effects of macro policies on income distribution and poverty" and "In formal models, the basic economic philosophy of

of the researcher determines the 'closure rule' adopted." The appropriate closure rules are not easily explored empirically because of the difficulty of nesting the alternatives within one larger framework in an empirically tractable manner.

4. If the country is a large enough actor in any international market to affect international prices, there is a further question about the nature of that impact. There is not likely to be such an impact for most products for most developing countries since most of those countries are small relative to world markets. I maintain this "small country" assumption throughout this chapter.

5. For developed market economies, fiscal and monetary policies often are considered separately because monetary authorities are thought to be able to act in well-developed financial markets with some independence from fiscal authorities. Monetary authorities are not thought to have such independence in most developing economies, in part because of poorly developed financial capital markets. Therefore I consider fiscal and monetary policies together here.

6. The equilibrium price level is more likely to increase the greater is the shift to the left of the supply curve versus the demand curve and the steeper are both curves at the initial equilibrium.

7. The 1985 Argentinean "Austral" adjustment program and the 1986 "Crusado" Brazilian program attempt to avoid such asymmetries and to break inflationary expectations by freezing (or at least reducing radically changes in) all prices, wages, etc. In these countries prior to these programs indexation of prices, wages, etc. was so pervasive that it created tremendous inertia opposing any anti-inflationary efforts.

8. There is some controversy in the economic literature about whether households are better modeled as having unified preferences of an altruistic household head or as having bargaining among the various members of the household with each having different preferences and control over assets. From the point of view of casual observation, the bargaining approach probably seems more realistic. But for most purposes, given available data, one cannot distinguish between the alternative approaches. The problem in identifying which approach is preferable from reduced-form estimates with most existing data is that if a certain outcome (e.g., child health) depends on, say, women's wages, one cannot be sure to what extent that dependence reflects the value of women's time versus the strength of their bargaining position (both of which their wages may be representing). See, for example, Becker (1981), Behrman (1986, 1987), Folbre (1986), Jones (1983), Rosenzweig and Schultz (1982b, 1984), Manser and Brown (1980), McElroy and Horney (1981).

9. I do not find this interpretation persuasive. But, in any case, they do not find a positive tradeoff.

10. In the 1960s and early 1970s, however, most emphasis was on longer-run macroeconomic planning models. See Blitzer, Clark and Taylor (1975) for a state-of-the-art survey as of the mid-1970s, which devotes almost no attention to macroeconometric and other short-run modeling approaches necessary for the evaluation of economic adjustment policies.

11. Preliminary studies by others also suggest that the use of category-specific price indices and comparison with a longer-run trend rather than just the previous year may weaken the extent to which social sectors appear to be favored, but such adjustments do not seem to lead to the conclusion that the social sectors are cut significantly more than the average.

12. Many observers claim that economic adjustment programs in general and food subsidy cuts in particular lead not only to protests and riots, but to more fundamental political instability in developing countries. Bienen and Gersovitz (1985: 37) however, analyze recent experience and conclude that such subsidy cuts "do not appear more fundamental as a cause of instability than many other short run factors . . ."

13. Unless the cheap food policies involved consumer subsidies with arbitrage precluded between consumer and producer prices.

14. Of course there generally are leakages to other household members in the latter type programs. Beaton and Ghassemi (1979), for example, reviewed over 200 reports on food distribution programs targeted towards young children and found that the net increase in the food intake of the targeted children was 45–70 percent of the food distributed. The other 30–70 percent of the food distributed increased the real income of the rest of the household, perhaps with nutrition and health benefits.

15. Pinstrup-Andersen and Alderman (1986) and Rodgers (1986) discuss in some detail targeting approaches.

16. In their simulation of targeting, they assume that the basic and additional rations are discontinued for all but the poorest 25 percent of the population, that this part of the population also received an additional coarse flour ration, and that bread at the current fixed nominal price is available only in the poorest 20 percent of urban neighborhoods (p. 28).

17. But not including those such as basic education and some types of preventive medical care for which the benefits are considerable to society as a whole (i.e., there are large externalities).

18. Based on cross-country estimates, Behrman and Deolalikar (1986b) report a drop on the average of 8 percent for every 10 percent drop in income, with a somewhat larger (smaller) drop for poorer (richer) populations.

19. In many societies even rice is a fairly aggregate food group in the sense relevant for this discussion since the price per calorie may vary substantially in a given locale due to different qualities (e.g., broken versus whole heads, color and length of grains, taste and aroma, degree of processing).

20. For some other nutrients—namely proteins, iron, thiamine and niacin—the decreases are about the same or smaller. For beta-carotene and vitamin C, they are about 4 percent. For calcium it is 7 percent and for fat, 8 percent. Because the Food and Agriculture Organization (FAO) calculates the nutrient data from fairly aggregate data, all of these estimates may overstate the actual nutrient responses since they ignore intra food category responses.

21. The use of nutrients directly as the dependent variable typically results in data construction in which much more of the substitution among sources due to relative price per nutrient variation is captured than if expenditure or quantity is used as the dependent variable at typical levels of aggregation (see Behrman and Deolalikar, 1985).

22. One might ask why direct income transfers would be preferable. Pinstrup-Andersen (1985a) argues that food subsidies are more politically acceptable.

23. Preston (1980) also notes that the case of South Korea, nicely reviewed by Sang Mok Suh in the Jolly and Cornia volume, scarcely is mentioned in the editors' introduction and summary even though South Korea has had rapid gains in child growth, child survival and school enrollment gains as well as high economic growth and relatively great success in adjusting to world economic fluctuations. Preston goes on to state, "There is a certain irony when a strategy of economic development is so successful that one's social successes get discounted. But survey countries like South Korea are instructive when setting the broad parameters of social economy policy."

24. This statement should *not* be misinterpreted to mean that health and nutrition policy improvements should be considered only in the long run after all the short-run problems are resolved. As Frances Stewart observed at the symposium, economies always have short-run problems, so to postpone a particular action until the short-run problems are resolved is to postpone it forever. What is meant by the statement in the text is that the payoff does not appear to be high to tying health and nutrition

policies and analysis to short-term economic adjustment policies that will be reversed when the economic conditions change. They should be a more permanent part of the policy package.

References

Abbott, G. C. "Debt and the Poorer Developing Countries," *Development Policy Review* 2 (1984): 181–189.

Addison, T., and L. Demery. "Macro-Economic Stabilisation, Income Distribution and Poverty: a Preliminary Survey." Overseas Development Institute, 1985.

Ahluwalia, M. S., and F. J. Lysy. "Employment, Income Distribution and Programs to Remedy Balance of Payments Difficulties," in William R. Cline and Sidney Weintraub, eds., *Economic Stabilization in Developing Countries*. Washington, D.C.: The Brookings Institution, 1981, pp. 149–190.

Ahmed, R. "Foodgrain Supply, Distribution, and Consumption Policies Within a Dual Pricing Mechanism: A Case Study of Bangladesh," Research Report 8. Washington, D.C.: International Food Policy Research Institute, 1979.

———. "Agricultural Price Policies Under Complex Socioeconomic and Natural Constraints: The Case of Bangladesh," Research Report 27. Washington, D.C.: International Food Policy Research Institute, 1981.

Adelman, I., and S. Robinson. *Income Distribution Policy in Developing Countries: A Case Study of Korea.* Stanford, CA: Stanford University Press, 1978.

Alderman, H., and J. von Braun. "Egypt: Implications of Alternative Food Subsidy Policies in the 1980s." Washington, D.C.: International Food Policy Research Institute, 1985.

———. "The Effects of the Egyptian Food Ration and Subsidy System on Income Distribution and Consumption," Research Report 45. Washington, D.C.: International Food Policy Research Institute, 1982.

Alderman, H., J. von Braun, and S. A. Sakr. "Egypt's Food Subsidy and Rationing System: A Description," Research Report 34. Washington, D.C.: International Food Policy Research Institute, 1982.

Barro, R. J. "Money and Output in Mexico, Colombia, and Brazil," in Jere R. Behrman and James A. Hanson, eds., *Short-Term Macroeconomic Policy in Latin America.* Cambridge, MA: Ballinger Publishing Company, 1979, pp. 177–200.

Bartel, A., and P. Taubman. "The Impact of Specific Diseases on Earnings," *Review of Economics and Statistics* (February 1979).

Beaton, G. H., and H. Ghassemi. "Supplementary Feeding Programmes for Young Children in Developing Countries," report prepared for UNICEF and the ACC Subcommittees on Nutrition, 1979.

Behrman, J. R. *Macroeconomic Policy in a Developing Country: The Chilean Experiences.* New York: North-Holland Publishing Company, 1977.

———. "Intrahousehold Allocation of Nutrients in Rural India: Are Boys Favored? Do Parents Exhibit Inequality Aversion?" Philadelphia: University of Pennsylvania, 1986.

————. "Nutrition, Health, Birth Order and Seasonality: Intrahousehold Allocation in Rural India," *Journal of Development Economics*, 1987.

———— and A. Deolalikar. "Determinants of Health and Nutritional Status of Different Family Members in Rural India: A Latent Variable Approach." Philadelphia: University of Pennsylvania, mimeo, 1986a.

————. "Is Variety the Spice of Life? Implications for Nutrient Responses to Development." Philadelphia: University of Pennsylvania, mimeo, 1986b.

————. "Health and Nutrition," in H. B. Chenery and T. N. Srinivasan, eds., *Handbook on Development Economics*. Amsterdam: North-Holland Publishing Co., 1987a.

————. "Will Developing Country Nutrition Improve with Income? A Case Study for Rural South India," *Journal of Political Economy*, 1987b.

———— and J. A. Hanson, eds. *Short-Term Macroeconomic Policy in Latin America*. Cambridge, MA: Ballinger Publishing Company, 1979.

———— and J. R. Vargas. "A Quarterly Econometric Model of Panama," in Behrman and Hanson, 1979.

———— and B. L. Wolfe. "More Evidence on Nutrition Demand: Income Seems Overrated and Women's Schooling Underemphasized." *Journal of Development Economics* 14:1–2 (January-February 1984): 105–128.

Beltran del Rio, A., and Ramy Schwartz. "Bibliography of Latin American Macroeconomic Models." Philadelphia: Wharton Econometric Forecasting Associates, mimeo, 1986.

Bhagwati, J. *Anatomy and Consequences of Exchange Control Regimes*. Cambridge: Ballinger, National Bureau of Economic Research, 1978.

Bienen, Henry S., and Mark Gersovitz. "Consumer Subsidy Cuts, Violence, and Political Instability." Princeton: Princeton University, mimeo, 1985.

Black, S. W. "The Impact of Changes in the World Economy on Stabilization Policies in the 1970s," in William R. Cline and Sidney Weintraub, eds., *Economic Stabilization in Developing Countries*. Washington, D.C.: The Brookings Institution, 1981, pp. 43–81.

Blitzer, C. R., P. B. Clark, and L. Taylor. *Economy-Wide Models and Development Planning*. Oxford: Oxford University, 1975.

Bouis, H. "Rice Policy in the Philippines," unpublished Ph.D. thesis, Stanford University, 1982.

Brodersohn, M. S. "The Phillips Curve and the Conflict Between Full Employment and Price Stability in the Argentine Economy, 1964–1974," in Behrman and Hanson, 1979, pp. 201–225.

Buffie, E. F. "Financial Repression, the New Structuralists and Stabilisation Policy in Semi-Industrialised Economies," *Journal of Development Economics* 14:13 (April 1984): 305–322.

Chambers, R., R. Longhurst, and A. Pacey. *Seasonal Dimensions to Rural Poverty*. London: Frances Pinter Publishers Ltd., 1981.

Cline, W. R., and S. Weintraub, eds. *Economic Stabilization in Developing Countries*. Washington, D.C.: Brookings Institution, 1981.

Davies, R., D. Saunders, and R. Loewenson. "Stabilization Policies and the Health Status of Children: The Case of Zimbabwe," mimeo, 1986.

deMelo, J., and S. Robinson. *General Equilibrium Models for Development Policy*. Cambridge: Cambridge University Press, 1982.

Diaz-Alejandro, C. F. *Exchange Rate Devaluation in a Semi-Industrialized Country: The Experience of Argentina 1955–1961*. Cambridge, MA: MIT Press, 1965.

———. "Southern Cone Stabilization Plans," in Cline and Weintraub, 1981.

Edirisinghe, N. "Preliminary Report on the Food Stamp Scheme in Sri Lanka: Distribution of Benefits and Impact on Nutrition." Washington, D.C.: International Food Policy Research Institute, February 1985.

Fernandez, R. B. "The Short-Run Output-Inflation Tradeoff in Argentina and Brazil," in Behrman and Hanson, 1979, pp. 133–167.

French-Davis, R. "The Monetarist Experiment in Chile: A Critical View," *World Development* 11 (November 1983): 905–926.

Folbre, N. "Cleaning House: New Perspectives on Households and Economic Development," *Journal of Development Economics* 22:1 (June 1986): 5–40.

Foxley, A. "Stabilisation Policies and their Effects on Employment and Income Distribution: A Latin American Perspective," in Cline and Weintraub, 1981, pp. 191–234.

———. *Latin American Experiments in Neo-Conservative Economies*. Berkeley: University of California Press, 1983.

Gavan, J. D., and I. S. Chandrasekera. "The Impact of Public Foodgrain Distribution on Food Consumption and Welfare in Sri Lanka," Research Report 13. Washington, D.C.: International Food Policy Research Institute, 1979.

George, P. S. "Public Distribution of Foodgrain in Kerala—Income Distribution Implications and Effectiveness," Research Report 7. Washington, D.C.: International Food Policy Research Institute, 1979.

Hanson, J. A. "The Short-Run Relation between Growth and Inflation in Latin America: A Quasi-Rational or Consistent Expectations Approach," *American Economic Review* 70:5 (December 1980).

Helleiner, G. "The IMF and Africa in the 1980s," *Essays in International Finance* 152 (Princeton, July 1983).

Hicks, N., and A. Kubisch. "The Effects of Expenditures Reductions in Developing Countries." Washington, D.C.: World Bank, mimeo, 1983.

———. "Cutting Government Expenditures in LDCs," *Finance and Development* (September 1984).

Isenman, P. "Basic Needs: The Case of Sri Lanka," *World Development* 8 (1980): 237–258.

Islam, S. "Devaluation, Stabilization Policies and the Developing Countries: A Macroeconomic Analysis," *Journal of Development Economics* 14:1–2 (January-February 1984).

Jolly, R. "Adjustment with a Human Face." New York: UNICEF, pamphlet, 1985.

Jolly, R., and G. A. Cornia. *The Impact of World Recession on Children: A Study Prepared for UNICEF*. Oxford: Pergamon Press, 1984.

Jones, C. "The Mobilization of Women's Labor for Cash Crop Production: A Game Theoretic Approach," *American Journal of Agricultural Economics* 65:5 (December 1983): 1049–1054.

Jimenez, E. "Pricing Policy in the Social Sectors: Cost Recovery for Education and Health in Developing Countries." Washington, D.C.: The World Bank, mimeo, 1984.

Johnson, O., and J. Salop. "Distributional Aspects of Stabilization Programs in Developing Countries," *IMF Staff Papers* 27:1 (1980): 1–23.

Kaldor, N. "Devaluation and Adjustment in Developing Countries." *Finance and Development* 20:2 (June 1983): 35–37.

Kanbur, S. M. Ravi. "Poverty: Measurement, Alleviation and the Impact of Macroeconomic Adjustment." Princeton: Princeton University, mimeo, 1985.

Katseli, L. T. "Devaluation: A Critical Appraisal of the IMF's Policy Prescriptions," *American Economic Review* 73:2 (May 1983).

Khan, M. S. "Exchange Rate Responses to Exogenous Shocks in Developing Countries." Washington, D.C.: The World Bank, mimeo, 1986.

Khan, M. S., and M. D. Knight. "Some Theoretical and Empirical Issues Relating to Economic Stabilization in Developing Countries." *World Development* 10:9 (September 1982).

Killick, T., ed. *The Quest for Economic Stabilization: The IMF and the Third World.* London: Heinemann/ODI, 1984a.

———, ed. *The IMF and Stabilization: Developing Country Experiences.* London: Heinemann/ODI, 1984b.

Knight, J. B. "Devaluation and Income Distribution in Less-Developed Economies," *Oxford Economic Papers* 28:2 (July 1986): 200–227.

Knudson, O.K., and P. L. Scandizzo. "The Demand for Calories in Developing Countries," *American Journal of Agricultural Economics* (February 1982): 80–86.

Krueger, A. O. "The Political Economy of the Rent-Seeking Society," *American Economic Review* 64 (June 1974).

———. *Foreign Trade Regimes and Economic Development Liberalization Attempts and Consequences.* Cambridge, MA: Ballinger, NBER, 1978.

Krugman, P., and L. Taylor. "Contractionary Effects of Devaluation," *Journal of International Economics* 8 (1978).

Kumar, S. K. "Impact of Subsidized Rice on Food Consumption and Nutrition in Kerala," Research Report 5. Washington, D.C.: International Food Policy Research Institute, 1979.

Lau, L. "A Bibliography of Macroeconomic Models of Developing Economies." Palo Alto: Stanford University, mimeo, 1975.

Leslie, Joanne, Margarette Lycette and Mayra Buvinic. "The Crucial Role of Women in Health: Weathering Economic Crises" Chapter 13 of this volume.

Levinson, F. J. *Morinda: An Economic Analysis of Malnutrition Among Young Children in Rural India.* Cambridge, MA: Cornell/MIT International Nutrition Policy Series, 1974.

Levy, S. "Short Run Responses to Foreign Exchange Crisis," Discussion Paper 66. Boston: Boston University, Center for Latin American Development Studies, mimeo, 1985.

Lucas, R. "Some International Evidence on the Output-Inflation Tradeoff," *American Economic Review* 63 (June 1973): 326–334.

Manser, M., and M. Brown. "Marriage and Household Decision-Making: A Bargaining Analysis," *International Economic Review* 21:1 (February 1980): 31–44.

Mateus, A., et al. "Morocco: Compensatory Programs for Reducing Food Subsidies." Washington, D.C.: World Bank, mimeo, 1986.

McElroy, M. B., and M. J. Horney. "Nash-Bargained Household Decisions: Toward a Generalization of the Theory of Demand," *International Economic Review* 22:2 (June 1981): 333–350.

McKinnon, R. I. "Foreign Trade Regimes and Economic Development: A Review Article," *Journal of International Economies* 9 (1979): 429–452.

Mellor, J. "Food Price Policy and Income Distribution in Low-Income Countries," *Economic Development and Cultural Change* 1 (1978): 1–26.

Mohammed, A. F. "The Case by Case Approach to Debt Problems," *Finance and Development* (March 1986: 27–30.

Murty, K. "Consumption and Nutrition Patterns of ICRISAT Mandate Crops in India." Hyderabad, India: ICRISAT, Economics Program Progress, Report 53, 1983.

Murty, K. N., and R. Radhakrishna. "Agricultural Prices, Income Distribution and Demand Patterns in a Low-Income Country," in Robert E. Kalman and J. Martinez, eds., *Computer Applications in Food Production and Agricultural Engineering.* Amsterdam: North-Holland Publishing Company, 1981.

Nashashibi, K. "Devaluation in Developing Countries: The Difficult Choice," *Finance and Development* 20:1 (March 1983): 14–17.

Nelson, J. M. "The Political Economy of Stabilization: Commitment, Capacity, and Public Response," *World Development* 12:10 (October 1984): 983–1006.

Nugent, J. B., and Glezakos, C. "Phillips Curves in Developing Countries: The Latin American Case," *Economic Development and Cultural Change* 30:2 (January 1982): 321–334.

Pastor, M. "The IMF in Latin America: Debate, Evidence and Case Study." Mimeo, 1985.

Payne, P. "Public Health and Functional Consequences of Seasonal Hunger and Malnutrition." London: London School of Hygiene and Tropical Medicine, mimeo, 1985.

Payne, P., and P. Culter. "Measuring Malnutrition: Technical Problems and Ideological Perspectives," *Economic and Political Weekly* 25 (August 1984): 1485–1491.

Pinstrup-Andersen, P. "Food Prices and the Poor in Developing Countries," *European Review of Agricultural Economics* 12:1–2 (1985a).

———. "The Short-Term Impact of Macro-Economic Adjustment Policies on the Poor with Emphasis on the Nutrition Effects: The Need for Research." Washington: IFPRI, mimeo, 1985b.

———. "Assuring Food Security and Adequate Nutrition for the Poor During Periods of Economic Crisis and Macroeconomic Adjustments: Policy Options and Experience with Food Subsidies and Transfer Programs." Washington: IFPRI, mimeo, 1986a.

———. "Macroeconomic Adjustment Policies and Human Nutrition: Available Evidence and Research Needs." Washington: IFPRI, mimeo, 1986b.

——— and Harold Alderman. "The Effectiveness of Consumer-Oriented Food Subsidies in Reaching Rationing and Incomes Transfer Goals," in Per Pinstrup-Andersen, ed., *Consumer-Oriented Food Subsidies: Benefits, Costs and Policy Options.* Baltimore: Johns Hopkins University Press, 1986.

——— and E. Caicedo. "The Potential Impact of Changes in Income Distribution of Food Demand and Human Nutrition," *American Journal of Agricultural Economics* 60:3 (1978): 402–415.

———, R. de Londonno, and E. Hoover. "The Impact of Increasing Food Supply on Human Nutrition: Implications for Commodity Priorities in

Agricultural Research and Policy," *American Journal of Agricultural Economics* (May 1976): 131–142.

——— and T. Uy. "Seasonal Fluctuations in Food Consumption and Incomes in Northern Nigeria" (research in progress). Washington, D.C.: International Food Policy Research Institute, 1985.

Pitt, M. M. "Food Preferences and Nutrition in Rural Bangladesh," *Review of Economics and Statistics* 65:1 (February 1983): 105–114.

——— and M. R. Rosenzweig. "Health and Nutrient Consumption Across and Within Farm Households," *Review of Economics and Statistics* 65:1 (February 1983): 105–114.

Porter, R. C., and S. I. Ranney. "An Eclectic Model of Recent LDC Macroeconomic Policy Analyses," *World Development* 10:9 (September 1982): 751–766.

Preston, Samuel H. "Review of Richard Jolly and Giovanni Andrea Cornia, editors, *The Impact of World Recession on Children*," *Journal of Development Economics* 21:2 (May 1986): 374–376.

Pyatt, G., and J. I. Round. "Social Accounting Matrices for Development Planning," *Review of Income and Wealth* 23:4 (1979).

Pyatt, G., and E. Thorbecke. *Planning for a Better Future.* Geneva: International Labour Office, 1976.

Radhakrishna, R. "Distributional Aspects of Caloric Consumption: Implications for Food Policy," in K. T. Achaya, ed., *Interfaces between Agriculture, Nutrition and Food Science.* Tokyo: The United Nations University, 1984, pp. 231–240.

Rao, V. K. R. V. "Investment, Income and the Multiplier in an Underdeveloped Economy," *The Indian Economic Review* (February 1952).

Rogers, Beatrice Lorge. "Design and Implementation Considerations for Consumer-Oriented Food Subsidies," in Per Pinstrup-Andersen, ed., *Consumer-Oriented Food Subsidies: Benefits, Costs and Policy Options.* Baltimore: Johns Hopkins University Press, 1986.

Rosenzweig, M. R., and T. P. Schultz. "Child Mortality and Fertility in Colombia: Individual and Community Effects," *Health Policy and Education* 2. Amsterdam: Elsevier Scientific Publishing Co., 1982a, pp. 305–348.

———. "Market Opportunities, Genetic Endowments, and Intrafamily Resource Distribution: Child Survival in Rural India," *American Economic Review* 72:4 (September, 1982b): 803–815.

———. "Market Opportunities and Intrafamily Resource Distribution: Reply," *American Economic Review* 74 (June 1984).

Sahn, D. "Analysis of Food Consumption Patterns and Parameters in Sri Lanka," 1984. Washington, D.C.: International Food Policy Research Institute, pending publication.

Seckler, D. "Small but Healthy: A Basic Hypothesis in the Theory Measurement and Policy of Malnutrition," in P. V. Sukhatme, ed., *Newer Concepts in Nutrition and Their Implications for Policy.* India: Maharashtra Association for the Cultivation of Science Research Institute, 1982.

Selowsky, M. "Target Group-Oriented Food Programs: Cost Effectiveness Comparisons," *American Journal of Agricultural Economics* (December 1979).

——— and L. Taylor. "The Economics of Malnourished Children: An Example of Disinvestment in Human Capital," *Economic Development and Cultural Change* 22:1 (October 1973): 17–30.

Sen, A. K. "Family and Food: Sex Bias in Poverty," in *Resources, Values and Development*. Oxford: Basil Blackwell, 1984, pp. 346–368.

Shah, C. H. "Food Preference, Poverty and the Nutrition Gap," *Economic Development and Cultural Change* 32:1 (October 1983): 121–148.

Shepard, Donald S., and Elisabeth Benjamin. "User Fees and Health Financing in Developing Countries: Mobilizing Financial Resources for Health," Chapter 16 of this volume.

Srinivasan, T. N. "Malnutrition: Some Measurement and Policy Issues," *Journal of Development Economics* 8:1 (1981): 3–19.

————. "Malnutrition in Developing Countries: The State of Knowledge of the Extent of its Prevalence, its Causes and its Consequences," mimeo, 1985.

Strauss, J. "Joint Determination of Food Consumption and Product in Rural Sierra Leone: Estimates of a Household-Firm Model," *Journal of Development Economics* 14:1–2 (January-February 1984): 77–104.

Sukhatme, P. V., ed. *Newer Concepts in Nutrition and Their Implications for Policy*. India: Maharshtra Association for the Cultivation of Science Research Institute, 1982.

Tanzi, V. "LDC Fiscal Policy Responses to Exogenous Shocks." Washington, D.C.: International Monetary fund, mimeo, 1985.

Taylor, L. "Short-Term Policy in Open Developing Economies: The Narrow Limits of the Possible," *Journal of Development Economics* 1 (1974): 85–104.

————. *Macro Models for Developing Countries*. New York: McGraw-Hill, 1979.

————. *Structuralist Macroeconomics*. New York: Basic Books, 1983.

————. "Macro Effects of Myriad Shocks: Developing Countries in the World Economy." Chapter 2 of this volume.

Taylor, L., and F. J. Lysy. "Vanishing Income Redistributions: Keynesian Clues About Model Surprises in the Short Run," *Journal of Development Studies* 6 (1979).

Timmer, C. P., and H. Alderman. "Estimating Consumption Parameters for Food Policy Analysis," *American Journal of Agricultural Economics* 61 (1979): 982–987.

Trairatvorakul, P. "Effects on Income Distribution and Nutrition of Alternative Rice Price Policies in Thailand," Research Report 47. Washington, D.C.: International Food Policy Research Institute, 1985.

UNICEF. "The Impact of World Recession on Children: A UNICEF Special Study," in *State of the World's Children 1984*. Oxford: Oxford University Press, 1984.

van Wijnbergen, S. "Stagflationary Effects of Monetary Stabilization Policies: A Quantitative Analysis of South Korea," *Journal of Development Economics* 10 (1982): 133–169.

Williamson-Gray, C. "Food Consumption Parameters for Brazil and their Application to Food Policy," Research Report 32. Washington, D.C.: International Food Policy Research Institute, 1982.

Wolfe, B. L., and J. R. Behrman. "Determinants of Child Mortality, Health and Nutrition in a Developing Country," *Journal of Development Economics* 11:2 (October 1982): 163–194.

————. "Is Income Overrated in Determining Adequate Nutrition?" *Economic Development and Cultural Change* 31:3 (April 1983): 525–550.

World Food Council. *Improving Access to Food by the Undernourished.* Report by the Executive Director to the Eleventh Ministerial Session. Paris, June 10–13, 1985 (WFC/1985/4).

Zulu, J. B., and S. M. Nsouli. "Adjustment Programs in Africa," *Finance and Development* (March 1984).

PART II

APPROACHES TO FOOD AND NUTRITION POLICY

6

Assuring Food Security and Adequate Nutrition for the Poor

Per Pinstrup-Andersen

The impact of macroeconomic adjustment programs on food security and nutritional status of the poor is not well documented. However, there are signs that it has been positive for some groups, particularly small farmers, while it has been negative at least in the short run for certain other groups of the poor. The various ways in which positive or negative impact may come about and the complexities involved are discussed elsewhere (Behrman, 1986; Pinstrup-Andersen, 1986) and will not be repeated here. Suffice to mention that macroeconomic adjustments in many countries appear to have resulted in large decreases in real incomes of the poor as consumers and wage earners. This has come about through rapidly increasing prices of food and other commodities that are usually traded internationally (tradeables); reduced wages and employment in the production of goods and services that are not usually traded internationally (non-tradeables); and government efforts to maintain little or no growth of the wage rates in the production of tradeables. Those poor who produce a marketed surplus of tradeables, on the other hand, may have benefitted.

Increased employment in the production of tradeables may have partially compensated for negative effects on real incomes, but available evidence does not support the notion that the poor have been fully compensated in the short run. Furthermore, macroeconomic adjustment programs often include measures to reduce government spending on food and housing subsidies, transfer programs, and various other social programs such as public health. Thus, two key variables for

147

nutrition—real incomes of the poor, including government transfer, and their access to health facilities—are usually affected.

Because the poor spend a large share of their budget on food and other basic necessities, their purchasing power is strongly correlated with their ability to meet nutritional needs; even small decreases may have serious nutritional consequences. An increasing number of institutions and individuals are responding at least partially to this by expressing concern about the need to protect or compensate certain groups of low-income households when macroeconomic adjustment programs are introduced. Such protection or compensation may be provided in many different ways. This chapter summarizes the evidence from studies of and experience with the most common programs and policies which may be considered, and discusses the principal lessons for the design of future programs and policies. Only food-related programs and policies will be discussed.

Performance of the Most Common Programs and Policies

What policy and program options does a government have for assuring that the poor have economic access to sufficient food to avoid a deterioration of their nutritional status during periods of economic crises and macroeconomic adjustments, and what has been the performance of these policies and programs in the countries where they have been tried?[1] These options are discussed in three groupings: (1) food price subsidies, (2) food-linked income transfer programs, and (3) income-generation programs.

Food Price Subsidies

Most governments attempt to influence the price consumers pay for food. In low-income countries, they frequently aim to reduce consumer food prices below a free market level, thus providing a subsidy to the consumer. The goals of subsidy programs and policies vary among countries and over time. They may include, among others, improving the real purchasing power of all or certain groups of consumers, reducing or eliminating energy and nutrient deficiencies in low-income population groups, maintaining low urban wages, and assuring social and political stability.

The design of subsidy policies and their implementation procedures vary widely among countries and include explicit price subsidies targeted to selected population groups and/or food commodities as well as explicit or implicit general price subsidies with little or no targeting.

In some countries, consumer-oriented food subsidies are large and widespread and place a heavy financial burden on either the government[2] or food producers while in others, subsidy costs are small and of little consequence to the government and/or farmers. Similarly, the benefits from food subsidies and their distribution as well as their cost-effectiveness vary among countries. Some subsidy programs greatly enhance poor people's purchasing power and nutritional status, while others primarily benefit middle and upper income population groups. In some countries, consumer-oriented food subsidies are of such magnitudes that they exercise considerable influence over foreign trade, inflation, and the performance of the agricultural and other sectors as well as economic growth and equity in general.

Policy and Program Characteristics. Case studies undertaken by the International Food Policy Research Institute (IFPRI) and national collaborators in eleven countries represent the variety of policies and programs that may be referred to as consumer-oriented food price subsidies.[3]

Consumer prices below open market or border prices for one or more commodities are a common feature of the programs. Wheat and rice are the commodities most commonly subsidized. Some of the programs provide explicit subsidies, i.e., the costs are borne by the government, while others provide implicit subsidies. The latter are usually maintained through low producer prices. Rice price subsidies in Thailand and Egypt are totally financed by rice producers through low producer prices, while the majority of the wheat subsidies in Egypt and Brazil are financed by public funds. As a general rule, it appears that the more the program is targeted, the less the agricultural sector contributes relatively, to meeting subsidy costs. This relationship occurs because implicit subsidies are most conveniently enforced through government intervention in market prices while targeted programs are often based on imported food, including food aid.

Some program components provide subsidies for a specified household ration only, e.g., sugar, rice, tea, and edible oil subsidies in Egypt, while others subsidize the total quantity marketed of a particular commodity, e.g., wheat subsidies in Sudan, Egypt, and Brazil, and rice subsidies in Thailand.

A few of the programs are narrowly targeted to certain population groups, e.g., milk subsidies for children in Mexico, while others make subsidized commodities available to all, e.g., rice price subsidies in

Thailand and wheat subsidies in Brazil. A strong urban bias is common, e.g., wheat subsidies in Sudan and rice and wheat subsidies in Bangladesh, although not universal, e.g., Egypt and Sri Lanka.

Impact on Real Incomes of the Poor. Food price subsidies have significantly increased real incomes of the poor in a number of countries. Thus, the subsidized ration scheme which existed in Sri Lanka until 1979 contributed 16 percent of total incomes of the poorest decile of the population in 1978–79 (Gavan and Chandrasekera, 1979). Research on the food ration shops in Kerala, India, shows that about one-half of total incomes of low-income families was accounted for by ration income. George (1979) concludes that "the removal of rationing would have a very serious impact on these low-income consumers." In a study of the ration shops in several Indian states, George (1985) concludes that for India as a whole, about two-thirds of the subsidies are obtained by households with annual incomes below 3,600 rupees (US $300), which is about one-sixth of the average income for the country. In Kerala, the poorest 59 percent of the population received 87 percent of the subsidies, while in Tamil Nadu, the poorest 65 percent received only one-half of the subsidies, or less than their proportional share. Thus, the relative share of the benefits obtained by the poor may vary even within a given country.

The benefits received from food price subsidies may vary among groups of poor households. Thus, removal of the implicit price subsidy in Thailand would result in large losses for the urban and certain groups of rural poor, while other groups of rural poor would gain (Trairatvorakul, 1984). In Pakistan, the urban poor obtained more than 10 percent of their incomes from subsidized food rations during the mid-1970s while the impact on the incomes of the rural poor was negligible (Rogers, 1987a).

Ahmed (1979) found that subsidized food rations contributed significantly to the real incomes of the urban poor in Bangladesh while benefits to the rural poor were very limited. A strong urban bias was also found in food subsidies in China, where it is estimated that only 10 percent of the benefits were obtained by the rural population (Lardy, 1983).

However, a number of food price subsidy programs, including the ration shop schemes in Sri Lanka and Kerala, were not biased toward the urban population. Furthermore, the distribution of benefits from the Egyptian food price and subsidy policies as a whole is slightly biased toward the rural sector (Alderman and von Braun, 1984). The net value of all food subsidies captured by the poorest quartiles of the urban and rural population in Egypt was estimated to be 13 and 17 percent of their incomes, respectively. The richest urban quartile experienced a small net loss primarily because of large producer subsidies for meat and dairy products and correspondingly high consumer prices. Landless labor and small farmers were the principal beneficiaries in the rural sector.

The effect of food price subsidies on real incomes of the poor depends on the nature of the subsidy scheme, including the degree of targeting, the choice of commodities to be subsidized, and the design and implementation of the distribution scheme. Targeting is a particularly important consideration because it reduces the fiscal costs of untargeted subsidies without reducing the benefits obtained by the target group. Very few of the existing food price subsidy schemes are targeted to low-income households. Some of the schemes are targeted to urban households, either explicitly through the issue of ration cards or implicitly by limiting the distribution of subsidized commodities to urban areas. Thus, as further discussed in a subsequent section, there are opportunities for reducing the costs of existing schemes without negative effects on the poor.

The choice of commodity and commodity quality is important in price subsidies, as illustrated by evidence from studies in Brazil, Egypt, Mexico, and Pakistan. In the Brazil study it was found that a shift of existing explicit subsidies from wheat to rice would lower incomes to the rich, increase incomes of the middle-income group slightly, and slightly lower incomes of the poor. Shifting the subsidy to milk would result in a large decrease in incomes of the poor and a corresponding increase for the rich. The opposite would occur if the subsidy were shifted to cassava (Williamson-Gray, 1982). Thus, if the goal is to transfer purchasing power to the poor through a fixed government outlay on food price subsidies, the choice of commodity is important. Similarly, as further discussed below, commodity choice is important if nutritional improvements are a goal.

Findings from the Egypt study show that subsidies on bread are more beneficial to the urban poor than subsidies on wheat flour, while the opposite is the case for the rural poor (Alderman and von Braun, 1984). A study of Bangladesh concluded that distribution of sorghum at the ration shops would provide larger relative gains to the poor than currently distributed rice and wheat, because sorghum is acquired almost exclusively by the poor (Karim, Majid, and Levinson, 1980).

A study of maize subsidies in Mexico provides further insights into the importance of the choice of product to be subsidized (Lustig, 1986). In Mexico, maize prices to producers are supported through a policy of government price guarantees, while consumer prices of tortillas—a commonly consumed processed maize product—are subsidized. The price of unprocessed maize for final consumption purposes, however, is not subsidized. Although maize is a basic staple for both urban and rural households, the former usually buy subsidized tortillas while the latter make tortillas at home and thus do not benefit from the subsidy.

Limiting price subsidies to products that are perceived to be inferior or of low quality offers another possibility for altering the transfer patterns in favor of the poor. Distribution of subsidized wheat flour with a high extraction rate in Pakistan is a case in point (Rogers and Levinson, 1976).[4] In a study of wheat flour consumption in Rawalpindi City, Khan (1982) found that although it was available to all consumers, poor households purchased more than thirty kilograms of subsidized wheat flour from ration shops per month compared to about twenty kilograms for the highest income households, while purchases of non-subsidized wheat flour from the open market was about sixteen kilograms per month for the poor and fifty-eight kilograms per month for the highest income group. Thus, the perceived low quality of the subsidized commodity resulted in some degree of self-targeting to the poor.

In conclusion, there is ample empirical evidence that food price subsidies in the countries studied have significantly contributed to higher real incomes of the poor, particularly, but not exclusively, the urban poor. In several of the programs analyzed, the value of the food subsidies received by low-income households accounted for 15–25 percent of their total real incomes. As a general rule, better-off households received larger absolute benefits than poorer ones. However, benefits as a percent of current incomes were larger for the poor. Both the value and the distribution of benefits varied among program types and countries. This variation offers opportunities for increasing benefits or reducing costs of consumer-oriented food price subsidies through appropriate program choice and design, as further discussed below.

Impact on Food Security and Nutrition Among the Poor. Nutrition goals are important determinants of the design of some programs, such as the milk subsidies in Mexico. However, as opposed to food supplementation programs, use of an explicit nutrition criterion is not common in the design of consumer-oriented food price subsidies.

Household-level food security concerns are more commonly found among the goals of subsidy programs. Thus, programs currently found in many developing countries were initiated for the purpose of assuring consumers—usually but not always urban consumers—access to a specified amount of one or more food staples at prices fixed by the government. Many of these programs were introduced during wartime or following poor harvests or extreme foreign exchange crises. They were frequently based more on quantity planning than on price policy. The ration shop schemes in India, Pakistan, Bangladesh, and Sri Lanka fall into this category along with some of the food subsidies in Egypt. The initial principal purpose of these schemes was clearly to reduce the uncertainty at the household level of acquiring a certain minimum amount of basic staples.

These programs frequently provide basic rations to households irrespective of income level and are important components of local marketing infrastructure. Food rations in Egypt have reached more than 90 percent of the population in urban as well as rural areas (Alderman and von Braun, 1984). The subsidized food distribution system in Kerala, India is designed to provide a fixed allowance of rice to every individual, except food grain producers, at a subsidized price irrespective of income level (Kumar, 1979). Similarly, up until recently, sugar rations were available to virtually all households in Pakistan (Rogers, 1987a).

Ration schemes have also been used as part of policies to stabilize prices and insulate the domestic economy from price fluctuations in the international market. Thus, when international wheat and rice prices skyrocketed during 1973–74, the price of wheat and rice rations in Bangladesh increased much less. As a result, the ration price of rice fell to about 24 percent of the open market price as compared to 37 percent the year before and more than 70 percent during the mid-1970s (Ahmed, 1979). Sugar prices in Egypt provide another illustration: the domestic sugar prices to the Egyptian consumer, while constant in nominal terms, varied from 22 percent of the international prices in 1974 to approximately parity in 1977, to 144 percent in 1978, and back to 29 percent in 1980 (von Braun and de Haen, 1983).

Assuring all households access to a certain amount of food at constant or "reasonable" prices may entail large fiscal costs in periods of rapidly increasing food prices, as illustrated by the programs in Egypt during the last half of the 1970s.

How successful have consumer food subsidy programs been in reaching rationing or household food security goals? In general, programs providing fixed quantity rations, whether fixed per person or per household, have been successful in reaching the population groups toward which they were directed and in providing these groups with a constant supply of the rationed food at low prices. In many cases this is achieved by using the private sector as the final outlet in the distribution network, as exemplified by the Egyptian and Pakistani ration schemes. Some programs reached the population groups most in need while others did not. For example, food subsidies in Bangladesh primarily benefited urban consumers, although a large majority of the absolute poor is found in rural areas. On the other hand, wheat flour rations in Pakistan appear to have been most beneficial to low-income households due to low perceived quality (Khan, 1982). In some cases, including rural Pakistan and Bangladesh, the poor do not always draw the full quota to which they are entitled. This likely reflects cash constraints and the costs of visiting ration centers.

Findings from the case studies show that it is difficult for one program to achieve both universal household food security (rationing) and income transfer goals in one program in a cost-effective manner. The reason is that targeting, which is essential to achieve cost-effective income transfer, by definition excludes non-target households from food security provided by the program. This conflict may be overcome if food security is sought only for those households targeted for transfers. However, this has not been the case in most subsidized rationing schemes.

The effect of food price subsidies on nutrition is a function of the real incomes embodied in these subsidies and captured by households with members who are malnourished or at risk of becoming malnourished. Thus, the findings regarding income transfers and targeting have implications for nutrition.

Both income and price elasticities for staple foods tend to be large in absolute value among the absolute poor (Alderman, 1986; Pinstrup-Andersen, 1985). This implies that food price subsidies—whether limited to certain rations or not—are likely to result in increasing household food consumption. This is borne out by empirical evidence from the case studies.

The subsidized ration shop scheme in Sri Lanka increased daily energy consumption by sixty-three calories per capita on the average and by 115 calories among the poorest decile (Gavan and Chandrasekera, 1979). A pilot food price subsidy scheme in the Philippines increased average daily calorie consumption per adult equivalent unit by 130 calories (Garcia and Pinstrup-Andersen, 1986). Ahmed (1979) estimated that low-income urban consumers in Bangladesh consumed about 250 calories more per person daily due to the rations and George (1985) estimated that the poorest Indian consumers increased their calorie consumption up to 18 percent. Finally, data from a study by Rogers (1981) in Pakistan illustrate the differential impact in urban and rural areas of programs that are urban-biased. She found that the Pakistani ration shop scheme contributed an increase of 114 calories to the daily per capita calorie consumption of the urban poor but only sixteen calories for the rural poor.

The choice of commodity as a carrier of the subsidy is important, as Williamson-Gray (1982) showed for Brazil. She found that the current wheat bread subsidies caused a slightly lower total calorie consumption by the poor because the increased bread consumption was associated with larger decreases in the consumption of rice and other foods. Shifting the current government outlays on wheat subsidies to rice would greatly increase total calorie consumption by the poor.

There is very little direct empirical evidence on the effect of food subsidies on the nutritional status as measured by anthropometrics. Kumar (1979) found that the weight-for-age of children in Kerala would fall by 8 percent if the ration scheme was discontinued. Similarly, results from a pilot food price subsidy scheme in the Philippines showed a positive effect on the weight-for-age of pre-schoolers (Garcia and Pinstrup-Andersen, 1986).

The extent to which increases in household calorie consumption leads to improved nutrition depends on the degree to which malnourished household members share in the increase and the relative importance of food deficiencies versus health and sanitation factors in the existing nutrition problems. In Egypt, for example, calorie consumption levels are high and the critical constraint to improved nutrition appears to be poor sanitation and high frequency of diarrhea occurrence rather than lack of food. The importance of diarrhea as a cause of malnutrition is shown by Leslie (1982) for Northeast Brazil and by Pinstrup-Andersen (1984b) for the Cauca region of Colombia.

Evidence concerning the impact of subsidy schemes on food consumption by children is available from Mexico (Kennedy, 1987) and the Philippines (Garcia and Pinstrup-Andersen, 1986). In both cases, the impact was positive and significant. In the case of Mexico, the increase in the consumption of milk—the subsidized commodity—by children was partially offset by decreased consumption of other commodities. Furthermore, in both cases, calorie consumption by other household members increased significantly due to the subsidies. In the Philippines a disproportionally large share of the net increase in household food consumption went to adults, although the goal of the program was to increase food consumption by preschoolers, Although this implies large "leakages" from the point of view of program goals, the households that received the subsidies were very poor and all household members, including adult males, were calorie deficient.

In summary, it appears that food price subsidies have had significant and positive effects on food consumption by poor households and high-risk household members. This appears to have reduced malnutrition among children although the empirical evidence of impact on anthropometrics is limited.

Fiscal Costs. The magnitude of government expenditures and deficit spending is a key consideration in most macroeconomic adjustment programs. Thus, the feasibility of a program is determined in part by its fiscal cost.

The fiscal cost of a subsidy program depends on the magnitude of the total subsidy and the distribution of cost between the government and the agricultural sector. Untargeted explicit consumer-oriented food subsidies are usually very expensive, and subsidy costs increased considerably during the 1970s in several countries. The fiscal cost of the Egyptian food subsidies increased drastically during the 1970s, to about U.S. $2,000 million in 1981, i.e., about 18 percent of total government expenditures. Rapidly increasing fiscal costs also occurred for the Sri Lankan food ration shop scheme up through the first half of the 1970s, reaching U.S. $1,000 million in 1975, or around 15 percent of total government expenditures. Changes in the subsidy programs during the second half of the 1970s, including a shift to food stamps with a fixed nominal value, rapidly increasing food prices, and exclusion of about one-half of the population from the program, reduced fiscal costs to the current five percent of government expenditures (Edirisinghe, 1986).

The Sri Lankan experience illustrates two approaches to reducing fiscal cost with very different effects on the poor. One is targeting the poor and the other is reducing the real value of the subsidy. While both may be very effective in reducing fiscal costs, the latter results in reduced benefits for the poor while the former need not. These reductions may be severe, as illustrated in Sri Lanka where the real value of the food stamps has decreased rapidly since 1979 due to large price increases and a fixed nominal value of the stamps. The negative impact on food consumption and nutrition among the poor has been severe (Edirisinghe, 1986; and Sahn, 1986).

Impact on the Agricultural Sector. The impact on the agricultural sector varies greatly among the programs, depending on agricultural price and procurement policies, price depressing effects of imports and food aid, degree of targeting, supply response, and a series of fiscal and macroeconomic relationships. While food grain subsidies in India and Bangladesh were supported in part by domestic procurement at relatively low prices, the ration shop schemes in Sri Lanka were managed alongside relatively high producer prices, thus requiring higher rates of government subsidies. In Egypt, rice price subsidies are financed totally by the producers, while the Egyptian government and consumers are financing meat and livestock subsidies to the producers.

The study of the Egyptian food subsidies found that while the gross fiscal support of the agricultural sector increased with increasing fiscal costs of the food subsidies during the 1970s and early 1980s, the share of public investment in agriculture was reduced. Implicit taxation of producers through low procurement prices was reduced in the late 1970s and early 1980s, while food subsidies grew along with the improved foreign exchange situation. The burden of financing low food prices for the consumers was gradually shifted from agriculture to the government. It is hypothesized that this shift will be reversed if the foreign exchange situation worsens and/or the availability of external food aid is reduced.

In general, explicit consumer food subsidies need not have adverse effects on agricultural incentives. On the contrary, such subsidies enhance the purchasing power of consumers who in turn increase their demand for food and thus provide opportunities for increasing prices to the producers. Implicit consumer food subsidies, on the other hand, are likely to be harmful to producers because they are usually maintained through artificially low producer prices. Countries having explicit subsidies frequently also have implicit ones, and the impact of each of these on agricultural incentives is often confused. Finally, a negative impact may occur if governments spend money on explicit subsidies that would otherwise have been spent on public investment in agriculture, e.g., agricultural research and technology, irrigation, infrastructure, etc.

Macroeconomic Implications. While some food subsidy programs are of very limited magnitude, others are large enough to have important macroeconomic implications. Corresponding to about 8 percent of GNP, the Egyptian program is an example of the latter. On the assumption that the program is financed through deficit spending at the margin, i.e., changes in the fiscal costs of subsidies would be reflected in similar changes in deficit spending, increasing subsidy costs would fuel inflation. Increasing subsidy costs would also cause an increase in foreign liabilities and a devaluation of the free market exchange rate for Egyptian currency (Scobie, 1983).

Import demand for food in Egypt is very inelastic. This is in large measure caused by the subsidy program and the high priority on maintaining stable and relatively low food prices for the Egyptian consumers and the government monopoly on food imports, which makes it easier for government to control import quantities. As a consequence, changes in either the price of imported food or the supply of foreign exchange are likely to be reflected primarily in the importation of industrial goods. Scobie (1983) estimated that a fall of one dollar in foreign exchange would reduce imports of food and other consumer goods by only sixteen cents, while the importations of industrial raw materials, fuel, and chemicals would fall by forty cents, and capital goods by thirty-four cents.

This has important implications for real output and investment in the industrial sector. Thus, the study estimates that a fall in foreign exchange supplies of 10 percent reduces real industrial output by 4 percent and investment by 6 percent. Similarly, a 10 percent rise in the cost of imported food would result in a fall of 1 to 2 percent in industrial output as importation of raw materials is reduced to provide more foreign exchange for food imports (Scobie, 1983).

Food-Linked Income Transfer Programs

Food Stamps. Food-linked income transfer programs take many forms, of which food stamps and food supplementation programs are the most common. Both types of programs are attempts to transfer incomes to families or individuals in target groups in the form of food or food purchasing power, in order to assure that dietary intakes increase. The most common arguments for transferring food or food-linked incomes rather than cash are that the marginal propensity to consume food may be higher when food and food-linked incomes are transferred than when the transfer is cash income, or that food is available to the government at a cost below market prices, that is, as foreign food aid or surplus production.

In many cases transfers are limited to specified rations smaller in quantity than those that would be acquired without subsidy—that is, the quantity is inframarginal. This implies that the nutritional effect would be expected to be no different from that of a transfer of cash income equal to the real income embodied in the transfer.

But food-linked income transfers need not be inframarginal. One way to design transfer programs that will have an effect on the acquisition of food beyond the income effect is to require the household to pay an amount close to that which it now spends on food in order to obtain food stamps that will cover a larger quantity. Such a "purchase requirement" was included in the U.S. food stamp program until 1979. Programs designed in this fashion are likely to have a greater effect on the acquisition of food by a household because in addition to the income effect, they make food cheaper at the margin.

Purchase requirements are difficult to implement in a socially just manner. If the amount to be paid for the food stamps is based on the average expenditures for food by the target group, the program will tend to be regressive among target households and may exclude the neediest from participating because the amount may exceed what they are able to pay. On the other hand, in most societies it is impossible to extract a different amount from each household on the basis of the ability to pay.

But even if food-linked income transfers do not influence nutrition any differently than cash transfers of the same magnitude, the former may be politically feasible when the latter are not. Better-off population groups are generally more willing to support income transfers aimed at the alleviation of overt human misery, such as extreme and highly visible malnutrition, than general income transfers for which the spending decisions related to the transfers are left in the hands of the recipient households. For this reason, income transfers to the poor may be politically desirable or feasible only if earmarked for alleviation of extreme human misery, even though the final result is not different from that obtained from transfers that are not earmarked.

Two developing countries—Sri Lanka and Colombia—have had food stamp programs. In the absence of a purchase requirement and with the value of stamps appreciably less than prestamp food expenditures, the Sri Lankan program has served primarily as an income transfer. The average increase in calorie intake attributed to this transfer came to 15 percent of total calories for the poorest decile in 1981. This percentage declined to 5 percent of the calories consumed by the fifth income decile (Edirisinghe, 1987).

The Colombian food stamp program, which was discontinued in 1982, was part of a larger food and nutrition plan, including nutrition education and growth monitoring of children. The program was targeted to low-income regions, and within those regions to households with preschoolers and pregnant and lactating women. The value of the food stamps was very low—less than 2 percent of average incomes of participating households—and it was not possible to detect any impact on the nutritional status of the target individuals (Pinstrup-Andersen, 1984b). The impact on household food consumption was not significantly different from the impact of wage incomes of the same magnitude. Thus, like the Sri Lanka food stamp program, no difference was detected in the marginal propensity to consume food from food stamp and other income.[5]

There is evidence from other studies, however, that the marginal propensity to consume food varies with income source. Thus, a Philippine study indicates that the income transfer embodied in food subsidies for inframarginal rations has a larger impact on household calorie consumption than an equal amount of wage income (Garcia and Pinstrup-Andersen, 1987). Similarly, Kumar (1979) found that in Kerala, India, the marginal propensity to consume food varied among women's incomes, men's income, and incomes in kind from home gardens. One possible explanation for different marginal propensities among income sources is that the intrahousehold budget control is a function of the source of income and that the marginal propensity to consume food varies among members of a household. This is an area where more research is needed.

Food Supplementation. While food stamps usually transfer incomes to target households while relying on private distribution channels for redemption of the stamps, supplementary feeding programs distribute foods through public agencies to pregnant and lactating women, infants, and preschoolers.[6] School feeding programs providing food for school children may also be considered under this category.

Three types of delivery systems are generally used for supplementary feeding. These include on-site feeding, take-home feeding, and nutrition rehabilitation centers (NRC). NRCs include both residential facilities and programs in which children are cared for during the day but return home at night.

In two recent reports data from more than 200 supplementary feeding projects have been reviewed (Anderson et al., 1981; Beaton and Ghassemi, 1979). The results indicate that many supplementary feeding programs have had a significant and positive effect on prenatal and child participants. In studies conducted in Guatemala, India, Colombia, Mexico, Canada, and the United States, it has been found that supplementation during pregnancy improves neonatal outcome (Lechtig et al., 1975; Iyenger, 1967; Mora et al., 1979; Chavez, Martinez, and Yaschine, 1975; Higgins, Crampton, and Moxley, 1973; Kennedy et al., 1982). Women in four villages in Guatemala who received a supplement of more than 20,000 calories during pregnancy, for example, had babies of higher mean birth weight than women in the lower supplementation group; the incidence of babies of low birth weight—those weighing less than 2,500 grams—was decreased by half in the highly supplemented group (Lechtig et al., 1975). Similarly, in India, birth weights of infants born to women who received a daily protein-energy supplement of 700 calories and twenty grams of protein were significantly higher than those of infants born to a nonsupplemented control group (Iyenger, 1967).

Studies of infants and children have shown that supplementary feeding programs are often associated with improved growth, decreased morbidity, or improved cognitive development (Gopaldas et al., 1975; Freeman et al., 1980).

It seems clear that many studies of supplementary feeding programs show some benefit. However, the benefits are usually small. Increments in birth weights attributed to the supplementary feeding programs are typically in the range of forty to sixty grams. Similarly, the increases in growth seen in preschoolers, although significant, are small.

A number of reasons are given for these small but significant effects. First, it appears that only a part of the food given is actually consumed by the target population. Leakages of the supplemented foods occur when the food is shared by nontarget family members or when the food is substituted for other food that normally would be consumed. Beaton and Ghassemi (1979) have estimated that leakages can account for 30–80 percent of the food distributed. Partly because of these leakages, supplementary feeding programs usually fill only 10–25 percent of the apparent energy gap in the target population. Given this small net increment in energy, it is not surprising that the observed effect on growth is small.

Most studies have concentrated on growth as the sole measure of the outcome of supplementary feeding. Beaton and Ghassemi (1979) have suggested that physical growth may not be the only benefit nor even the most important benefit of supplemental feeding. In one study, an increase in voluntary activity was found as a result of the additional food; in children this increase in activity may affect cognitive development (Rutishauser and Whitehead, 1972).

Beaton and Ghassemi (1979) also make the point that any leakage in the food supplement is seen as inefficiency in the distribution program. It cannot be assumed, however, that the energy unaccounted for provides no benefit to the family or community. Attention needs to be focused on a better assessment of the potentially wide range of benefits that can be produced by supplementary feeding. Given the magnitude of reported food leakage, the effect on household income may be substantial and the resultant effect on the nutritional status of nontarget members of the family may also be significant. Few studies have documented the potential effects of supplementary feeding on income maintenance.

In addition to the quantity of food distributed, factors such as the timing of supplementation, duration of participation, and nutritional status of recipients influence the effectiveness of supplemental feeding. These are further discussed in Kennedy and Pinstrup-Andersen (1983).

In conclusion, it appears that food supplementation schemes may be effective means for protecting or compensating high-risk members of poor households from potentially negative effects of macroeconomic crises and adjustments—provided the substitution between the supplement and food from other sources, as well as sharing among household members, are taken into account when designing the schemes and deciding on the size of the supplement. Failure to do so will yield disappointing results and only partial compensation will be provided. In view of the substitution and sharing that is likely to occur within the household, efforts to target individuals rather than households cannot always be justified.

Income-generating Programs

Food subsidies and transfer programs are not the only ways to protect the poor and their nutritional status in periods of economic crisis and macroeconomic adjustments. Improvements in the efficiency of food production through technological change, improved rural infrastructure, and expanded input use, as well as improved marketing efficiency, offer great opportunities for reduced consumer prices for food without adverse effects on producers.

Enhancing the capacity of the poor to generate sufficient incomes to meet their requirements for food and other demands is the most appropriate long-term means to meet welfare goals. Consumer food subsidies or alternative transfer programs should be viewed as temporary but important means to assure that the poor are able to acquire sufficient food to meet nutritional requirements in the interim while such capacity is being created.

Successful economic development should pursue a dual objective of expanded economic growth and reduced poverty through a strategy which enhances the income-generating ability of the poor. To achieve this objective, development activities and policies should focus on expanding the demand for goods and services that the poor can provide and enhancing the ability of the poor to supply these goods and services.

The most important asset possessed by the poor is their labor. Thus, emphasis should be on expanding the demand for labor. Depending on the degree of unemployment and the nature of the labor market, this will result in increased employment and/or increasing wages. Many of the poor are employed in the so-called "informal sector," providing various locally produced goods and services. Activities that result in increased demand for these goods and services, therefore, will be more appropriate than those resulting in increased demand for goods and services produced by capital-intensive enterprises. Past and ongoing research at IFPRI show strong linkages between incomes of agricultural households and the demand for locally produced non-agricultural goods and services. The kinds of consumption goods and services demanded are typically produced by small labor-intensive enterprises.

Efforts to enhance the ability of the poor to supply goods and services are another important consideration. Of greatest importance in this regard are the quality of the human resource, entrepreneurship, and ownership of productive resources. Improvement of the human resource requires education—both formally and through development of skills—as well as improved health and nutrition. Public investment in education, training, health, and nutrition generally has a very high payoff and should not be viewed merely as consumption or welfare programs. This results not only in higher productivity in wage labor and hence potentially higher earnings, but is also likely to enhance entrepreneurship. The importance of the latter among the poor is grossly underestimated in many developing countries. What is called the "informal sector" consists primarily of more or less successful small-scale entrepreneurs who, if provided more support, could greatly expand employment and output at the same time as a larger number of the poor would successfully pursue entrepreneurship activities. Such support includes credit, technical assistance, certain elements of physical infrastructure, and institutional support that protects small enterprises from unfair competition and promotes small-scale capital accumulation. There are many examples of successful programs providing such support, including the Grameen Bank in Bangladesh which provides loans to small-scale entrepreneurs without collateral. However, development efforts often ignore the large potential contributions of small-scale entrepreneurship to output and well-being among the poor.

It is of paramount importance that the above considerations be taken into account in the design of macroeconomic adjustment programs. Although some of the appropriate activities, such as investment in employment-intensive industry, education, cost-reducing technology for food production, and reduced costs of food marketing, may have a payoff for the poor only in the longer run, it is important that macroeconomic adjustments are designed to achieve such long-run poverty reductions. Transfer programs to correct acute problems should not be used as an excuse for not following a development strategy aimed at the alleviation of poverty and malnutrition. For example, the large reductions in public investment in primary education in many countries during the last ten years are likely to hurt severely the future income-earning capacity of the poor.

Among income-generating programs with immediate effects, public works programs are the most common. The major advantage of conveying income to the target households through wage labor rather than through transfer programs is that the former generates an output—e.g., physical infrastructure—and can be self-targeting (Reutlinger, 1987). Food is frequently used as partial or total payment to workers in public works programs primarily because food is available to governments either free or at a cost below its market or cash value through external food aid.

Food-for-work programs have been successful in augmenting incomes of low-income households—primarily rural ones—and creating infrastructure in several countries, notably India and Bangladesh. The impact on nutrition has been studied in only a few projects, and the results are mixed. In a study of a food-for-work project in Bangladesh, Kumar (BIDS/IFPRI, 1983) found no significant difference in food consumption between participants and non-participants. Those most heavily involved in the project were found to have a marginally higher level of food consumption. Although energy expenditures were not measured in this study, it may be hypothesized that they increased with participation in the project. Thus, it is possible that the net impact on the energy adequacy rate of the worker was negative or, alternatively, the energy consumption of other household members was reduced.

Follow-up studies were made in the project areas to assess the nutrition effects of the infrastructure generated by the food-for-work project. It was found that household energy consumption was slightly higher and the prevalence of stunting among children lower in the project areas than the control areas (Kumar and Chowdhury, 1985). Thus, it appears that the project resulted in long-term improvements in the area over and above any immediate effects on project workers.

However, until more research is completed on the matter, it is very difficult to derive generalizable conclusions regarding the nutrition effects of food-for-work projects. What is clear, however, is that such projects, when properly designed and implemented,[7] can have a significant impact on incomes of the poor while generating much needed infrastructure.

Reutlinger (1987) suggests that explicit government subsidies to enhance employment of the poor in the private sector may be a more promising approach than public works programs. Such subsidies could be directed to labor-intensive enterprises in the formal sector as well as the self-employed in the informal sector.

Lessons for the Design of Policies and Programs

Targeting

The most useful lesson for the design of policies and programs to alleviate negative nutritional effects of macroeconomic crises and adjustment programs undoubtedly is that food subsidy and transfer programs can be cost-effective in reaching this goal provided they are appropriately targeted. Lack of appropriate targeting results in unsustainably large fiscal costs in cases of general, untargeted explicit subsidies or large economic costs in cases of implicit subsidies in the form of depressed producer prices. Furthermore, inappropriately targeted subsidies and transfers, e.g., those available to all urban but no rural households, are not cost-effective in reaching the poor and malnourished because they include the better-off urban households and exclude the rural poor.

Appropriate targeting implies here the identification of those households that: (1) are poor, (2) have members who are either malnourished or at risk of becoming malnourished, and (3) have been or are likely to be adversely affected by macroeconomic crises and/or adjustment programs. The necessary information for such identification is not readily available. Real incomes of individual households or groups of similar households vary over time and are not usually known in most developing countries. Attempts to obtain reliable information on a periodic basis are likely to be expensive. Thus, the challenge is to identify proxies or indicators of poverty and malnutrition that are sufficiently reliable for targeting purposes and not excessively expensive to monitor. Many such indicators have been suggested (Rogers, 1987b). The appropriateness of each depends on a variety of country- and program-specific factors. Geographical targeting, which was successfully used in the Philippines (Garcia and Pinstrup-Andersen, 1986), offers great promise in cases where the poor tend to be concentrated in certain localities. In cases where the nutrition problem is principally found among preschoolers, growth monitoring may be an appropriate targeting mechanism. However, this approach is, strictly speaking, curative; ideally the programs would be preventive. Target households would be identified *before* the children become malnourished, not *after*.

A large number of other targeting mechanisms have been tried, some with success, others with failure. These include targeting by the nutritional status of household members, or by employment status, choice of inferior commodities or commodity qualities for subsidization, and targeting on certain periods of the year in cases where seasonal fluctuations in ability to acquire sufficient food are severe. The most appropriate choice among the various targeting approaches depends on the particular circumstances within which subsidies are introduced (Rogers, 1987b).

Since groups of poor households may be affected differently by macroeconomic crises and adjustment programs, identification of the poor and potentially malnourished is necessary but not sufficient. We must know which of these groups are likely to benefit and which are likely to lose from the macroeconomic changes. Furthermore, the magnitudes of losses should be estimated or predicted. Once the groups have been identified, policies and programs must be designed in such a way that the benefits are captured by those households while the costs are borne by others. The design and implementation of programs to reach them and exclude non-target households are extremely difficult. The difficulties are due to political and logistical factors as well as insufficient information. Non-target households will oppose successful targeting, in some cases to the point of threatening political and social stability. Furthermore, the cost of administering subsidy and transfer programs increases as the degree of targeting increases. This is of particular concern in those developing countries where trained manpower is very scarce.

Thus, for the above reasons, perfect targeting should not be attempted. There is a point beyond which increases in administrative costs, including the cost of identification of target households, exceed the cost savings from further reducing benefit leakages to non-target households. Furthermore, as a program gets more narrowly targeted, the risk of excluding target households increases due to insufficient information. Finally, a program narrowly targeted on the poor is likely to have little political support in all but the most enlightened societies and if implemented may have a short life, as exemplified by the Colombian food stamp program.

Choice of Program Type

The cost-effectiveness of food subsidy or transfer programs may also be improved by choosing the right program type for the particular circumstances. As discussed earlier in this paper, the most common types are price subsidies for specific rations or for unlimited quantities of food, food stamps, and food supplementation schemes. The income effects of price subsidies for inframarginal rations would not be expected to differ greatly from food stamps. However, the degree to which food security goals are achieved may vary greatly between the two program types. The critical issue is whether the household is assured a certain physical quantity, at a fixed price, or a certain monetary transfer. In the former, recipient households are assured a constant transfer in real terms while in the latter, price fluctuations and increases in the open market prices may erode the real purchasing power of the transfer, as illustrated by the food stamp program in Sri Lanka (Edirisinghe, 1986).

The issue of appropriate adjustments in subsidized food prices is particularly important in periods of devaluation of the local currency and/or rapid food price increases in the international market. Maintaining fixed nominal prices for food staples in such cases may result in large and unsustainable increases in the cost of food subsidies. On the other hand, fixing the nominal value of the transfers would rapidly reduce their real value.

While, as argued above, targeting needy households is essential to assure a high level of cost-effectiveness, it is less clear that attempts to target programs to individuals within these households would further improve the cost-effectiveness. Although available evidence is somewhat ambivalent, it appears that the additional benefits captured by the household members most at risk in many cases do not justify the additional costs of intrahousehold targeting unless complete feeding or clinical treatment are provided.

In cases of severe nutritional deficiencies, well designed food supplementation programs which target individuals appear to have been more cost-effective than similar size transfers to households (Knudsen, 1981;

Kennedy and Knudsen, 1985). The key is to be found in the degree of substitution between the food made available through the program and food consumed by the malnourished but obtained from other sources. Attempts to convince parents of malnourished children that the food supplement should be viewed as medicine for these children, together with a fixed duration of the feeding of a particular child determined by strict entry and exit criteria, are likely to reduce substitution (Kennedy and Knudsen, 1985). Active participation of the parents in measuring progress of the children during program participation—e.g., through growth monitoring—may also help assure low leakage.

A note of caution may be warranted at this point. As a general rule, it is not clear that society as represented by implementing agencies is better equipped to decide on food distribution within the household than the household itself. Usually, calorie and protein deficiencies are part of extreme poverty. The needs for other basic necessities and the strategy for long-run survival of the household may not always place highest priority on improving the nutrition of those household members targeted by program authorities. These matters are probably better decided upon by the household, provided it is informed about available options and the consequences of alternative action. Thus, providing appropriate information to the households, including nutritional education, is probably a better strategy than attempting to circumvent household decision making by targeting individuals.

Nutrition education is mostly needed when the poor are faced with large increases or decreases in real incomes or other unusual circumstances, such as shifts from subsistence to a cash economy. Nutrition education aimed at reallocating a given amount of real income or food in a household where no other changes have taken place is less likely to be successful.

The choice of program type should ideally be based on the relative cost of achieving the desired impact—i.e., the cost-effectiveness. However, deficiencies in available empirical evidence make comparisons among programs difficult. The deficiencies include lack of commonality among program evaluations, including lack of agreement about cost components to be included and the appropriate indicator of impact. A large proportion of ex-post evaluations show no statistically significant impact on anthropometric indicators while others do not measure the impact on food consumption by the malnourished. Failure to separate program effects from the effects of other factors is also common in many program evaluations and a full account of the various constraints to improved nutrition in the program population is often absent in evaluation reports. This issue is particularly important when the program attempts to alleviate constraints that are not the most limiting for

Table 6.1 Cost Effectiveness of Selected Programs

Programs	Annual Cost per Intended Beneficiary (Year) (US$)	Energy Embodied in Transfer (Cal./Person/Day)	Net Increase in Cal Cons./Person/Day	Percent "Leakage"	Cost of Transferring 100 Calories/Person/Day for One Year (US$)	Cost of a Net Increase of 100 Calories/Person/Day for One Year (US$)	Source
Food Subsidy Programs							
Brazil	1980	21.32[a]	300	n.a.	n.a.	7.11	n.a.	World Bank (1984)
Colombia	1981	35.04[b]	n.a.	296	n.a.	n.a.	11.84	World Bank (1984), Pinstrup-Andersen (1984)
Egypt	1982	41.60[a]	626	n.a.	n.a.	6.65	n.a.	Alderman (1984), Kennedy and Alderman (1986), and author's calculations
Mexico	1982	14.68[a]	95	100	−5.3	15.38	14.68	Kennedy et al. (1984) and Kennedy (personal communication)
Mexico	1982	38.16[b]	248	58	76.6	15.38	65.79	Kennedy et al. (1984) and Kennedy (personal communication)
Philippines	1984	9.18[a]	272	136	50.0	3.38	6.75	Garcia and Pinstrup-Andersen (1986)
Philippines	1984	14.35[b]	454	34	92.5	3.38	42.21	Garcia and Pinstrup-Andersen (1986), and author's calculations
Sri Lanka	1982	8.60[a]	228	98	57.0	3.77	8.77	Edirisinghe (1986)
Supplementary Feeding							
Brazil	1980	46.48[b]	500	n.a.	n.a.	9.29	n.a.	World Bank (1984)
Colombia	1982	42.08[b]	305	165	45.9	13.80	25.50	Anderson et al. (1981), Kennedy and Alderman (1986), and author's calculations
Costa Rica	1982	160.72[b]	737	462	37.3	21.81	34.79	Anderson et al. (1981), Kennedy and Alderman (1986), and author's calculations
Dominican Republic	1982	24.48[b]	337	48	85.8	7.26	51.00	Anderson et al. (1981), Kennedy and Alderman (1986), and author's calculations
India (Tamil Nadu)	1982	33.10[b]	300	n.a.	n.a.	11.03	n.a.	World Bank (1984)
India	1982	24.51[b]	340	160	52.9	7.21	15.32	Anderson et al. (1981), Kennedy and Alderman (1986), and author's calculations
Indonesia	1982	56.01[b]	n.a.	n.a.	n.a.	n.a.	n.a.	World Bank (1984)
Pakistan	1982	39.97[b]	298	131	56.0	13.41	30.51	Anderson et al. (1981), Kennedy and Alderman (1986), and author's calculations

[a] All household members were intended beneficiaries. [b] Only selected household members, usually preschoolers, were intended beneficiaries.

improved nutrition, such as food supplementation for children that are heavily affected by infectious diseases or other non-food factors.

In spite of these and other deficiencies in available empirical evidence, an attempt is made in Table 6.1 to make comparisons among the cost-effectiveness of various programs. Since relatively few programs show significant effects on anthropometric indicators, the calorie consumption effects are used as the indicator of impact.

As shown in Table 6.1, the cost of a net increase of one hundred calories per intended beneficiary per day varies greatly among programs. Because of the above-mentioned data deficiencies, it is not possible to provide a complete explanation of these variations. In general, it may be concluded that the "leakage"—i.e., the difference between the amount of calories transferred and the net increase in energy consumption—is large in most of the programs.

The leakage in programs aimed at all members of target households is due to substitution between program food and food from other sources. When programs are targeted on individual household members, such as preschoolers, one additional source of leakage—i.e., consumption of program food by non-target household members—is present. Thus, it is not uncommon to find leakage above 50 percent. The largest leakage is found in food subsidy programs targeted on households but for which only certain household members are considered intended beneficiaries—i.e., benefits captured by other household members are not considered. In such cases, attempts to target specific household members—something usually done in food supplementation schemes—result in higher cost-effectiveness. If, on the other hand, the aim of the program is to transfer energy to poor households irrespective of how food consumption by individual household members is affected, then household-targeted food stamp and food price subsidy programs are much more cost-effective.

Thus, if the purpose is to protect or compensate low-income households for negative effects on real income due to economic crises or macroeconomic adjustment programs, it appears that programs which transfer the desired energy or nutrients to these households at the lowest cost should take priority over programs targeted on individual household members.

Implementation

Several lessons were learned regarding program implementation. Rogers (1987b) discusses these, and only the most relevant ones will be discussed here. Most importantly, it appears that the use of private sector distribution channels for subsidized food can be very cost-effective and often more so than public distribution schemes. Food stamps which may be redeemed in private stores are an obvious example. However, even when the subsidy is embodied in a lower price for a certain commodity ration, it is not clear that a separate public distribution network can operate at a lower cost or a lower degree of corruption and abuse of the program. Private distribution channels have been successfully used in a number of countries, including the Philippines and Egypt, at a relatively low cost. However, government officials in several countries have expressed the view that a public distribution network for food and other necessities is needed to cope with natural disasters, political or social instability, and other emergencies to avoid serious disruptions in the availability of these goods. Thus, it appears that household food security goals may not be fully achieved through the private distribution network in countries where a strong competitive market environment is absent and/or where the risk of political or social instability is high.

Source of Financing

Deficit government spending is usually an important element of macro-economic crises and adjustment programs usually attempt to reduce such deficits. Depressed prices to farmers are also a common component of economic crises and higher agricultural prices are often pursued as part of adjustments. Therefore, fiscal as well as economic costs are important considerations in the choice and design of policies and programs to protect or compensate the poor. Efforts to cut government spending appear to focus more on explicit subsidies on consumer goods and services than explicit and implicit subsidies to public enterprises, including energy and air transportation. More in-depth analysis of the consequences of alternative ways to cut deficit spending might in some cases result in more favorable outcomes for the poor.

Alternative sources of revenue to cover the cost of subsidy and transfer programs might also be explored. These would include the possibility of using external aid either in the form of food or cash as currently done in Jamaica. Food aid has played a major role in financing food subsidies and supplementation schemes in many developing countries, such as Egypt and Bangladesh. Innovative ways of integrating external aid for alleviating adverse short-term nutrition effects into more traditional macroeconomic adjustment programs may assure the achievement of short-run welfare goals for the poor as well as long-run growth objectives.

Notes

1. Only a summary of the most important issues and findings can be presented here. More details may be found in Kennedy and Pinstrup-Andersen (1983), Kennedy and Alderman (1986), Beaton and Ghassemi (1979), and Pinstrup-Andersen (1987).

2. Governments, in turn, may cover the costs from a variety of sources including taxes, income from public enterprises, foreign aid, and deficit spending (see Scobie, 1987, for a discussion of this matter).

3. The countries are: Bangladesh (Ahmed, 1979 and 1981), Brazil (Williamson-Gray, 1982, and Calegar and Schuh, 1986), Egypt (Alderman, von Braun, and Sakr, 1982; Alderman and von Braun, 1984; Scobie, 1983 and 1985; von Braun and de Haen, 1983; Alderman and von Braun, 1986), India (Kumar, 1979, George, 1979 and 1985), Mexico (Kennedy, 1984, and Lustig, 1986), Pakistan (ongoing), Philippines (Garcia and Pinstrup-Andersen, 1987), Sri Lanka (Gavan and Chandrasekera, 1979; Edirisinghe, 1987), Sudan (Pinstrup-Andersen et al., 1982), Thailand (Trairatvorakul, 1984), and Zambia (Kumar, 1987). In addition, case studies were done for food stamp programs in Colombia (Ochoa, 1987, and Pinstrup-Andersen, 1984b) and Sri Lanka (Edirisinghe, 1986, and Sahn, 1986).

4. A high extraction rate has an adverse effect on the appearance of the flour (it becomes darker) because a larger portion of the grain is converted into flour. However, the nutritional quality is not negatively affected.

5. The marginal propensity to consume food is a measure of the change in food consumption associated with a change in incomes of one unit of currency.

6. The discussion of food supplementation relies heavily on Kennedy and Pinstrup-Andersen (1983).

7. Some of the design and implementation issues are discussed in Kennedy and Alderman (1986), BIDS/IFPRI (1983 and 1985).

References

Ahmed, Raisuddin. *Agricultural Price Policies under Complex Socioeconomic and Natural Constraints: The Case of Bangladesh*, Research Report 27. Washington, D.C.: International Food Policy Research Institute, 1981.

———. *Foodgrain Supply, Distribution, and Consumption Policies within a Dual Pricing Mechanism: A Case Study of Bangladesh*, Research Report 8. Washington, D.C.: International Food Policy Research Institute, 1979.

Alderman, Harold, Joachim von Braun, and Ahmed Sakr. *Egypt's Food Subsidy and Rationing System: A Description*, Research Report 34. Washington, D.C.: International Food Policy Research Institute, 1982.

Alderman, Harold and Joachim von Braun. "Egypt's Food Subsidy Policy: Lessons from the Past and Options for the Future." *Food Policy* 3:11 (August 1986), pp. 223–237.

———. *The Effects of the Egyptian Food Ration and Subsidy System on Income Distribution and Welfare.* Research Report 45. Washington, D.C.: International Food Policy Research Institute, 1984.

Alderman, Harold. "The Effect of Income and Food Price Changes on the Acquisition of Food by Low-income Households." Washington, D.C.: International Food Policy Research Institute, 1986.

Anderson, Mary Ann, et al. *Nutrition Intervention in Developing Countries, Study I: Supplementary Feeding*. Cambridge, Massachusetts, 1981.

Bangladesh Institute of Development Studies and International Food Policy Research Institute. *Development Impact of the Food-For-Work Program in Bangladesh*. Technical papers submitted to the World Food Programme. Dhaka: BIDS, and Washington, D.C.: IFPRI, 1985.

———. "Characteristics and Short-Run Effects of the WFP-Aided Food-for-Work Programme in Bangladesh." Dhaka: BIDS, and Washington, D.C.: IFPRI, mimeo, 1983.

Beaton, George H. and Hossein Ghassemi. *Supplementary Feeding Programs for Young Children in Developing Countries*. New York: United Nation's Children Fund, 1979.

Behrman, Jere R. 1986. "The Impact of Economic Adjustment Programs," Chapter 5 of this volume.

Calegar, Geraldo M. and Edward Schuh. "Costs, Benefits, and Food Consumption Impact of the Brazilian Wheat Price Policy." Washington, D.C.: International Food Policy Research Institute, mimeo, 1986.

Chavez, A., C. Martinez, and T. Yaschine. "Nutrition, Behavioral Development, and Mother-Child Interaction in Young Rural Children," *Federation Proceedings* 34 (1975): 1574–1579.

Edirisinghe, Neville. "The Food Stamp Program in Sri Lanka: Costs, Benefits, and Policy Options." Washington, D.C.: International Food Policy Research Institute, Research Report 58, March 1987.

Freeman, H. E., et al. "Nutrition and Cognitive Development Among Rural Guatemalan Children," *American Journal of Public Health* 70 (1980): 1277–1285.

Garcia, Marito and Per Pinstrup-Andersen. "Pilot Food Subsidy Scheme in the Philippines: Impact on Income, Food Consumption, and Nutritional Status." Washington, D.C.: International Food Policy Research Institute, 1987 (forthcoming research report).

Gavan, James and Indrani Sri Chandrasekera. *The Impact of Public Foodgrain Distribution on Food Consumption and Welfare in Sri Lanka*, Research Report 13. Washington, D.C.: International Food Policy Research Institute, 1979.

George, P. S. *Some Aspects of Procurement and Distribution of Foodgrains in India*, Food Subsidies Working Paper 1. Washington, D.C.: International Food Policy Research Institute, 1985.

———. *Public Distribution of Foodgrains in Kerala: Income Distribution Implications and Effectiveness*. Research Report 7. Washington, D.C.: International Food Policy Research Institute, 1979.

Gopaldas, T., et al. *Project Poshak*, vol. 1. New Delhi: CARE, 1975.

Higgins, A., E. W. Crampton, and J. E. Moxley. "Nutrition and the Outcome of Pregnancy," in R. O. Scow, ed., *Endocrinology*. Amsterdam: Excerpta Medica 1973, pp. 1071–1077.

Iyenger, L. "Effect of Dietary Supplementation Late in Pregnancy on the Expectant Mother and Her Newborn," *Indian Journal of Medical Research* 55 (1967): 85–89.

Karim, Rezaul, Manjur Majid, and James F. Levinson. "The Bangladesh Sorghum Experiment," *Food Policy* 5 (1980): 61–63.

Kennedy, Eileen T. "Alternatives to Food Subsidies as a Means of Achieving Nutrition Objectives," in Per Pinstrup-Andersen, ed., *Consumer-Oriented Food Subsidies: Benefits, Costs, and Policy Options*. Washington, D.C.: International Food Policy Research Institute, 1987.

————. "Determinants of Family and Preschooler Food Consumption." *Food and Nutrition Bulletin* 5:4 (1983): 22.

Kennedy, Eileen T., et al. "Effect of a Milk Subsidy on the Distribution of Benefits Within the Household." Washington, D.C.: International Food Policy Research Institute, mimeo, 1984.

————. "Evaluation of the Effect of WIC Supplemental Feeding on Birth Weight." *Journal of the American Dietetic Association* 80 (1982): 220–227.

Kennedy, Eileen T. and Harold Alderman. *Comparative Analysis of Nutritional Effectiveness of Food Subsidies and Other Selected Food-Related Interventions*. Washington, D.C.: International Food Policy Research Institute, 1986.

Kennedy, Eileen and Odin Knudsen. "A Review of Supplementary Feeding Programmes and Recommendations on their Design," in Margaret Biswas and Per Pinstrup-Andersen, eds., *Nutrition and Development*. New York: Oxford University Press, 1985.

Kennedy, Eileen T. and Per Pinstrup-Andersen. *Nutrition-Related Policies and Programs: Past Performances and Research Needs*. Washington, D.C.: International Food Policy Research Institute, 1983.

Khan, Riaz Ahmad. *Issues of Food Distribution in Pakistan*, Staff Paper AE-101. Islamabad, Pakistan: Pakistan Agricultural Research Council, 1982.

Knudsen, Odin. *Economics of Supplemental Feeding of Malnourished Children: Linkages, Costs and Benefits*, Staff Working Paper 451. Washington, D.C.: World Bank, 1981.

Kumar, Shubh K. "The Design, Income Distribution, and Consumption Effects of Maize Pricing Policies in Zambia," in Per Pinstrup-Andersen, ed., *Consumer-Oriented Food Subsidies: Benefits, Costs, and Policy Options*. Washington, D.C.: International Food Policy Research Institute, 1987.

————. *Impact of Subsidized Rice on Food Consumption and Nutrition in Kerala*, Research Report 5. Washington, D.C.: International Food Policy Research Institute, 1979.

Kumar, Shubh K. and Omar Haider Chowdhury. "The Effects on Nutritional Status," in *Development Impact of the Food-For-Work Program in Bangladesh*. Technical Papers submitted to the World Food Programme by The Bangladesh Institute of Development Studies, Dhaka, and International Food Policy Research Institute, Washington, D.C., 1985.

Lardy, N. R. *Agricultural Prices in China*, Staff Working Paper 606. Washington, D.C.: World Bank, 1983.

Lechtig, Aaron, et al. "Effect of Food Supplementation During Pregnancy on Birth Weight," *Pediatrics* 56 (1975): 508–520.

Leslie, Joanne. "Child Malnutrition and Diarrhea: A Longitudinal Study from Northeast Brazil." Ph.D. thesis, Johns Hopkins University, 1982.

Lustig, Nora. *Food Subsidy Programs in Mexico*, Food Subsidies Working Paper 3. Washington, D.C.: International Food Policy Research Institute, 1986.

Mora, J. O., et al. "Nutrition Supplementation and the Outcome of Pregnancy," *American Journal of Clinical Nutrition* 32 (1979): 455–462.

Ochoa, Mario. "The Colombian Food Stamp Program," in Per Pinstrup-Andersen, ed., *Consumer-Oriented Food Subsidies: Benefits, Costs, and Policy Options*. Washington, D.C.: International Food Policy Research Institute, 1987.

Pinstrup-Andersen, Per, ed. *Consumer-Oriented Food Subsidies: Benefits, Costs, and Policy Options*. Washington, D.C.: International Food Policy Research Institute, 1987.

Pinstrup-Andersen, Per. "Macroeconomic Adjustment Policies and Human Nutrition: Available Evidence and Research Needs." Prepared for the ACC/SCN 12th Session, Tokyo, April 7–11, mimeo, 1986.

———. "Food Prices and the Poor in the Developing Countries," *European Review of Agricultural Economics* 12 (1985): 69–85.

———. "Food Subsidies: The Concern to Provide Consumer Welfare while Assuring Producer Incentives." Prepared for IFPRI Workshop on Food and Agricultural Policy, Elkridge, Maryland, April 29–May 2, 1984a.

———. "The Nutritional Impact of the Colombian Food and Nutrition Program in the State of Cauca, Colombia." Report to Colombian Government. Washington, D.C.: International Food Policy Research Institute mimeo, 1984b.

Pinstrup-Andersen, Per, et al. "Impact of Changes in Incomes and Food Prices on Food Consumption by Low-income Households in Urban Khartoum, Sudan, with Emphasis on the Effect of Changes in Wheat Bread Prices." Report submitted to Sigma One Corporation. Washington, D.C.: International Food Policy Research Institute, 1982.

Reutlinger, Shlomo. "Supply Side Income- and Employment-Augmenting Interventions and the Intrinsic Value of Food Supply Self-Sufficiency for Enhancing Food Consumption Among the Poor," in Pinstrup-Andersen, 1987.

Rogers, Beatrice Lorge. "Pakistan's Ration System: The Distribution of Costs and Benefits," in Pinstrup-Andersen, 1987.

———. "Design and Implementation Considerations for Consumer Food Price Subsidies," in Pinstrup-Andersen, 1987.

———. "Pakistan: Nutrition Sector Assessment." Washington, D.C.: World Bank, mimeo, 1981.

———. *Consumer Food Price Subsidies and Subsidized Food Distribution Systems in Pakistan*. MIT International Nutrition Planning Program Discussion Paper 6. Cambridge, MA: Massachusetts Institute of Technology, 1978.

Rogers, Beatrice Lorge and James F. Levinson. *Subsidized Food Consumption Systems in Low-income Countries: The Pakistan Experience*. MIT International Nutrition Planning Program Discussion Paper 6. Cambridge, MA: Massachusetts Institute of Technology, 1976.

Rutishauser, I. H. E. and R. Whitehead. "Energy Intake and Expenditure in 1 to 3 Year Old Ugandan Children Living in a Rural Environment." *British Journal of Nutrition* 28 (1972): 145–152.

Sahn, David E. "Food Consumption Patterns and Parameters in Sri Lanka." Washington, D.C.: International Food Policy Research Institute, mimeo, 1986.

Scobie, Grant M. "Macroeconomic and Trade Implications of Consumer Food Subsidies," in Pinstrup-Andersen, 1987.

———. *Food Subsidies and the Government Budget in Egypt*, Food Subsidies Working Paper 2. Washington, D.C.: International Food Policy Research Institute, 1985.

———. *Food Subsidies in Egypt: Their Impact on Foreign Exchange and Trade.* Research Report 40. Washington, D.C.: International Food Policy Research Institute, 1983.

Timmons, Robert J., Roy I. Miller, and William D. Drake. "Targeting: A Means to Better Intervention." Ann Arbor: Community Systems Foundation, mimeo, 1983.

Trairatvorakul, Prasarn. *The Effects on Income Distribution and Nutrition of Alternative Policies in Thailand.* Research Report 46. Washington, D.C.: International Food Policy Research Institute, 1984.

von Braun, Joachim and Hartwig de Haen. *The Effects of Food Price and Subsidy Policies on Egyptian Agriculture.* Research Report 42. Washington, D.C.: International Food Policy Research Institute., 1983.

Williamson-Gray, Cheryl. *Food Consumption Parameters for Brazil and Their Application to Food Policy.* Research Report 32. Washington, D.C.: International Food Policy Research Institute, 1982.

World Bank. "Nutrition Review." Washington, D.C.: World Bank, mimeo, 1984.

7

Food Policy and Economic Adjustment

C. Peter Timmer

Economic adjustment to pressures from world recession, high debt, and low prices for traditional commodity exports has the potential to threaten the quantity and quality of nutrient intake among the world's poor. Lack of growth in employment opportunities, lower incomes, and pressures on real wages keep urban and rural nonfarm workers from maintaining access to food in local markets. And lower commodity prices, by causing farm incomes to fall, threaten food consumption in farm households. Lower food prices might help those who still have adequate incomes—but when the entire domestic economy is undergoing structural adjustment to the changed external economy, most of the poor are caught with reduced opportunities to earn income. When the world economy was booming the poor were threatened by high food prices; when the world economy is in crisis the poor are threatened by lack of access to the abundant food supplies.

It is always important to find ways to improve the nutritional status of the poor, and especially during economic recessions. But the financial resources then are more limited, and policymakers tend to focus on more pressing macroeconomic issues. To understand this problem, policymakers need a capacity to analyze the nutritional and health problems of the poor as they relate to the macroeconomic environment. The analysis of food policy—the attempt to understand how food intake is affected by macroeconomic forces through the workings of the entire food system—has received increasing attention since the world food crisis in the mid-1970s. Although the problems then were different, the analytical needs are the same: to understand how the food system works in order to trace links through it from the macroeconomy to food intake by poor consumers.[1] This chapter briefly reviews the current economic environment, summarizes the elements of food policy analysis, and concludes by discussing the implications for design and choice of policy interventions of the problems of economic adjustment.

Food policy provides a framework for relating society's objectives for its food sector to the technical, economic, and political constraints facing decisionmakers in the food system. From the process of balancing objectives and constraints emerges a set of policies and programs that reflect the government's efforts to build an environment for decisionmakers, public and private, that is conducive to meeting society's objectives. These objectives usually have four basic dimensions:

1. efficient growth in the food and agricultural sectors
2. improved income distribution, primarily through efficient employment creation
3. satisfactory nutritional status for the entire population through provision of a minimum subsistence floor for basic needs
4. adequate food security to ensure against bad harvests, natural disasters, or uncertain world food supplies

Food policy analysis has the task of improving the efficiency of a government's efforts to find a satisfactory balance between these objectives and the many constraints in the food system. In the mid-1980s, the constraints on implementation of an effective food policy seem to have multiplied. Not only must the traditional constraints on a broadly focused food policy be overcome—the urban bias that is characteristic of many governments in the developing world, the lack of adequate market infrastructure, and the weak budgetary base for government-financed activities, for example—but a combination of international forces now adds to the pressures on governments seeking to enhance the welfare of the poor.

This volume examines these new international constraints as they affect health. The virtual collapse of commodity markets for the traditional exports of many developing countries, the debt burden from borrowing of recycled petro-dollars, and the rising protectionism in rich countries seeking to protect their own workers from competition for markets in industrial products place new and complex burdens on the design of food policies that promote growth in agricultural output and farm incomes while improving the nutritional status of the poor. This chapter explains the food policy framework that can be used to evaluate the tradeoffs and organize the complexities for sensible deliberation by a country's policymakers.

Four basic issues for food policy are raised by the new international setting. Are the macroeconomic reforms proposed by the IMF, the World Bank, and other international agencies likely to help or hinder the development of an effective food policy? If the macro reforms force a cut in direct or indirect food subsidies, can special programs be set up to protect the vulnerable but not wreck the budget? If current low world prices for food grains are passed on to domestic farmers and consumers, will food policy objectives be enhanced or harmed? Should farmers and consumers be protected from instability in world commodity markets, even though the long-run trend in prices is eventually reflected in the domestic economy?

These four issues can be resolved only in specific country settings. Programs that improve nutritional status through better income distribution in the context of rapid and secure growth in food output do not come to agencies pre-designed. In addition, experience with the development process shows that these objectives are not automatically satisfied by a free-wheeling market economy turned loose to reward the already affluent or the most able. Policymakers can learn from the successes and failures of other societies, but most learning about which food policies will work and which will not must come from an honest attempt to implement policies and programs and a willingness to analyze their consequences.

Analysis is the key to preventing this process from degenerating into simple trial and error. The analysis of a country's food policy starts with food consumption patterns, food production potential, and the effect of the macro policy environment on both. These three sectors are connected by the domestic food marketing sector and influenced by the international economic environment. In the relatively open economies characteristic of all but the very largest developing countries, the domestic macroeconomy is strongly influenced by the international macroeconomy. There is relatively little impact felt in the opposite direction, which is one reason developing countries have never regarded interdependence as a key policy issue; the fact of dependence remains much more powerful. Food prices are a critical link joining the interconnected production, consumption, marketing, and macro sectors. Unfortunately, price links tend to cut two ways—high prices help producers but hurt consumers, and vice versa. The analysis sketched out here emphasizes this pervasive and double-edged role of food prices as an important element providing coherence to an analytical framework for understanding the entire food system.

Understanding the Food System:
A Perspective for Food Policy Analysts

Getting Started

This chapter places food consumption and nutrition issues within a food policy framework that specifically incorporates the macro linkages to the current crises in the world economy. Getting started on such a complicated task is always difficult because everything seems to need to be addressed first. One way to start is to focus on the hunger problem directly and then to proceed through the linkages to the macroeconomy. The food policy framework is essential with this starting point, however, because it is easy to become involved in the myriad details and personal tragedies that describe the hungry. With the framework of linkages established first, the analyst runs less risk of losing sight of the ultimate policy goals. Finding answers to four basic questions about nutrient intake and hunger will start the analyst on the right path:

1. Who are the individuals most vulnerable to hunger and malnutrition and where are they located geographically? Much of this information is available from household budget surveys, nutrition surveys, or even reports from regional hospitals and clinics. The information can be assembled to reveal the nature and prevalence of hunger, and it can then be linked to the functional significance of the problem. How important is it to the individual, to the family, and to society to intervene? The evidence will almost certainly suggest that certain vulnerable groups—infants, children, and pregnant or lactating women—are more likely to suffer than adult males or women in the formal work force. The extent to which this is true, and especially the extent to which overall food resources at the household level make it true, strongly conditions the nature and cost of intervention options.

2. How do the poor change their food consumption patterns, for the household and for individuals within the household, when incomes and prices change, whether by policy or through economic crisis? The first question requires descriptive evidence. The second question requires analysis of that evidence to achieve an understanding of how protein-calorie intake changes when incomes change, when food commodity prices change, either in tandem relative to nonfood prices or relative to each other, or when family size, place of residence, health status, or season of the year might change. Such disaggregated food consumption analysis is essential to further analysis of food policies. The analysis tends to be complicated, but there is significant potential for borrowing and carefully adapting an understanding of basic food consumption parameters from other societies.

3. What policies and programs are available to improve household food consumption and nutritional status? Efforts to change food consumption decisions span a wide range: food stamp programs, fair price shops, school lunch programs, general price subsidies, nutrition education, and amino acid fortification of basic cereals. The scope of possible interventions is enormous. Each program has inherent problems and costs relative to its benefits. Whether the costs are worth paying depends on the actual results of the program in a particular circumstance. Evaluation can be done only on a case-by-case basis, but analysts can be prepared for economic crises by maintaining an inventory of potential interventions that can be implemented on relatively short notice.

4. How are the consumption intervention policies and programs connected? It is necessary to ascertain the linkages among the various consumption programs themselves. There are sure to be synergistic and competitive elements that reinforce successes and failures. In addition, it is essential to determine how the consumption programs are linked to the rest of the food sector—the effects on production, on the marketing sector, and even on the macroeconomy and international trade. An important ingredient in such analysis is a consistent framework for understanding these linkages within the food system and for predicting the potential repercussions of macroeconomic crises on the health and nutritional status of the population (see Timmer, Falcon, and Pearson, 1983).

Consumption

For the analysis of food policies, food consumption is the variable of proximate concern. Nutritional status is strongly influenced by water and sanitation conditions, health status, food preparation techniques, and a host of other variables that intervene between how much food enters the household and how well nourished the household members are. But in most circumstances, it is the quantity of food consumed within the household that determines whether hunger is a significant factor in their lives. Consequently, major analytical attention is focused on food consumption patterns.

Two separate analyses must be conducted and ultimately reconciled. First, it is necessary to generate an understanding of the major parameters of market demand for basic foodstuffs. When average GNP per capita rises, how much is market demand for rice likely to increase?

Market demand for wheat? For cassava, for maize, for meat? How much meat is from grain-fed livestock and what effect will rising demand for meat have on demand for grain? How sensitive is market demand to absolute and relative food prices? If all food grain prices rise relative to nonfood prices, how much does demand drop? When the price of maize rises, does consumption of wheat rise, while that of maize falls?

Answering these questions is important because the resulting income, own-price, and cross-price elasticities provide necessary linkages from macro price policy and macroeconomic performance to food consumption and, through the food marketing sector, to incentives for agricultural production. In short, these parameters provide the *initial* link between the current world economic crisis and health consequences in individual countries. Obtaining these aggregate parameters of market demand with a high degree of confidence is seldom easy. Time series data are frequently short and of dubious accuracy when domestic food grain production makes up a significant part of total consumption. Mechanical regression analysis seldom gives plausible parameters. A combination of intuitive judgment, talks with traders, evidence from household surveys, simple graphical and statistical analysis of available data, and familiarity with similar parameters in other countries is frequently the best that can be achieved. Economic theory suggests some basic consistency relationships; reality suggests that parameters can change from year to year because of changing expectations, if for no other reason. Aggregate demand parameters are important, but they must be used with care.

The second step in food consumption analysis is to disaggregate the first step. The motivation for this step is quite different from the need to know aggregate parameters of market demand to understand the macro linkages in the food sector. Now we need to trace the effects of various changes in prices and incomes, whether transmitted from the international economy or from domestic policies, on the food intake of the poor.

The starting point is to discover what the poor actually eat. Everyone knows that they eat less food than do the rich. But in virtually all societies the composition of foods the poor eat is also significantly different from the diets of middle-income and wealthy groups. The point can usually be demonstrated and suitably quantified by preparing separate food balance sheets for three or four income classes in a society and comparing them with the aggregate food balance sheet that is published by most governments. The information needed to do this is normally available from household expenditure surveys, which, if not published, are likely to be in the file drawers of the statistical bureau. Any country that publishes a cost of living index has such data, although the base year may not be recent. Failing this, careful interviews with a dozen representative consumers in each income category will substitute and will not fail to provide fascinating perspectives on the variation in food habits across income classes.

Food policy analysis should always go this far in understanding disaggregated food consumption patterns. It is critical to get the commodities and the amounts right. Whether it is then possible to disaggregate the demand parameters by income class depends on data availability, computer facilities, and analytical capacity. With the right combination of these factors, as in Indonesia, the Philippines, Brazil, and Thailand, powerful analysis of the determinants of food intake by income class can be done. Using extremely large household expenditure surveys conducted by statistical bureaus for other purposes, researchers can carry out such analysis commodity by commodity and income class by income class. Only the analytical costs are attributable to food policy analysis.

The results of the analyses that have been completed show rough patterns across income classes that seem to hold from one country to another (Alderman, 1986; Timmer, 1981; Waterfield, 1985). Intuitive prior judgments that the poor are significantly more responsive to economic signals, both income and price signals, are strongly borne out in the analysis. The analysis has also demonstrated significant variations in levels of food consumption and in parameters of change by geographic region, by age and gender, and especially by season of the year. It does not help malnourished children to have enough food on average for the year if they starve during a three-month, preharvest "hungry season."

Production

What should society ask of its food production sector? The question is harder to answer than it seems. Most people's immediate instinct is that the domestic food-producing sector should satisfy the society's food consumption "needs." But then the thoughtful hedges begin. The United States should not grow all of its sugar and bananas, Kenya need not grow all of its wheat, nor should Europe grow all of its soybeans.

Farm income generated by efficient agricultural production is the productivity base from which all other production objectives can be discussed. Without efficient income generation, the entire rural sector acts as a drag on both macroeconomic performance and the ability of policymakers to deal with hunger and malnutrition. Knowing which crops, which new technologies for crops, which size of farms, which investments in rural infrastructure, and which production techniques will generate increases in agricultural productivity and employment is partly the responsibility of policy analysis, public investment, and macro price policy and partly the responsibility of millions of farmers who typically make rational decisions within the constraints of their own household and resource environment.

When tight budgets cause government spending on construction projects to be reduced, or weak (and heavily protected) world markets limit industrial exports, the agricultural economy may offer the only short-run hope for increases in employment and value added. Depressed world markets for agricultural commodities threaten this source of growth if the world prices are passed on to domestic farmers. While this is inevitable for export crops when budgets do not allow subsidies, price policy for imported commodities has more degrees of freedom.

Government intervention in prices of basic food commodities is pervasive but has widespread consequences that are poorly understood (Timmer, 1986). Nearly all price policies face an inherent dilemma—higher prices for producers mean lower welfare for consumers, at least in the short run. Unfortunately, the poor live in the "short run"; they have little capacity to tighten their belts and wait for higher investments and increased productivity to reach them. However, policy that always focuses only on such short-run concerns runs the real danger of forfeiting investment and productivity gains, thus endangering the long-run welfare of the poor as well.

From the point of view of balancing the short-run interests of consumers with the long-run need for investment and productivity gains, protection of farmers from low-cost imports has two appealing features: it generates tariff revenue (or trading profits) and raises farm incomes. When the imported commodity is also an important foodstuff, such as wheat or rice, the higher domestic price has negative consequences for nutrition. The task then becomes one of finding the types of interventions discussed in the final section of this chapter: those that alleviate the nutritional impact while capturing the output and employment effects.

Food production policy has three major tasks: (1) ensuring the availability of efficient agricultural technology for the various agro-climatic zones of the country; (2) providing a set of macro price policies—prices for capital, labor, foreign exchange, and rural goods (relative to urban goods)—which at the least do not actively discriminate against the rural sector and which ideally would provide more positive incentives for food production; and (3) providing the infrastructure for a rural marketing system for inputs and outputs with equal access for all classes of farmers, at a minimum, and preferential access for small farmers as an ideal. Each of these public policy roles with respect to efficient food production has an implicit or explicit consequence for income distribution. The ideal policies build a concern for income distribution specifically into the design of policies and programs. The evidence suggests that rural income distribution can worsen in the context of efficient growth in agricultural production without such specific attention (see Hayami and Kikuchi, 1982).

Food production analysis must ask many of the same kinds of questions asked about food consumption. For each of the major agro-climatic zones in a country, what yields are farmers actually producing on their fields? What is the seasonal pattern of land use relative to temperatures, rainfall, or water availability? Are crops grown in monoculture stands or are they extensively intercropped? What are the possibilities for alternative crops for any given season? Nothing may compete with growing paddy rice in the rainy season, but soybeans, peanuts, maize, or cassava may be possibilities for the same plot immediately after the rice harvest. When rice prices change, little change in areas planted to rice is likely in such an environment, whereas farmers may show extreme sensitivity to prices of soybeans relative to those of peanuts.

What prices are farmers receiving at the farm gate for their output, and how do such prices compare with international prices that are suitably discounted to local levels? The answer to this question is quite revealing about the extent of incentive or disincentive to domestic farmers for their respective crops. If farmers are receiving high prices for their crops but are achieving very low yields, both by world standards, then a visit to the local agricultural experiment station is in order. It is possible that the farmers simply do not know how to use available crop technology very efficiently. Then a vigorous agricultural extension program is called for. But historically such circumstances have been explained by an absence of a high-yielding crop technology that worked, with available inputs, reliably on a farmer's field.

How these three empirical questions—about farmer's yields, price incentives at the farm-gate level, and available technology—relate to each other provide strong clues to the agricultural policies on which the government should focus its attention. Most developing countries have provided their farmers with very poor incentives and, until recently, little modern biological technology. For most countries, this record of neglect and discrimination must be reversed if the domestic food production sector is to play a dynamic role in the overall modernization process, if income distribution between urban and rural areas is to be more equal, and if domestic food security is to be improved without increasing resort to unstable world markets. Providing improved incentives to farmers was "easy" in the world market environment of the mid-1970s because prices were high. It is much more difficult in the

1980s when prices are low. Food policy is constantly striving for a balance of interests between the short-run welfare concerns of the poor and the need to create a dynamic rural economy that will provide the jobs to raise them out of poverty. In the mid-1970s, the balance was upset by high commodity prices; in the mid-1980s, it is upset by low commodity prices. Intervention in both circumstances is needed to reach food policy objectives. Free trade in basic food commodities is not sufficient.

Marketing

Marketing is the invisible sector of the food system. Farmers receive "low" prices for their produce, consumers pay "high" prices for their food, and the middlemen in between get rich by speculating on the margin. Even in normal times, most governments seek ways to squeeze the private traders who carry out food marketing. In economic crises when governments look desperately for ways to protect consumers and producers, at least the favored ones, sweeping price controls designed to eliminate the profits of speculators and traders are very popular. They are nearly always disastrous to the welfare of small farmers and poor consumers because government officials—as well as the general population—lack an understanding of the productive tasks that must be carried out by the marketing sector.

Since foods as consumed are usually different in time, place, or form from foods as produced, nearly all foods must be marketed in the technical sense. Not all foods must enter the marketing system, however; the farm household itself often transports grain from the field to the house, stores it, and processes it before consumption—that is, performs the three marketing functions. Economic modernization raises the opportunity cost of such household activities. The marketing system tends to supply an ever-larger share of these services relative to household production. For food policy analysts, the important questions about the marketing system involve its static efficiency with respect to transformations in time, space, and form and its dynamic capacity and flexibility to handle varying and especially larger quantities.

Market efficiency is a measure of how the marketing system equates costs of storage, transportation, and processing with the associated price differences. High marketing margins do not denote inefficient markets if costs are commensurately high. High costs typically reflect inadequate physical and institutional infrastructure in the marketing system: poor roads accessible to trucks only in the dry season, lack of central marketplaces where price formation is competitive and resulting prices publicly announced and broadcast to farmers, shortage of fertilizer godowns close to the point of fertilizer use, or inadequate milling facilities. Public policy should normally focus on investments with a high payoff that improve the physical capacity of the marketing system. Greater capacity usually means lower short-run marginal costs when supplies increase sharply, and the flexibility of the system to respond to shocks is also improved. It is too late to create a responsive, low-cost marketing system when an economic crisis strikes, but policies that fragment markets and raise costs can only make matters worse.

The marketing system must transmit price signals efficiently as well as serve as the arena for price formation for many agricultural commodities. Most countries have national food price policies for their basic staple grain (and frequently for many other commodities). Such policies are normally implemented by special trade arrangements at the international border with respect to imports and exports of the commodity. Even with such a macro food price policy, the marketing system must still transmit the desired price signals up to consumers and down to farmers, generating price margins that reflect marketing costs along the way. For other commodities that frequently are very important for farm income (fruits, vegetables, livestock, and pulses), the marketing system must provide the price formation arena itself. The institutions by which governments encourage or discourage this activity heavily influence the net returns to farmers and the retail prices to consumers.

For income distribution, the consequences of inefficient price formation or poor transmittal of policy-determined price signals are almost uniformly bad. High marketing costs do not imply high incomes for the "middleman," but they do tend to imply high returns to those who can take the risks of a costly marketing venture. Even in efficient and low-cost marketing systems, many middlemen who transport and store grain tend to make windfall profits when food prices rise suddenly and unexpectedly. Although no one notices their losses when food prices fall unexpectedly, speculative profits on holding food grain during a shortage seem antisocial, if not criminal, and many societies have treated the middleman as both. Honest profits are to be made in food marketing. Public policy can see to it that such profits, and only such profits, are a normal component of the cost of providing food to consumers.

Food Policy Analysis and the Macroeconomic Environment

Agricultural policy analysis has traditionally focused on the farm sector *per se*, and there has been relatively little emphasis on the consequences for consumption of changes in farm policies. Marketing has been treated as an adjunct to farm output rather than a separate productive economic activity with its own unique set of risks and returns and opportunities for employment creation. Food policy analysis integrates the consumption, production, and marketing sectors of the food system into a consistent framework for understanding tradeoffs involved in reaching society's objectives with respect to reducing hunger, improving food security, and raising farm productivity.

These objectives usually cannot be reached with policy instruments available to the ministry of agriculture alone, even when there is no crisis in the world economy impinging on farm prices or causing major reductions in government budget allocations to farm subsidies, irrigation investments, and salaries for extension workers. In normal circumstances the macro policy context is at least as important to effective design and implementation of food policy objectives as specific food and agricultural policies themselves. In the crisis atmosphere induced by forced economic adjustments, both the short run *and* long run objectives for the food system can be sidetracked unless these objectives are set squarely in the context of the macroeconomic debate.

Domestic Macro Policy

Domestic macro policy, in combination with conditions in the world economy, determines the environment in which a food strategy is designed and implemented. As the main theme of this conference demonstrates, this macro environment is frequently hostile to several of the objectives of a food strategy, especially the critical one of efficient growth in agricultural production. At other times, the macro environment can be hostile to the achievement of nutritional objectives. Some macro environments are so bad that they are hostile to *all* food policy objectives at the same time.

Macro policy has three essential components from the perspective of the food system. The first is fiscal, budgetary, and monetary policy. Fiscal policy encompasses the overall tendency toward expansion or contraction of the economy, budget policy entails the actual sectoral allocations of the fiscal total, and monetary policy tends to be the instrument that accommodates fiscal policy when tax revenues fall short of budgetary expenditures. Monetary policy can be operated independently of fiscal policy, but in most cases the money supply tends to expand to fill fiscal deficits. The inevitable result is chronic, and frequently rapid, inflation. Thus many countries develop a food strategy in a macro policy context of significant price inflation.

The second essential component of macro policy is the real level of an economy's macro prices—wages, interest rates, and the urban-rural terms of trade (or food prices). All three macro prices tend to be biased against efficient agricultural production, at least to the extent that governments are able to implement their policy intentions. Since prices are meant to signal relative scarcity to decision makers in the economy, policy-dictated macro prices that are sharply at variance with actual scarcity values tend not to be widely applicable as actual decision variables. Low interest rates, even negative real interest rates, can be maintained for a few preferential customers through a rationing system and an accommodating monetary policy. But such rates depress savings and force informal credit rates, especially in rural areas, to higher levels than otherwise. High minimum wages can be enforced in large industries, but they reduce the demand for labor and force wages lower in the much larger informal labor market, also heavily rural. And low food prices, if enforced only by statute, tend to generate a black market where nonpreferred customers, especially the poor, must pay much higher prices for their food. Forced market deliveries from food surplus areas depress agricultural incentives. A set of such distorted macro prices, although perfectly understandable as a political reaction to the very difficult pressures of economic modernization, places a very heavy burden on an effective food strategy.

Low food prices can also be maintained, usually more effectively, by government policies that control food imports or exports. Restricting food exports or subsidizing imports has the effect of reducing domestic prices of food. Because restricting food exports usually provides a surplus for the government budget, as in Thailand, it is a doubly popular policy with urban-based government officials. Subsidizing imports requires a budget allocation, and so the costs of such a policy for low food prices are more apparent.

The third component of macro policy, however, typically hides some of these costs behind an overvalued exchange rate. The foreign exchange rate (also a macro price because it is set and defended by the Central Bank) measures the price of a unit of foreign exchange in terms of the number of units of domestic currency required to purchase it—for example, the U.S. dollar in terms of the Indonesian rupiah. Indonesia's exchange rate between August 1971 and November 1978 was 415 rupiahs per U.S. dollar, after which its rate was changed to 625 rupiahs per dollar. From 1974 to 1978, the rupiah became increasingly overvalued as domestic inflation ran much faster than that of its trading partners. Domestic prices of food were kept low, not by large budget subsidies on imports, but by large imports valued at an overvalued exchange rate. The burden on rural producers and the benefits to urban consumers came through the overvalued exchange rate (permitted in this instance by petroleum revenues), which made imported commodities appear cheaper to the domestic economy than they should have. The sharp devaluation in 1978 eliminated this bias, and the costs of maintaining low food prices were transferred directly to the budget. The visibility of such costs changes the nature of food policy discussions from one of trying to explain that a bias exists to one of examining the costs and benefits of the bias; this helps account for the usual insistence by the IMF that the domestic currency be devalued as a condition for lending its assistance. A devaluation also tends to increase sharply the terms of trade for rural commodities that are not specifically subsidized by domestic macro price and trade policy. Rural areas almost always benefit from a devaluation of the domestic currency, which reflects long-run scarcity more accurately.

Broad-based macroeconomic reforms encompassing all three components of macro policy—fiscal, budgetary, and monetary policy; macro prices for labor, capital, and food; and the foreign exchange rate—are not likely to be carried out at the behest of food strategists. But they should be carried out in any case if a country is concerned about growth and equity. Food strategists should be on the right side rather than the wrong side of the macro policy debate.

What is the right side of this debate? Although approaches obviously vary according to the economic and political structure of a country, macro policy reform nearly always has both significant short-run consequences for food consumption and large political costs. This is true whether the reforms are instigated by foreign donors or by governments trying to keep their economy in balance without losing sovereignty to foreign donors and banks. If effective government programs to deal with the consumption consequences for the poor are in place before a major reform is implemented, then they do not have to be assembled in a scramble after problems begin to appear. Facing the political costs of macro reform is easier if the virility of the society has not been repeatedly identified with the existing exchange rate, negative interest rates, and heavy protection of domestic industry. Food policy cannot resolve either the dilemma over food consumption or the political consequences of economic hard times, but it can help make a complicated situation more understandable to policy makers and to the general public. One of the most important roles of macro food policy analysis, then, is not in immediate policy changes, but in generating an understanding of the need for consumption interventions and assisting in their design, while building the political constituency for a macro policy environment more favorable to rural areas.

With these steps taken, the components of effective macro policy are fairly straightforward, even classical: (1) a reasonably balanced budget with restrained monetary growth leading to stable prices by the standards of international trading partners; and (2) macro prices set to reflect long-run opportunity costs of the factors of production (determined by their marginal productivity in producing tradeables at an equilibrium exchange rate). Such opportunity costs should not be read from international prices with a narrow, short-run, or mechanical vision. If interpreted too narrowly, environmental costs are left out. A short-run view fails to take into account temporary fluctuations in highly leveraged international markets, especially for sugar and food grains. To follow international prices mechanically implies that some formula can translate border prices into appropriate domestic price policy (see Timmer, 1986). But with these provisos, such a macro policy reform will end up reflecting the reality of the domestic economy rather than the shadows of planners' wishes.

International Elements in a Domestic Food Strategy

Few countries have tried and even fewer have succeeded in isolating themselves from the international economy. The opportunity for most countries to trade in the international economy means it can serve as the standard by which domestic resource allocations are made, at least before consequences for income distribution and the impact of instability are factored into the policy decision. Tradeable goods, especially most goods from the rural sector, can be imported or exported at the margin. The international marginal cost relative to domestic costs of production indicates the efficiency in income generation of a domestic project.

If international opportunity costs are to serve as a standard of comparison to domestic production (and consumption) costs, some understanding of the long-run functioning of major international commodity markets is essential to the analysis of a country's food policy. Such commodity markets are interconnected by technical and economic relationships, primarily through the livestock feeding industry. Cassava, maize, wheat, and soybeans are linked through these mechanisms. Wheat and rice, for example, are linked by China through a calorie arbitrage implemented by shifting food demand patterns with its urban rationing system for grain. Understanding commodity interdependence is the essence of understanding international markets. But such understanding does not produce easy answers. When world commodity prices are high, it is expensive for domestic policy to keep food prices cheap within a country; when world prices are low, it is expensive to provide greater price incentives for the country's farmers.

Several international instruments of assistance are available to domestic food strategy planners. None is important enough that it should influence the basic strategic design for the food sector. Food aid can be useful as a short-run support (on the consumption side) to a bridge linking existing food price policy with greater long-run price incentives to the domestic agricultural sector. The World Bank and other assistance agencies can provide useful funding and design assistance for critical urban and rural infrastructure. Their support of the international agricultural research institutes is absolutely critical for developing the long-run technological base for rapid improvement in domestic agricultural productivity. And last, analytical assistance is available for the design of effective food strategies. This design process is highly complex and requires personnel trained to think creatively about such complexity.

Food Consumption and Nutrition Interventions in a Food Policy Context

How can food policy analysis lead to better designs of food and nutrition interventions that will also improve implementation? The answer—"do good analysis"—is not as simple as it might seem. Policymakers the world over complain that they get good advice on policy design, but no one seems able to help them when it comes to implementation. The standard reason given is that policy design can rely on basic theoretical principles, while implementation must deal with the messy details of the real world—bureaucratic politics, vested interests, tight budgets, lack of commitment, and so on. This misses the point. The analysis must *incorporate* these issues if it is to be genuinely useful. For this reason the food policy framework focuses on the linkages among the various sectors of the food sector and how each of the decision makers in the sectors will respond to policy initiatives. Food policy analysis leads to better design *and* implementation of food and nutrition interventions when it uses the results of these responses in program design as well as in the macro policy debate.

Because food policy analysis must be grounded in the realities of local situations and environments, no concrete, general guidelines for intervention design can be offered here. The best that can be done is to survey the landscape and remind analysts of where the pitfalls and quicksand are likely to be hidden. Food and nutrition interventions are strewn across the entire landscape; they are available over the widest imaginable range of categories and diversity. For example, an overvalued exchange rate for a food-importing country gives all its food consumers a significant subsidy. Because many poor countries with food deficits tend to maintain overvalued exchange rates, the most prevalent food consumption intervention, and probably the most important in terms of aggregate impact on protein-calorie intake, is precisely via this macro price (the foreign exchange rate). This is the broadest and least-targeted food consumption intervention and hence usually has the most devastating short-run impact on the society when it is removed in a crisis environment. Totally at the opposite end of the spectrum is hyperalimentation through intravenous feeding. Hospital patients can be kept alive, even healthy, for extended periods of time without any resort to the gastrointestinal tract. All required nutrients for maintenance and growth can be supplied directly to the bloodstream without prior eating or digestion. This is certainly the ultimate in targeted nutrition intervention.

Table 7.1 breaks this wide spectrum of potential interventions into a 2 × 2 matrix of categories: food as opposed to nutrition interventions, and targeted as opposed to nontargeted interventions. Both distinctions are blurred at best, but they do provide ends of spectrums along two important dimensions. This matrix provides a starting point for the discussion of what has been called "an endless and seamless web." Like general equilibrium, where everything depends on everything else,

Table 7.1
Categories of Food and Nutrition Interventions

	Food	*Nutrition*
Targeted	Food stamps with means test Fair-price shops with means test and geographic or commodity targeting Targeted ratio programs Supplementary feeding programs for women, children, or other vulnerable groups Price subsidies for inferior food commodities Food-for-work programs	Maternal and child health clinics with means tests or geographic targeting Targeted nutrition education Targeted weaning foods Vitamin and mineral supplements for deficit populations Malnutrition wards in hospitals for severe cases
Nontargeted	*Direct (program)* General food ration schemes Fair-price shops for primary food-stuffs and unrestricted access *Indirect (policy)* Overvalued exchange rate for imported food General food price policy or subsidy Food production input subsidies (fertilizer, water, credit, seed, machinery)	Nutrition education on radio and television and through other general media General fortification schemes (for example, iodized salt) Basic policies encouraging breast-feeding or discouraging infant formula Public health interventions (water, sanitation, innoculations)

Source: Timmer, Falcon, and Pearson, *Food Policy Analysis.* Johns Hopkins University Press for the World Bank, 1983.

seamless webs have the disadvantage of no starting points. If everything must be understood and implemented simultaneously, there is little hope of actually beginning. Table 7.1 provides a rough toehold for the assault.

The first important distinction is between food interventions and nutrition interventions. Many nutrition planners consider all interventions that ultimately might affect nutritional status as "nutrition interventions," but a much narrower view of the field is taken here. Specifically, nutrition intervention projects (NIPs in the jargon of the trade) are restricted to those activities that accomplish nutritional objectives without using changed intake of basic staple foods as the primary operator causing the nutritional changes. Hence nutrition education, development of calorie-dense weaning foods, vitamin and mineral supplementation or fortification, encouragement of breast-feeding, and public health measures can each have significant impact on nutritional status when there are no significant changes in staple food intake.

The other major category of interventions includes the possibilities for improving the distribution or intake of basic food staples and hence reducing the extent and severity of chronic hunger. This category of interventions is the main focus of food policy analysis, not because nutrition interventions are unimportant, but because they can be so much more efficient and effective in an environment where significant protein-calorie deficits have been eliminated. This is a controversial assessment, especially when broad-scale food interventions are set against broad-scale public health interventions that focus on the synergistic impact on nutritional status of clean water, adequate sanitation facilities, and basic treatment of infections and gastrointestinal disease.

However this debate is resolved in any particular empirical setting, it should be made clear what the debate is not about. In the context of widespread protein-calorie deficits, nutrition interventions in the narrower sense (nutrition education, malnutrition wards in hospitals, food fortification, and even child feeding or school lunch programs) have not been very successful at improving nutritional status among the recipient population. Such narrower nutrition intervention projects usually can be effective only when household food intake is sufficiently above a threshold that all family members potentially have access to adequate protein and energy for growth and body maintenance.

The second major distinction is between targeted and nontargeted interventions. Targeting refers to the intended recipient group. If an intervention is specifically designed so that virtually all the benefits reach a particular specified group, then it is targeted. If the benefits are broadly distributed among an entire population, the program is nontargeted. But targeting is not an all or nothing property. Intent must be clearly distinguished from distribution of actual benefits. For example, a food stamp program may be intended as highly targeted because of an income test for qualification. But if most people lie about their incomes and no independent data can be used to verify the report, a food stamp program may actually be relatively nontargeted. On the other hand, a shop selling subsidized food in the center of a very poor section of town may be freely accessible to all buyers, but in fact, because of the targeted location (and possible restrictions on quantities that may be purchased at any one time—no truckload lots), the food subsidy may accrue almost entirely to food-deficit households.

Targeting can be judged only by result, not by intent. One of the major purposes for doing disaggregated food consumption analysis is to provide the necessary descriptive and analytical understanding of the food consumption patterns of the poor in order to predict actual results. Knowing what the poor eat and why, and knowing how those patterns will change when their external environment changes (especially in an economic crisis), is absolutely essential to designing targeted food interventions that target in fact as well as in intent. Since most food interventions take the form of an implicit or explicit subsidy (and hence alter either the price facing the consumer or transfer real income to the household), the necessity to have disaggregated price and income elasticities for important food staples is obvious.

But why is targeting so important a topic? Why not use fairly simple international trade instruments, such as imports with subsidies, to provide cheap food to the entire food-consuming population? Such broad subsidies, although quite effective if implemented widely and with vigor, as in Egypt and Sri Lanka until 1979, are extremely expensive and may have powerful disincentive effects on the producing sector. Targeting consumer subsidies to just those households in greatest need may provide most of the nutritional gains of the broader subsidies without the enormous fiscal burden or the production disincentives. But the *intent* to target is no guarantee of impact. The food stamp program in Sri Lanka that replaced the universal food distribution was neither targeted effectively nor maintained in real purchasing power for the poor, and the evidence is now compelling that the switch in macro policy in 1978 to a more open trade regime with domestic prices reflecting international prices was accompanied by a significant deterioration in nutrient intake of the poor, with increases in infant and child mortality observed in some localities (Goldman and Timmer, 1982; Sahn, 1986; Samarasinghe, 1987).

Two basic sets of linkage issues complicate the design and implementation of food and nutrition interventions. First is the set of factors that raises or lowers the efficiency and effectiveness of any single intervention when other interventions are introduced simultaneously or sequentially. A second set of connections is apparent when an intervention has ramifications on other sectors of the food system and on the macro economy at large. For example, the impact of generalized food subsidies through low food prices clearly has potential negative effects on food production. The mechanisms by which subsidies and food price policies are implemented usually have enormous impact on the food marketing sector. And an overvalued exchange rate that is maintained especially for its impact on holding food costs down can have widespread ramifications on the entire growth strategy and speed of development. Consequently, the effect of individual food and nutrition interventions can be extremely important both for program effectiveness in related interventions and for the rest of the economy.

Integrated conceptual design of food and nutrition interventions pay high dividends through greater cost-effectiveness of individual programs and greater opportunities to sense and capture program synergies. Since the possible range of food and nutrition interventions is extremely wide, one major task of food policy analysis is to identify all the interventions underway (whether advertised as such or not) and to quantify, however roughly, their actual impact on energy deficits (and other nutritional problems).

With the understanding gained from the food sector analysis outlined above, the analyst can identify intended targeting mechanisms that do not work effectively and suggest other forms of targeting that will perform better. Much of the improved performance comes from intersecting targeting, for example, by geographic region at particular times of year, and selecting specific commodities consumed primarily by the poor. Significant synergy might also be expected from programs that intersect: maternal and child health clinics that provide staple foods, birth control services, and maternal and child health care may raise the effectiveness of all three programs (see Johnston and Clark). The integration of the delivery of such diverse services does not come free, however. The managerial and organizational complexity of such integrated programs seems to rise according to some power of the tasks being performed. If managerial and organizational talent is not a free good, the true costs and actual ability to deliver through such integrated schemes must be considered.

This chapter has attempted to explain how the food consumption sector of a country responds to an economy threatened by domestic or international macroeconomic crisis. One important objective of public policy in such circumstances is to alleviate the likely increase in energy deficits among the poor. The government interventions that ultimately achieve that result will almost certainly not be restricted to narrow sectoral interventions designed to deliver more food to hungry people. A reduction in hunger, even in the context of macroeconomic crises, will most likely come from a coordinated effort involving many sectors and using a complicated array of policies which might have partially conflicting objectives and effects. Understanding this, and working to reduce the conflicts while enhancing the nutritional effects, is the role of food policy analysis. Knowledge of food consumption patterns is the first step in such analysis. But as the other sessions at this conference indicate, it is certainly not the only step.

Notes

1. The integrating framework described in this chapter was initially developed in *Food Policy Analysis*, by Timmer, Falcon, and Pearson during the late 1970s and early 1980s.

References

Alderman, Harold. "Survey of Methodologies for Estimating Disaggregated Food Consumption Parameters." Washington, D.C.: International Food Policy Research Institute, 1986.

Goldman, Richard, and C. Peter Timmer. "The Scope and Limits of Food Price Policy in Sri Lanka." HIID Development Discussion Paper no. 136. Cambridge, MA: Harvard Institute for International Development, June 1982.

Hayami, Yujiro, and Masao Kikuchi. *Asian Village Economy at the Crossroads: An Economic Approach to Institutional Change.* Tokyo: University of Tokyo Press, 1981, and Baltimore: Johns Hopkins University Press, 1982.

Johnston, Bruce F., and William C. Clark. *Redesigning Rural Development: A Strategic Perspective.* Baltimore: Johns Hopkins University Press, 1982.

Sahn, David. "The Impact of Economic Liberalization on Nutrient Intake in Sri Lanka." Washington, D.C.: International Food Policy Research Institute, April, 1986; processed.

Samarasinghe, S. "Sri Lanka: A Case Study from the Third World," Chapter 3 of this volume.

Timmer, C. Peter. "Is there 'Curvature' in the Slutsky Matrix?" *Review of Economics and Statistics* 62 (1981): 395–402.

———. *Getting Prices Right: The Scope and Limits of Agricultural Policy.* Ithaca: Cornell University Press, 1986.

Timmer, C. Peter, Walter P. Falcon, and Scott R. Pearson. *Food Policy Analysis.* Baltimore: Johns Hopkins University Press for the World Bank, 1983.

Waterfield, Charles. "Disaggregating Food Consumption Parameters." *Food Policy* 10 (1985): 337–351.

8

The Special Case of Africa

Andrew M. Kamarck

Sub-Saharan Africa is the poorest region in the world and the one that is making least economic progress. The UN has classified thirty-four countries in the world as being among the world's poorest; of these, twenty-nine are in sub-Saharan Africa. That is, almost two-thirds of the forty-five independent countries, other than South Africa, south of the Sahara (on the continent and nearby islands) are among the world's poorest. In contrast, in Latin America only Haiti ($300 per capita GNP in 1984) is classified among the world's poorest countries. In Africa Haiti would be average; that is, almost half the countries are poorer than Haiti and half richer.

Since 1960, the average standard of living in sub-Saharan Africa has fallen. While output has grown slowly, stagnated or even dropped, the rate of population growth has accelerated over this period. The population growth rate has increased to an average of around 3 percent, now the highest in the world. In other areas it has gone down, in Asia below 2 percent, in Latin America to around 2 percent (United Nations, 1985, pp. 44–45). If the current growth rate continues, the total population of sub-Saharan Africa, now 350 million, will surpass 500 million by the year 2000.

African exports are about 10 percent of the world total. Twenty years ago they were about 17 percent. This rough statistic is an indication of how African growth has lagged behind that of the rest of the world. Part of the lag is due to external causes and is explained by the fall in real prices of exports of primary commodities in the 1980s due to the global recession and slow growth in the industrialized countries. These external factors affected countries on other continents also, but they were able to at least partially compensate. Most African countries faced special, greater obstacles, as we shall see below, and were not able to compensate.

The disappointing economic progress of sub-Saharan Africa also characterizes and affects the food and nutrition sector. Low export earnings, for example, hurt agriculture. Farmers are deprived of needed inputs purchased from abroad—even hoes in some countries are hard to come by. Processing and transport capacity break down. The goods that farmers would like to buy are scarce, and they lose the incentive to produce crops to sell on the market.

Tropical Africa (continental sub-Saharan Africa and the nearby islands) is likely to have food and nutrition problems for several generations to come. There is no easy solution since the problems are complex and deep-rooted; they involve both human institutions and nature; and, in large part, they are so specific to the African environment that the mere transfer of existing knowledge and techniques from other continents does not respond to the imperfectly understood African needs. Most of the obstacles arise from Africa's history, institutions, and climatic and geographic factors and can only be overcome or bypassed in the long run. Some, however, are due to current government policy and are susceptible of correction within a reasonable period of time.

This chapter, after briefly indicating the main outlines of the long-term production crisis in agriculture, concentrates on analyzing the main elements that affect progress here: current government policies and the international consensus on the reforms needed in them; the longer-term natural obstacles from climate; and the political and sociological impediments.

Food and Nutrition Position

Agriculture is by far the most important economic sector in sub-Saharan Africa: it has over half of the labor force in most countries and it produces about 40 percent of the Gross Domestic Product (GDP). In spite of this, sub-Saharan Africa has trouble feeding its peoples. The 1984–85 famine which affected at least twenty-four African countries merely dramatizes the situation. Per capita food production over the last twenty years has decreased, whereas in Latin America and Asia it has increased (World Bank, 1984). Output of the basic food cereals has grown considerably more slowly in sub-Saharan Africa (averaging less than 2 percent per year) than population growth. This result, it should be recognized, is not entirely due to a shortfall in output: imported food is regarded by many urban dwellers as a "superior" good. Consequently, when income permits—often subsidized by an over-valued exchange rate—bread from wheat is bought by consumers in place of the traditional cassava, millet or sorghum. Although the region is still not highly urbanized, the rate of growth of urban population in the region has been among the highest in the world: over the last twenty years the proportion of people in cities has gone from one-tenth to around one-fifth of the total.

Hunger was a problem even prior to the 1984–85 famine. In 1980, based on World Bank data, the indications are that a quarter to almost half of the total population, or around 90 million to 150 million people, in sub-Saharan Africa were not able to secure adequate food for nutrition. The lower estimate of 90 million is people who were not able to secure a caloric consumption that would prevent serious health risks and stunted growth in children. (This caloric standard is defined as being below 80 percent of the FAO/WHO requirement.) If the consumption standard used is "enough calories to enable an active working life (or at least 90 percent of the standard FAO/WHO requirement)" then the estimate of the number of people in sub-Saharan Africa normally having inadequate nutrition rises to 150 million (Reutlinger, 1985). Since 1980, the situation has further deteriorated.

The coarse grains—maize, sorghum, millet—and the primary grains—rice and wheat—are the main foods in sub-Saharan Africa. One or another of the coarse grains is grown over most of the region outside of the rain forest area; rice is principally grown along the far western coast but is also an import; wheat, aside from Kenya, is almost wholly an imported food. As Table 8.1 shows, African consumption since 1960 has been shifting from the coarse grains towards the primary grains. The increase in consumption of primary grains represents at the same time an increase in the reliance on imported foods. African dependence on outside food sources has been growing at a rapid rate: commercial imports of grain have increased at an annual rate of 9 percent over the past twenty years. In Nigeria, as some incomes rose after its oil boom, consumption of imported wheat grew from 1 percent

Table 8.1
Percentage of Coarse Grains, Rice and Wheat in Total Grain Consumption in Sub-Saharan Africa

	1960	*1970*	*1980*
Coarse grains	84	81	76
Rice	10	10	13
Wheat		9	11

Source: US Foreign Agricultural Service in Mitchell, 1985.

of total grain consumption in 1960 to 12 percent in 1980 (Mitchell, 1985).

Government Policy

Most of the governments have done little to help modernize small-scale agriculture. Price policies favor the city dwellers and discourage investment in the land by farmers and pastoralists. Producer prices typically have been set by governments at levels which discourage the use of quality seeds and fertilizers. Marketing arrangements and the setting up of marketing organizations are regularly efficient only in providing relatively well-paid jobs for the politically well-connected.

The example of Nigeria, which has from one-fourth to one-third of the total population of sub-Saharan Africa, is instructive. During the 1970s, Nigeria profited greatly from the oil boom. Oil revenues boosted domestic incomes and prices in Nigerian cities. The exchange rate of the Naira was kept low so foreign imported goods became relatively cheaper. Consumption of food in the cities shifted from the local yams and cassava to imported "superior" foods such as rice and wheat. At the exchange rate, imported palm oil from Asia became much cheaper than the domestic palm oil and practically destroyed the industry which previously had met Nigerian consumption needs and had been one of Nigeria's principal exporters (*The Economist*, 1986).

The Marxist influence on government policy in agriculture in many countries has been damaging. Most governments organized highly inefficient state-run, centralized, marketing and services organizations, and even state farms in some instances. These wasted resources, provided poor services, and discouraged small farmers. Even in a moderate country like Tanzania, President Julius Nyerere's policies were directed by the desire to build an African socialism. The major policy objective of the government was ujamaa villagization—that is, concentrating the rural population into villages farming communally. By the end of the 1970s most of the rural population had been resettled into the villages, in some cases forcibly. At the same time, the government centralized the buying of crops and the import and provision of goods for the farmers into parastatal organizations. The farmers, separated from their fields and with the inefficient parastatals unable to handle crop purchasing effectively or to provide needed goods, cut back their production just to feed themselves or what they could sell across the border in Kenya. Agricultural production for local consumption and for export suffered a catastrophic drop.

Investment in sub-Saharan Africa has concentrated disproportionately in urban areas. Roads and bridges in many rural areas have broken down and over large regions of some countries like Zaire have vanished altogether; many farmers who had become involved in a market economy have had to revert to subsistence to survive.

Investment in agriculture has been neglected, in part, because the type of project needed tends to be given low priority in the process of choosing investments in African countries. The bulk of the economic literature on investment choice in the LDCs is irrelevant to what happens in practice. African governments do not have a wide array of projects to which they apply Social Benefit Cost Appraisals and then pick the ones that have the highest returns. The governments are organized along sectoral lines; there is a tremendous uncertainty about what is best to do for development and a lack of knowledge as to which investment proposals or ideas (which is what the decisionmakers have initially to choose from) are the best. Policy makers are overburdened, inexperienced and have limited time and attention to devote to decisions. Under these circumstances, investment decisions are made first on an intersectoral basis and then work is done on preparing projects within the favored sectors. Agriculture loses out, unless there is some spectacular large project that can get attention (Leff, 1985).

Since most African countries are not democracies, the votes of farmers have little weight. The farmers are scattered over the countryside and cannot apply direct pressure, while urban dwellers are concentrated and usually live mostly in the capital city. The people in the city also include the army officers and top bureaucrats who are the ruling class in most of the countries. Thus the needs of farmers in the authoritarian African countries inevitably get less weight than those of the city dwellers.

Tropical Climatic Obstacles in Agriculture

The natural obstacles to progress in agriculture in sub-Saharan Africa are immense (see Kamarck, 1976). Africa is *the* tropical continent. Sub-Saharan Africa is wholly in the tropics except for Swaziland and Lesotho. The lack of knowledge of how to cope with the tropical climate was and is a major obstacle to development. It has held back agriculture and weakened farmers' productivity through the diseases it abets. The existing advanced technology that has been developed to handle the problems and characteristics of agriculture in the temperate zones is mostly inapplicable to sub-Saharan Africa. Except in the case of a few

204 · *Health, Nutrition and Economic Crises*

export crops, there is not a long history of research on how best to farm efficiently in the tropics.

Tropical Africa does not have a single homogeneous tropical climate. There is, in fact, a continuously variable succession of climates that blend and overlap. A wet equatorial climate, in which rain falls in all months, and averages 200 to 300 centimeters a year, is the rule across most of the center. North and south from this area there is an alternately wet and dry tropical climate, the dry periods tending to grow longer as one goes farther north or south. Finally, there is the dry tropical climate, characteristic of the Sahara and the Namibia deserts.

These varying tropical climates are alike in not being temperate, that is, moderate. Rainfall determines the season. Rainfall is either too much or too little. One can be certain only of its unpredictability and violence. In much of Africa the rains never came in the early 1970s, and from 1980 to 1985 some thirty-four countries have been afflicted by drought. Rains tend to be much more violent and prolific than in temperate zones. Yearly rainfall fluctuates tremendously. A tropical country with a given average annual rainfall has a much greater risk of drought than a temperate country with the same average annual rainfall.

If soil is exposed, the violent torrential rains crush its structure and leach out the essential minerals and trace elements. The soil also must be protected against the heat of the sun, which otherwise would burn away the organic matter and kill the vital microorganisms which maintain the fertility of the soil. When soil is exposed, it can become barren and kill any possibility of farmers making a living. Soils in the tropics, except volcanic or alluvial soils, are usually poor and thin. Where one sees lush vegetation it is because there is a precarious equilibrium with the plants taking and returning sustenance to the soil.

If the vegetation is cleared to make a cultivated field, the soil is soon exhausted by a few years of crops. For this reason, African farmers in the humid tropics developed "shifting" or semi-nomadic cultivation. A field is hacked out, cultivated for a few years, and allowed to revert to bush again to lay fallow, in some cases for as long as ten to twenty years.* This is why when tree crops, such as cacao, coffee, and bananas can be grown, this particular problem is avoided and farmers are able to achieve higher incomes than from annual crops.

Over a large portion of tropical Africa, exposed soil has become laterite. With the extensive leaching what is mostly left is oxides of iron or hydroxides of aluminum. When exposed, this becomes almost as hard as cement and useless for farming.

*See Chapter 9 on how this works in Zambia.

The pattern of the rainfall makes farming difficult. In temperate climates, snow during the winter brings and conserves moisture so that the soil can be cultivated before it is necessary to plant in the spring. When the plants start to come up they grow slowly at first and the farmer can cultivate and eliminate most of the weeds. In the tropics, before the rains the soil is hard and unworkable. When the rains come, everything has to be done at once: cultivate and plant. At the same time the insects, weeds and other pests also burst forth. (And at this point the farmer may be weakened with an attack of malaria.)

The absence of frost means that the enemies of man's crops and animals are not wiped out by winter. The heat keeps a multiplicity of species alive in intense competition for survival. The conditions are right for rapid evolutionary change as species adapt to new opportunities. Whenever a new source of food appears that can be exploited by a particular life form, it multiples very rapidly. Whenever man introduces a new crop in large enough numbers, some particular life form finds it edible and rapidly attacks it. It can be a bird, like the weaver birds in their millions, or an insect like the locust, or a worm like the nematodes, or a weed, or a virus.

Cultivated plants are threatened by weeds, parasitic fungi, insects, spider mites, eelworms, and virus diseases. After harvest, storage pests and rats move in. Gigantic swarms of desert locusts in western and eastern Africa and red locusts in southern, central and eastern Africa, and brown locusts in southern Africa are a major recurrent threat to crops. Rainfall in 1986 was good in the Sahel, and crops were good. However, an enormous horde of grasshoppers was expected to hatch to feed off the favorable crops, and extraordinary measures had to be taken to ward them off. Constant research and battles against new threats are therefore necessary if any major increase in agricultural output is to be achieved. The poor countries of tropical Africa have had little resources to devote to such research and have given it even less priority.

Diseases of domesticated animals also have a major impact on agriculture. To cultivate their fields, most African farmers have to depend on human muscle power—using a hoe rather than a plow. Over most of the area the historic transition to mixed farming based on ox- or horse-drawn cultivation is interdicted because of the prevalence of trypanosomiasis. This disease, spread by the tsetse fly, is deadly to horses and cattle. Over 4 million square miles—an area greater than that of the United States—is controlled by the fly. Where the fly has been pushed out, constant vigilance and control measures are necessary to keep it from coming back.

Where the fly is absent, there are innumerable other parasitic, infectious, nutritional, toxic, metabolic, and organic diseases that affect livestock. Intestinal parasites result in retarded development of young animals, reduce yields of meat and milk, and diminish the working capacity of draft animals.

The traditional African farming practices, based on extensive cultivation and long fallow periods and which represented a viable adjustment to the African tropical environment, are breaking down under the need to absorb more people in the same space. The physical environment is being degraded and the ecological deterioration is threatening Africa's future. Cultivation and grazing are being pushed into marginal areas and forests. In many countries, forest and other vegetation cover is being stripped away with severe damage to soil fertility, watershed protection, household fuel supplies, and perhaps even causing a decline in the amount of rainfall. The degradation of the environment takes its revenge in drought, the spread of deserts, malnutrition, famine and death.

So far, the emphasis has been on the disadvantages the African farmer faces. Existing agricultural technology was mainly developed to avoid the difficulties and to exploit the advantages of the cycle of temperate zone seasons. It cannot cope with the problems of African tropical agriculture or use the particular opportunities for farming in the tropics—and the latter do exist. Sunlight energy for plant growth is 60 to 90 percent higher than in humid temperate regions. Plants in tropical rain forests produce up to three to five times more organic matter in a year than plants in temperate forests. The absence of frost, if pests are controlled, extends the potential length of the growing season; with the provision of water, up to three or four crops can be grown in a year. The climatic conditions that speed up evolution can also help develop new and better varieties of crops and livestock.

The key to discovering and exploiting the potential of tropical agriculture is research. Twenty years ago economic development texts did not even recognize that tropical countries had special climatic obstacles to overcome. Until recently there was little research in tropical agriculture other than on some export crops and most recently on tropical wheat and rice. The success of the research on rice and wheat financed by the Rockefeller and Ford Foundations led the World Bank to take the initiative to organize the comprehensive Consultative Group on International Agricultural Research (CGIAR). CGIAR, co-sponsored by the World Bank, the Food and Agriculture Organization, and the United Nations Development Program has made notable progress since 1971 in organizing and financing international research institutes to work on tropical crops and livestock. The crops and livestock covered account for some three-quarters of the food supplies of less developed countries.

Improved maize varieties, together with better agricultural policies, have already led to grain surpluses in Kenya, Zimbabwe and Malawi. A new hybrid sorghum strain which is pest- and drought-resistant can double the yield of local strains in normal weather conditions. It made possible a surplus in the Sudan in 1986. An alternative to shifting cultivation is being developed at the International Institute of Tropical Agriculture in Ibadan, Nigeria. This new method, "alley cropping," retains the basic features of the old system but economizes on the use of land. Alley cropping consists of planting food crops between rows of leguminous trees or shrubs whose leaves are periodically cut to supply nutrients to the soil. The technique allows a farmer to grow crops for a long period without having to leave the land fallow to revert to bush. This avoids also the use of heavy equipment for land clearing and preparation which in the tropics leads to rapid degradation of the soil from humidity and high temperatures (*Ceres*, 1986).

While progress is thus being made through the international agricultural research institutes to improve African food crops and to learn how to cope with the African tropical environment, most of the African countries lack the in-country capability to profit from the advances that are beginning to be made. The micro-climates and environments vary so much from area to area in Africa that adaptive research is necessary before any findings of the international research institutes can be applied. The World Bank has only now established a budget to make grants for agricultural research in Africa on a regional basis. The African countries also lack training facilities to prepare the people needed to go into the local research, extension services and agricultural management. For a brief period after World War II and before the African countries became independent, there appeared to be attractive careers for Europeans in doing agricultural research on African problems. Since then there has been little incentive for good researchers from outside Africa to devote their lives to such purposes.

Sustained action is needed on the part of the African countries and the donor countries and organizations to commit resources to needed research and extension work that may take twenty to twenty-five years to pay off. The adjustment programs' recognition of the need for finance of research and extension work is helpful; this effort should be continued not for a few years but for a generation.

Agriculture in Africa will improve only when farmers have learned to apply the useful results of research. Given the great variations in African micro-climates and soils and the still small scientific base of knowledge applicable, progress is bound to be slow. Some areas are so unfavorable that human beings cannot live there on anything more than bare subsistence. To live appreciably better, they will have to move to more favorable environments.

Some success has already been attained in producing and making available improved strains of maize and sorghum. The African tree crops (bananas, cacao, coffee, oil palm, rubber and tea) have been able to profit from the long research on these in other continents. Tree crop cultivation also has advantages over crops: the plants shade and protect the soil and come close to achieving the same kind of equilibrium with the soil and climate that the original forest had. Tree crops also permit the establishment of permanent farms and, consequently, improvements in techniques can be communicated and exploited more easily.

Obstacles from Human Diseases

Diseases that affect the African farmer are also an important obstacle.* The farmer is too often weakened just when the onset of the rains demands extra effort. The African farmer has to work, usually relying only on human muscle power, coaxing crops out of a soil that is rapidly depleted of its nutrients and surrounded by the enormous fecundity of a huge variety of minute life trying to feed off big life. The average farmer in tropical Africa is infected by at least two different types of parasites and will usually have had, or be currently subject to, attacks of malaria or schistosomiasis or be harboring debilitating worms or other diseases.

A large part of the mortality and sickness that affects farmers in tropical Africa is caused by diseases that also plague temperate countries. However, many of these diseases are more difficult to control in the tropics because of the warm temperatures the year round. Since there is no frost or winter, large populations of insect vectors are able to live for most or all of the year. Insects also multiply much more rapidly than in colder climates. The house fly, for example, spreads bacillary dysentery and other diseases. It takes forty-four days for the fly to develop from egg to adult at 16 degrees Celsius (62° F) but only ten days at 30 degrees Celsius (88° F). The more rapid maturity of the fly in the higher temperatures means a difference in the potential birth of millions of flies. But that is only a part of the story. Parasites, such as malaria, which live part of their lives in an insect are also ecothermic. That is, the speed of their development and multiplication within the insect host varies directly with the temperature (Gillett, 1974).

*See Chapter 9 for more details on some of the diseases discussed here.

Most of the diseases that afflict African farmers have not been brought under control; in fact, the necessary research effort only barely started a few years ago. A coordinated international research effort began only in 1975. The Special Program on Research and Training in Tropical Diseases is co-sponsored by the World Health Organization, the United Nations Development Program, and the World Bank. It is concentrating on malaria, schistosomiasis, sleeping-sickness, filariasis (including river blindness), leishmaniasis, and leprosy.

Considerable progress has been made in controlling onchocerciasis (river blindness), which is spread by the black fly with the apt name Simuluum damnosum. In large parts of Africa, particularly in the west African savannah, the river valleys with their fertile alluvial soil were uninhabitable. The black fly, which needs running water to reproduce, transmits threadlike parasitic worms from person to person when the female fly bites to get the blood it needs to develop its eggs. The worms reproducing in the human being travel through the body and when they reach the eyes cause blindness. Some 30 million people suffered from the disease when an international effort begun in 1974 to control it in the Volta River Basin (parts of Benin, Burkina Faso, Ghana, Ivory Coast, Mali, Niger, Togo). The effort has been successful by eradicating the fly larvae in the rivers. Transmission of the disease has been stopped in 90 percent of the area, and the parasites still living in people are reaching the end of their life span. People are migrating back into the abandoned valleys from the barren hills and beginning to cultivate the more fertile river bottoms. The program is now being extended westward to new river valleys in Guinea, Guinea-Bissau, Sierra Leone, Senegal, western Mali and southern Togo, Benin and Ghana. A promising drug, Ivermectin, is now being field-tested to kill the baby worms (microfilariae) that move through the body to the eyes and cause blindness. There is still no effective drug to kill the adult worms (macrofilariae) or to provide immunity from the disease (Nawaz, 1986).

Simple, widely applicable tests have recently been developed to detect African sleeping sickness (trypanosomiasis). The disease may be curbed by protecting the patients from being bitten by the tsetse fly, which transmits it. Improved traps have also been developed to catch tsetse flies to interrupt the spread of disease. A new cure for the disease is also being tested; the chemical alpha difluoromethylornithine (DFMO) has had outstanding success in one trial in the Sudan—it cured ninety-seven out of one hundred sleeping sickness patients. It even succeeded in killing the tryps that had lodged in some patients' central nervous system and had sent the patients into the characteristic coma.

Preliminary tests indicate that DFMO may also be useful in killing the malaria parasite. Some progress is also being made on developing a vaccine against malaria, and trials are beginning of several different types. Even if a vaccine does work against malaria, problems remain in storing and transporting it in a hot, humid climate and in making it cheap enough to be used in a widespread campaign (Harvard Health Letter, 1986).

In schistosomiasis the research to date has not produced an effective means to control or eradicate the disease, although progress is being made. Good sanitary habits and the provision of safe water have been most successful so far. Safe drinking water would also eradicate guinea worm or dracunculiasis, a disease which can be contracted only by drinking water that contains a tiny crustacean (Cyclops) that is contaminated with guinea worm larvae.

Work is also being done on developing bacteria, fungi and nematode worms to attack insect vectors. Bacillus thuringiensis (B.t.) is a bacterium one of whose strains is being tried in pesticides for use in killing different mosquitoes that carry malaria. Another strain is being tried against the gnat Culex fatigans, which is the vector of a filarial parasite that results in elephantiasis. Mermithids, minute nemode worms, are being investigated for their effectiveness in killing mosquito larvae.

In short, the importance of combatting the diseases of the tropics has finally been recognized and some progress is being made. There is still a long road of research and application ahead, however.

Political Impediments

The political situation in most African countries is a major impediment to agricultural progress. African governments are fragile and without any established firm agreement, custom or tradition on how power should be legitimately transferred. Instability, changes in government by force, guerrilla fighting, wars, and civil wars plague Africa.

The African countries gained independence in the 1960s, when a small percentage of population were educated or literate and only a very small or minute number had absorbed modern industrial culture. The official language, in most cases, continued to be that of the former metropolitan power, but only a small portion of the people can speak the official language. Only in a few countries (the Sudan, Somalia, Kenya, and Tanzania) was a local language given official status. Elsewhere, the diversity of tribal languages made it impossible to choose any language other than the former colonial one.

Independence came so rapidly that the Africans had little time to gain administrative experience, to establish traditions and habits of orderly government, and to learn how to carry out peaceful transition in the transfer of power.

Colonial governments were paternalistic; the civil servants were trained to approach problems with administrative rules or laws rather than by modifying the structure of economic incentives. The new African governments often gained independence with leaders who were educated in the west or in eastern Europe and used the Marxist ideology they learned to prepare for their anti-colonial struggle. Whether educated in the east or west, they assumed that the welfare state developed in high-income industrialized economies should represent the minimum of government services. Whether Marxist or not, the new governments tried to create state services and enterprises more appropriate to a twentieth century industrialized economy than to the poor, primary-commodity-producing, largely subsistence economies they inherited. Without the trained manpower even to carry out the minimum of law and order, the over-ambitious governments soon suffered from widespread inefficiency and the growth of corruption as the effective means to secure decisions.

Unfortunately, instability has also been increased by the worldwide competition between Communist and non-Communist ideologies. Whereas in most of the world the frontiers between Communist and non-Communist oriented areas have stabilized, sub-Saharan Africa is still an area of contention. Even where the clash between Marxists and non-Marxists has not led to civil war and destruction, Marxist ideas and policy copied from the Russian example have substantially damaged agricultural production.

This conflict has been present in the twelve-year civil war in Ethiopia and in the eleven years of guerrilla wars in Angola and Mozambique that followed a generation of guerrilla fighting for independence. In guerrilla-torn Mozambique, the main rail line from the principal port of Beira to Malawi is closed and would take months to restore. Another to Zimbabwe works only by daylight and is guarded by Zimbabwean troops. There is nothing to buy in the shops. There is no reason for farmers to produce more than enough to feed themselves. In Angola, the Benguela railway has been closed for years. Guerrillas range freely over most of the area. The U.S. government is helping to arm the guerrillas who threaten the country's principal foreign exchange earner, the American-owned oil installations (Peterzell, 1986).

Zimbabwe has had only six years of peace after fifteen years of guerrilla war. While nationalism rather than communism was the principal force motivating the guerrillas, the Communist powers provided financial support and training. Since the Soviet Union and China supported two different forces based on the two main ethnic groups, the struggle did not develop a single nationalist movement, and latent and sometimes open violence has continued after independence.

Sub-Saharan Africa is also the site of another worldwide confrontation. This conflict harks back to the beginnings of militant Islam. In western Europe, the boundary between Islam and the non-Islamic world was stabilized at the Straits of Gibraltar in 1492 and in eastern Europe at the frontier of a shrunken Turkey in 1912–13. In Africa, Islam's frontiers are still not permanently established. This leads at times to civil or international war and sometimes to coup and counter-coup. The main frontier of Islam runs across the widest part of Africa and then down the coast to Kenya. North of the line the majority of the population is Moslem. This includes Mauritania, Mali, Senegal, the Gambia, Guinea, Burkina Faso, Niger, the northern halves of Nigeria, of Chad and of the Sudan, as well as nearly all the people of Eritrea and Somalia.

Islam has been a factor in the continuing war for independence of Moslem Eritrea from Christian Ethiopia for around thirty years, in the fighting between the south and north of the Sudan off and on for thirty years, in the back and forth war in the Chad for twenty years, and in the almost continuous border incidents and recurrent war between Somalia and Ethiopia. These latter include an undeclared Somali-Ethiopian war in the late 1960s; a Somali invasion, armed with Russian-supplied weapons, of Ethiopia's Ogaden region in 1977–78; repulse of the Somalis by Ethiopia with the help of Russian weapons and Cuban troops after the Russians changed sides; and Ethiopian occupation in 1982 of two salients of Somali territory, still held in 1986 (US Department of State, 1986).

Right-wing guerrillas in Mozambique have been reported to be partly financed by outside Islamic sources angered by the Marxist government's closing of mosques. Some of the coups and attempted coups in Nigeria and Sudan have involved Moslem-Christian rivalries as well as intra-Moslem conflicts in the latter. Uganda, one of the few African countries with large areas of good soil and good rainfall, has been cursed since 1970 with two successive governments which Amnesty International estimates murdered up to half a million people each and with an army that was out of control, preying on civilians and the civilian economy. Idi Amin, the first tyrant, was supported by Libya and is currently living in comfortable exile in Saudi Arabia because of his Moslem religion.

It took western Europe a thousand years to create national states from the collection of tribes and remains of the Roman Empire. With the spread of nationalism as the predominant secular religion in the last few centuries, permanent non-national minorities are increasingly less tolerated. Exchanges of population, driving minorities into exile, or out and out genocide have been the result. In the 1920s, for example, Greece and Turkey exchanged a million and a half people. After World War II, western Germany resettled over ten million Germans coming from Eastern Europe. There are still some ethnic Germans trickling in from Russia. This process is not completed, even in Europe where nationalism first began. The Turks and Greeks in Cyprus sorted themselves out into different parts of the island in the last decade, but a final division of the island between them is not yet agreed. There is no resolution of the Northern Ireland conflict and there are continuing tensions in multinational Yugoslavia. While Arabs and Israelis have exchanged refugees since 1948, the Israelis have settled the Jews from Arab countries but the Arab countries still refuse to settle the Arab refugees living in refugee camps.

With modern media and education, the nation-building process can go much faster in Africa than it did in Europe. This also means that the conflicts and tensions resulting from the process may grow more rapidly than they did in Europe. We have already seen massacres of some 20,000 Tutsi in Rwanda in 1959 and of an estimated 100,000 Hutu in Burundi in 1972. Millions of non-Nigerians have been expelled from Nigeria, hundreds of thousands of non-Ghanaians from Ghana, and tens of thousands of Asians from Tanzania and Uganda. These incidents, using the European pattern as evidence, may be only the beginning of a long list of similar hardships inflicted on minorities and disruptions to economic life that Africa will undergo in the years ahead. It is estimated that there are three to five million Africans who are at present refugees from their countries for political or ethnic reasons.

Even without civil war, expulsion or killing of minorities, stability in governments is rare. There have been seventy-three coups overthrowing governments from 1957 to the end of 1985. In other continents military coups are usually made by the top leaders. In Africa, the leadership of modern military forces is still so new that the habits of discipline are not yet fully ingrained. Consequently, almost any element of the army may decide to take independent action and carry out a coup. Coups have been led by generals, colonels, majors, captains, lieutenants (Ghana—Flight Lieutenant Rawlings), and even by sergeants (Liberia—Sergeant Doe) with a handful of men. Since independence in 1960, Nigeria, Africa's most populous nation, has had six military rulers and only nine years of civilian rule.

There are many motives for the coups: patriotic disgust at perceived mismanagement or corruption, desire for power, ethnic rivalry, ideology, etc. Islam has been a factor since 1966 in Nigeria, beginning with the Ibo coup against northern Moslem domination; its influence continued in the Hausa counter-coup and resulting civil war. The overthrow of the Ethiopian emperor was clearly influenced by the Marxist orientation of the military officers involved. There have been only three cases where a president retired voluntarily from office and in one of these, Cameroon, the retired president, Ahmadou Ahidjo, was subsequently accused of plotting to overthrow his successor.

The impact of insecurity is illustrated by the fact that of the eleven countries that the U.N. Office of Emergency Operations in Africa listed as still needing emergency food aid in 1986, five are presently involved in civil war (Angola, Chad, Ethiopia, Mozambique, Sudan) and five others (Burkina Faso, Cape Verde, Mali, Mauritania, Niger) have been subject to military coups. Only one, Botswana, has been immune to civil war and coups.

The net result of all these different political problems is that most African countries do not have sufficient security, stability, and assurance of equitable justice to encourage citizens or foreigners to invest in producing for the future.

Sociological Problems

The African societies and cultures developed over thousands of years within a context very different from the market-oriented economies of the industrialized West. Because of Africa's large size, its tropical climate, and its geography that until recently isolated sub-Saharan Africa from the rest of the world, it is only since 1900 that influences from the rest of the world have begun to be felt significantly in the area. Some persisting indigenous practices, customs and institutions which in the past were justified and necessary for survival now retard adaptation to new needs and opportunities.

Traditionally, there was no individual land ownership in sub-Saharan Africa. As Julius Nyerere has explained, "To us in Africa land was always recognized as belonging to the community. Each individual within our society had a right to the use of land. . . . But the African's right to land was simply the right to use it; he had no other right to it, nor did it occur to him to try and claim one" (Nyerere, 1968, p. 7).

The position today is complicated, confused and in evolution. In most of the region today there is still no individual ownership of land. Cadastral surveys and individual land titles in most countries do not exist. Customary law, which may vary regionally even within a country, still governs land tenure. Kenya and Zimbabwe are the leading exceptions, but even here individual ownership does not apply to all parts of the country. In some countries, where customary law still rules, depending on evolving practice and the penetration of the cash economy, it has become possible to varying extents to buy and sell certain "rights" to land. Such "rights" relating to a particular piece of land may pertain to cultivation, seasonal or continuous grazing, tree planting, tree produce collecting, or firewood gathering. This is obviously a subject where a great deal of research is needed.

Under these African conditions it is difficult—though not impossible—to achieve better agricultural productivity. Borrowing for improvements such as better implements, improved drainage, or fencing is more difficult and the incentive is weaker without a clear title to land. As discussed above, the consensus adjustment programs all rely on strengthening private incentives of farmers to secure an increase in farm output. This is important, but it must be recognized that the African farming sector is not structured to give private incentives full play. While there are many other factors also involved, it may not be entirely coincidence that the two countries in tropical Africa that do succeed in producing surpluses of food grains in good years are the two countries, Kenya and Zimbabwe, where farmers have individual land tenure.

Another similar societal problem in food and nutrition in tropical Africa arises from the custom in African society that it is the primary responsibility of women to raise the crops to feed the family. The growth of the cash economy has accentuated this problem. Men used to cooperate in some respects, particularly in helping to clear the land. Now, men increasingly devote their labor to working for wages or to growing cash crops. The cash income may be used to buy food to supplement homegrown crops during the hungry season. But as the cash economy has eroded previous habits of communal help, households without men now are much more subject to hunger before the crops come in.

The pattern of division of labor often means that at crucial times of year the nutrition of women and children suffers. When the rainy season comes, particularly in the areas that have a single rainy season, food from the preceding crop is scarce and men are fed first. During this "hungry season" the demands on the energy of the women for cultivating, planting, and weeding are greatest. Even if there is sufficient food, the demands of the seasonal farming labor peak needs leave women little time to gather and carry the firewood, to fetch water, to gather the green leafy vegetables needed to supplement the basic food, to cook, and to feed themselves and their children (Feierman, 1985).

Breastfeeding protects babies from disease and malnutrition. Since breastfeeding takes more time, mothers often disregard advice to breastfeed. Babies are fed from bottles, freeing the mothers to do their other essential work (*Economist*, May 31, 1986). In some areas in Burkina Faso, even though there is plenty of food available after good rains, Gretchen Glode Berggren of Save the Children Fund found that the custom of eating only one meal a day satisfies adults but leads to malnutrition in infants.

The solutions to the overload on mothers are not easy or obvious. Women need to get easier access to water; this will require digging wells, drilling bore holes or piping water to homes or settlements. The development and provision of fuel for cooking to save the time for searching and gathering firewood would also help greatly. But the most important change would be to change the division of labor among the sexes. This type of change may take a generation or two of education and enlightened leadership. Research on this subject is overdue.

The colonial period in sub-Saharan Africa, while relatively brief, still has an enduring impact on many important African institutions and practices. This is too big a subject to touch more than briefly in this paper. For our purposes, only one side of the picture needs to be mentioned. First, the urban bias of African governments (which now has a strong political basis) stems directly from the practice of colonial governments. These governments also left behind the expectation of urban dwellers to have a miniature Welfare State (largely financed by the rural sector): free medical services, free schools, free water, free or subsidized electricity, and subsidized housing. The new African leaders, trained in the modern industrialized countries, faulted the colonial governments only for being insufficiently generous in this regard. The colonial governments were governments of civil or military administrators and technocrats, and as such accustomed to achieve government ends by directive, laws or orders and not by structuring economic incentives. Cotton, for instance, was introduced into some areas of Uganda by simply ordering the local population to plant cotton. The present day African leaders, particularly the soldiers, in large part tend to have the same mind set.

Conclusions

Until recently, solutions for the African food crisis have focused largely on quick measures of providing food relief and on the need for changing short term policies. This was useful and necessary. As rainfall has improved in most places and famine survivors have returned to their home villages, the focus has shifted to the longer-term policies needed.

A meeting of the African heads of state in July 1985 at the annual Organization of African Unity summit meeting in Addis Ababa called attention to the adverse economic factors beyond their control, such as the decline in primary product prices, high interest rates, etc.* They then declared that in the past they had allocated too little domestic resources to "such high priority areas as agriculture, manpower, industry and . . . [too much to] "foreign consumer goods and nonproductive investment projects" (Kitchen, 1986).

Even as governments widely recognize the need for different policies, they find it difficult to grasp the need to change their approach to rural investment. This was evident from the results of the first African Environmental Conference held in Cairo, December 16–18, 1985, at which environment ministers and high ranking officials from forty-one African states were present. The Conference agreed to give priority to establish 150 model self-reliant villages in fifty African countries—that is, three villages per country—and to raise a $55 million fund to finance this plan over the next five years (Mpinga, 1986). In other words, the usual bias for spectacular show-piece investment continued to dominate. The investment needs of Africa are for a large number of small, unspectacular improvements on secondary or tertiary roads over wide areas, the provision of small quantities of inputs to millions of farmers, etc. The results, if favorable, are diffused over a large mass of people; the benefits, because they are hard to identify, do not easily win praise.

In early 1986 the World Bank and the IMF created a joint Structural Adjustment Facility of $3.1 billion to help countries develop three-year policy frameworks to restructure their economies and to start growing again. Governments were urged to streamline their tax systems, reduce the role of state-run ("parastatal") enterprises and reform price policies. Governments were expected to increase farmer incentives by increasing market prices of their crops or the producer prices set by marketing boards. This latter means that the government would give a larger share of the price paid by consumers back to the farmers and reduce the tax revenue of the government accordingly. In many cases it also means reducing the waste and extravagant spending of the marketing boards.

Where appropriate, governments also were to be encouraged to depreciate the exchange rate of their currencies and so encourage export crops by raising their prices. Persistent and large overvaluations of national currencies in a number of countries, coupled with high protection of domestic manufacturing or assembly operations, has shifted the domestic terms of trade against farmers. Government were also advised to discontinue other government interventions which discriminate against farming, such as protection of domestic industries that produce modern inputs (i.e., fertilizer) and explicit export taxes on rural exports.

*See Chapter 2.

Governments were urged to give a higher priority to public investment in research, extension, infrastructure in farming areas, soil conservation, land use planning, and credit to farmers (Stern, 1986; Jaycox, 1986; Schuh, 1986).

By June 1986 most African governments and the international aid community had reached a consensus on the policies that were needed. At the end of the special General Assembly session on the economic crisis in Africa the governments unanimously agreed on a "United Nations Program of Action for African Economic Recovery and Development 1986–1990." It states, "Primary focus will be on women farmers who contribute significantly to agriculture productivity."

The program declares:

> The main objective will be to give new impetus to agricultural development through:
>
> Raising substantially the level of investment in agriculture;
>
> Restoring, protecting and developing arable land and rendering it more productive;
>
> Establishing remunerative produce pricing policies, strengthening incentive schemes, and providing effective agriculture credit programs;
>
> Promoting reforestation;
>
> Putting in drought and desertification control programs.

The program also supports the rehabilitation and development of agro-related industries, the development of transport and communications, the improvement of distribution channels for domestic trade, favoring domestic goods over imports through price incentives. It specifically calls attention to the "pivotal role of women" in the production of food. It also calls on each African country to have a population policy that addresses "issues of high fertility and mortality, rapid urbanization and the protection of the environment." The Organization of African Unity estimated the cost of carrying out the program was around $128 billion over five years. It would require some $45 billion in external capital net of external debt service (now running at around $15 billion a year).

The World Bank is calling on the international community to provide around $11 billion a year in *concessional* aid to help finance the international payments and the adjustment policies to be undertaken by the poorest twenty-nine African countries. Bilateral concessional assistance to these countries is currently being disbursed at the annual rate of $8.5 billion, and the multilateral institutions hope to provide around $1 billion. The Bank calculated (1986) that this still leaves a gap of $1.5 billion to be filled from additional concessional aid by the donor nations.

Other sources of capital are needed to provide another $2 billion a year, of which $1 billion is hoped to come from commercial banks. Middle-income African countries are expected to need $7–10 billion a year (World Bank, 1986; *Economist*, June 7, 1986).

The program clearly recognizes most of the changes or "adjustments" in government policies that need to be made. The prescribed adjustment policies would reverse the past tilt towards urban populations. This implies that the decision makers will have to make sacrifices themselves as well as impose them on others—this may involve real political risks. If nothing is done to compensate for a shift in resources to the farmers, urban workers may not remain passive while their low standard of living is cut. If, however, raising food prices is accompanied by sufficient external aid to increase imports to restore local manufactures and to produce additional food supplies to maintain most of the real wage level, then the adjustment policies may succeed without riots, strikes or even new coups.

Some of the African governments have already acted on the prescriptions. Kenya, Nigeria, Zambia, and Zimbabwe have increased farm prices toward market levels and seen large increases in food produced. Ghana, Ivory Coast, Zambia and Zaire have allowed their foreign exchange rates to depreciate to better align their domestic price levels with the world market (Kitchen, 1986). Other countries like Mauritius, Malawi, Madagascar, Niger, Mali, Senegal and Mauritania have also taken various adjustment measures (Tillier, 1986).

While the African governments have problems in confronting the political costs of the consensus prescription, the donor governments have been reluctant to consider another part of the prescription. The external debts of the sub-Saharan African countries are estimated to have been between $90 and $125 billion at the end of 1985. The ratio of debt service to export earnings is at around an unsustainable 35 percent and amounts to around $15 billion a year (*Economist*, June 7, 1986). In accordance with the spirit of the times, much of the prescription advanced to the African governments can be summarized as advice to "rely on the market." The prescription quite properly insists on the importance of market discipline in Africa for promoting better allocation of resources and in encouraging output. On the other hand, it omits any suggestion that market considerations should enter into the treatment of the African external debts. During the 1970s there were many instances of bankers who pressed loans on Africans with little or no attention to creditworthiness or economic justification. There is no justification to grant immunity from the "discipline of the market" to bad banking decisions.

The prescriptions which are being advanced for Africa are undoubtedly useful; if carried out successfully, they should help improve food output and nutrition. Advice to get the economic incentives right is always useful and necessary. Better market adjustment policies, in addition to providing a short-term gain, create a more favorable reception to a flow of new productive technology as such technology is developed and the political and sociological environment improves.

The adjustment policy reforms are essentially agreed on by all the main actors concerned. With global economic recovery and an improvement in Africa's terms of trade the adjustment policies should result in a quick recovery in African agricultural productivity. The U.N. program goes beyond short-term measures designed to reduce current balance of payments deficits to policies and investments that would re-start or accelerate growth in Africa. If the program is substantially carried out it should provide a basis on which economic growth can resume. It should help to improve the quality of investment and expenditures in agriculture and the rest of the economy. In the longer term, the special African climatic, medical, political and sociological problems that were sketched above are severe obstacles to rapid progress on an agricultural growth path. These are, and can only be, partly addressed by a Program covering the next five years. It is in these areas that external help and initiatives in research could be most helpful.

References

Berg, Elliott. "The Potentials of the Private Sector in Sub-Saharan Africa," in Tore Rose, ed., *Crisis and Recovery in Sub-Saharan Africa*. Paris: Development Centre of the Organisation for Economic Co-operation and Development, 1985.

Ceres. "New Cropping System Reveals Promise for Low-Input Farming." *Ceres* (Food and Agriculture Organization) 19:1 (Jan.-Feb. 1986): 109.

Eagleburger, Lawrence S., and Donald F. McHenry, co-chairmen. *Compact for African Development*, Report of the Committee on African Development Strategies, a Joint Project of the Council on Foreign Relations and the Overseas Development Council. New York and Washington, 1985.

The Economist. "After the Ball, A Survey of Nigeria," *The Economist* 299:7448 (May 3, 1986): after p. 62.

———. "Primary Health Care Is Not Curing Africa's Ills," *The Economist* 299:7448 (May 31, 1986): 91–94.

———. "How Much Africa Needs," *The Economist* 299:7449 (June 7, 1986): 81.

Faber, Mike, and Reginald Herbold Green. "Sub-Saharan Africa's Economic Malaise: Some Questions and Answers," in Tore Rose, ed., *Crisis and Recovery in Sub-Saharan Africa*. Paris: Development Centre of the Organisation for Economic Co-operation and Development, 1985.

Feierman, Steven. "Struggles for Control: The Social Roots of Health and Healing in Modern Africa," *African Studies Review* 28:2/3 (June-September 1985): 73–148.

Gillett, J. D. "Direct and Indirect Influences of Temperature on the Transmission of Parasites from Insects to Man," in Angela E. R. Taylor and R. Muller, eds., *The Effects of Meteorological Factors upon Parasites*, Symposia of the British Society for Parasitology, Vol. 12. Oxford, London, Edinburgh, and Melbourne: Blackwell Scientific Publications, 1974.

Harvard Medical School, Department of Continuing Education. "Malaria," *The Harvard Medical School Health Letter* 11:3 (January 1986): 5–7.

Jaycox, Edward V. K. "Africa's Environmental Challenges and The World Bank's Response," *Finance & Development* 23:1 (March 1986): 21–22.

Kamarck, Andrew M. *Economics and the Real World*. Oxford: Basil Blackwell, and Philadelphia: University of Pennsylvania Press, 1983.

————. "The Resources of Tropical Africa," *Daedalus*, Journal of the American Academy of Arts and Sciences 111:2 (Spring 1982): 149–164.

————. *The Tropics and Economic Development*. Baltimore and London: Johns Hopkins University Press for The World Bank, 1976.

Kitchen, Helen. "Africa: Year of Ironies," *Foreign Affairs* 64:3 (1986): 562–582.

Leff, Nathaniel H. "Optimal Investment Choice for Developing Countries," *Journal of Development Economics* 18 (1985): 335–360. North-Holland.

Lipton, Michael. *Why Poor People Stay Poor*. Cambridge, MA: Harvard University Press, 1977.

Mitchell, Donald O. "Trends in Grain Consumption in the Developing World, 1960–80," *Finance and Development*, IMF and World Bank, 22:4 (December 1985): 12–13.

Mpinga, James. "To Renew the African Environment," *Development Forum* 14:2 (March 1986): 1, 10.

Nawaz, Shuja. "Riverblindness Controlled," *Finance and Development*, IMF and World Bank, 23:2 (June 1986): 32–34.

Nyerere, Julius K. *Ujmaa, Essays on Socialism*. Dar es Salaam, Nairobi, London, and New York: Oxford University Press, 1968.

Peterzell, Jay. "Angola: Reagan's Covert Action Policy VI," *First Principles* 2:3. Washington: Center for National Security Studies (January-February 1986): 1–10.

Reutlinger, Shlomo. "Food Security and Poverty in LDCs," *Finance and Development*, . IMF and World Bank, 22:4 (December 1985): 7–11.

Roemer, Michael. "African Economic Development in Africa: Performance since Independence, and a Strategy for the Future," *Daedalus* 111:2 (Spring 1982): 123–148.

Rose, Tore, ed. *Crisis and Recovery in Sub-Saharan Africa*. Paris: Development Centre of the Organisation for Economic Co-operation and Recovery, 1985.

Schuh, G. Edward. "Agricultural Policy Reform is High on the Bank's Agenda," *The Bank's World* 5:2 (February 1986): 13–14.

Stern, Ernest. "Africa: The World's Greatest Development Challenge," Remarks to Development Assistance Committee, *The Bank's World* 5:1 (January 1986): 11–12.

Tillier, Ellen. "Wanted for Africa: Funds to Boost Reforms, An Interview with Ramgopal Agarwala," *Bank's World* 5:4 (April 1986): 2–5.

United Nations. *World Population and Prospects*. New York: United Nations, 1985.

U.S. Department of State, Bureau of Public Affairs. "The Horn of Africa: U.S. Policy," *Gist* (February 1986): 1–2.

———. *Sub-Saharan Africa and the United States,* Discussion Paper. Washington, D.C.: U.S. Government Printing Office, Publication 9112, rev. December 1985.

World Bank. *Toward Sustained Development in Sub-Saharan Africa.* Washington, D.C.: World Bank, 1984.

———. *Financing Adjustment with Growth in Sub-Saharan Africa.* Washington, D.C.: World Bank, 1986.

9

Epidemiology of Hunger in Africa

Takateru Ohse

The causes of hunger in Africa—or in any other lesser developed area—are complex and intertwined. Much of the region's population is chronically hungry, and famines also occur. The causes of hunger are often compounded by the strategies and policies intended to solve them—and by demographic shifts and changes in cultivation patterns which occur in response to hunger.

In brief, a hunger disaster is caused by:

1. unavoidable climatic conditions, drought or flood
2. movement of people because of war, political instability or social unrest
3. mismanagement of the government in relief operations
4. weaknesses in domestic communication and transportation
5. agricultural policy priorities focusing on cash crops, with consequent neglect of food crop farming
6. quick deterioration of soil fertility in the tropical climate
7. desertification by uncontrolled population pressure

This chapter examines the interrelationships between the causes of famines and chronic hunger. It begins by describing the African ecosystem and factors, including diseases, that contribute to hunger. Then, sociological and political responses to the problem are analyzed and their interrelationships, as well as their effect on hunger, are examined. Based on this understanding of the epidemiology of hunger, suggestions

223

are offered to increase crop production without the negative effects of many other agricultural development strategies.

Bio-mass Production of the Environmental Ecosystem in Africa

Characteristics of Climate

Studies on the changes in climate of the African continent reveal two kinds of cycles: a long cycle and a short cycle. Long cycles of dry and rainy weather last tens of thousands of years. Approximately 180,000–200,000 years ago, a rainy period ended and was followed by a dry period. This lasted until the next rainy period, which began 60,000 years ago. A dry period followed, continuing until the next rainy period some 25,000 years ago. At the ice age 20,000 years ago the southern boundary of the Sahara was 480 km south of its present section. 10,000–5,000 years ago, there was another rainy period, after which the climate became drier; it has remained so to the present date. A second type of climatic cycle, lasting approximately eleven years, is related to the sunmacula. Measurement of water levels behind the Aswan High Dam of the Nile River recorded the lowest levels in 1973 (after the drought) and in 1984 (after the drought of 1980–1983). With our present scientific capabilities we cannot control or modify either type of change—the long cycle or the short cycle. The next low level of water of the Nile River is expected to occur in 1995 after a drought from 1991–1994.

As shown in Figure 9.1, the level of rainfall is not homogeneous throughout the continent. The magnitude of biomass production is greatest in the tropical rainforest area, where the annual precipitation is over 2200 mm, and the phytobiomass production decreases with the decrease of the rainfall. The area with an annual rainfall of less than 200 mm is almost a desert and its phytobiomass production is negligible.

Balance of Production and Consumption

The most primitive type of life, existing in a natural state without any modification of the ecosystem, is seen in the life of those groups of people who are hunter-gatherers. The Mbti Pygmy of the Ituri Forest of Zaire live in a tropical rainforest composed mainly of *Cynometra alexandrii, Brachystegia laurentii* and *Gilbertiodendron deweveii* trees and wild plants of approximately seventy-eight different kinds. One square kilometer of forest feeds 0.4 inhabitants. The main sources of food are gathering from plants (70 percent) and hunting animals (30 percent).

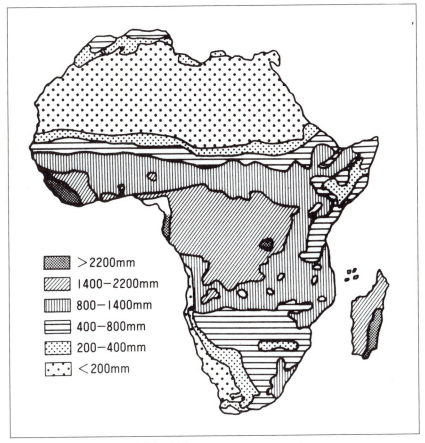

Figure 9.1. *Annual rainfall in Africa.*

The Bushmen in the Kalahari desert and savanna—which have Miombò flora—are also a hunting-gathering group. Their population density is 0.05–0.12/km^2; their sources of food are approximately 70 percent from plants and 30 percent from hunting animals.

These hunter-gatherers are omnivorous and never try to modify their environmental ecosystem. They neither cultivate plants nor graze animals. In general, the biomass production is ten times greater in the rainforest than in the arid savanna. The consumption of these two groups of hunter-gatherers is below the level of recycling of the environmental ecosystem and hence they do not damage the environmental balance. These small groups of people, however, will be gradually absorbed by the neighboring farmer-pasturalis tribes as the general population pressure becomes more intense.

Obstacles to Food Production

The Impact of Certain Endemic Diseases

Food production by means of agriculture requires water. At the present time, agricultural production is being carried out in areas where the natural rainfall is sufficient for the growth of crop plants. In these farming and grazing areas, certain water-associated endemic diseases such as malaria, schistosomiasis, trypanosomiasis and onchocerciasis impede the production of food crops and livestock farming.

In sub-Saharan Africa, a population of 370 million live in an area with malaria; every year, 100–150 million cases of malaria occur, and one million deaths of children under five years are reported. This disease

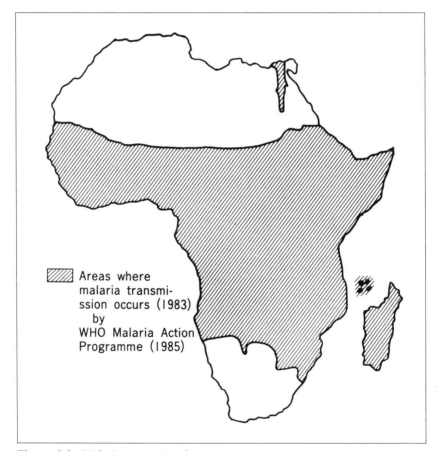

Areas where malaria transmission occurs (1983) by WHO Malaria Action Programme (1985)

Figure 9.2. *Malarious areas in Africa.*

greatly reduces the productive strength of workers (Figure 9.2). The most powerful vector mosquitos, *Anopheles gambiae* complex (*An. gambiae gambiae, An. arabiensis, An. melas, An. merus*) and *An. funestus*, are the greatest enemy.

Schistosoma mansoni and Schist. haematobium are endemic and becoming more highly endemic where new irrigation schemes are developing (Figures 9.3 and 9.4) as a result of the increase of breeding waters for vector snails.

African Trypanosomiasis, or sleeping sickness, is another enemy of nutrition. Figure 9.5 shows the Tsetse fly belt on the continent, covering an area of 10 million square kilometers—including most of the agricultural area of the continent. Thirty species of Glossina flies infest 37 percent of Africa in thirty-eight countries. This disease was once a

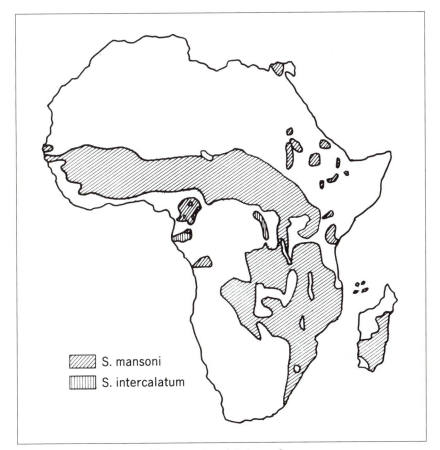

Figure 9.3. *Distribution of S. mansoni and S. intercalatum.*

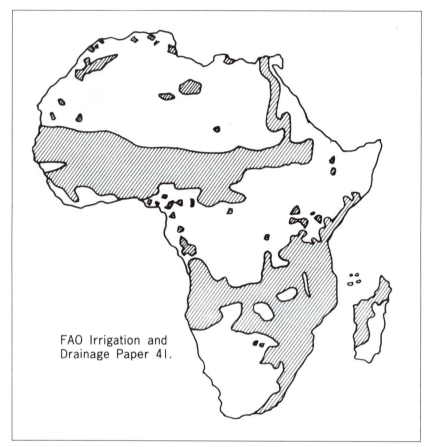

FAO Irrigation and Drainage Paper 41.

Figure 9.4. *Distribution of S. haematobium.*

dreaded human killer: even now, 45 million people are at risk, in East Africa by *Trypanosoma rhodesiense* and in West Africa by *Trypanosoma gambiense*. The control of human trypanosomiasis is progressing by means of newly developed conical traps which are impregnated with residual insecticides and by the application of Suramin and anti-di-fluoromethylornithine for treatment of patients (Figure 9.6).

Animal trypanosomiasis is a more serious and grave public health problem particularly in regard to nutrition. Domestic animals such as cattle, horse, sheep, goats, pigs, camels, dogs and cats are all vulnerable to trypanosomiasis. Within the tsetse fly belt, the supply of animal protein is extremely limited. At present, 20 million cattle are grazed in Africa; however, if the vector tsetse flies could be controlled, 120 million cattle could be raised and the supply of beef and milk would be greatly

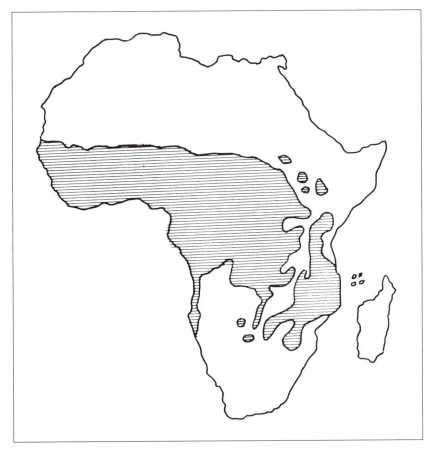

Figure 9.5. *Tsetse fly belt.*

increased. The existence of animal trypanosomiasis also restricts the use of animals in agriculture, limiting traditional farming practices such as horse-drawn plowing. To avoid this problem, the use of trypanotolerant N'Dama cattle in the Gambia is now under study.

Onchocerciasis (river blindness) is a kind of filariasis caused by the infection of *Onchocerca volvulus* and transmitted by black flies (*Simulium damnosum*) (Figure 9.7). In West African countries, people fearing loss of eyesight left the most fertile agricultural land and moved to less productive savanna areas where they are now starving. In 1974, the Volta River Basin Project (World Bank/UNDP/WHO) started to fight this disease. In Benin, Burkina Faso, Ghana, Côte d'Ivoire, Mali, Niger and Togo, helicopters and small planes are used for aerial insecticide spraying. Although this is a very expensive operation, it has been suc-

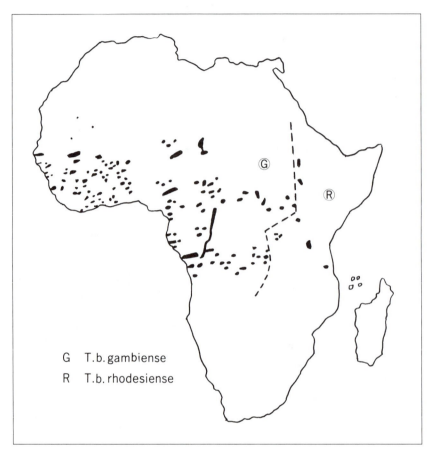

Figure 9.6. *African human trypanosomiasis: distribution of foci.*

cessful in freeing a large area from this disease. The population has resettled and agricultural development is going on. The neighboring area, including Guinea, Guinea Bissau, Sierra Leone, Senegal, West Mali, Benin and South Togo, will be the next target. This area has 30 million cases of river blindness and an at-risk population of 900 million. In several years, the area will be cleared from the danger of river blindness, and the most fertile parts of these countries will become the main productive areas for agriculture.

Causes of Desertification of Ecologically Fragile Arid Areas

In the rainforest area, in spite of the poorness of the soil, an equilibrium is maintained by the recycling of dead plants and fallen leaves. If land

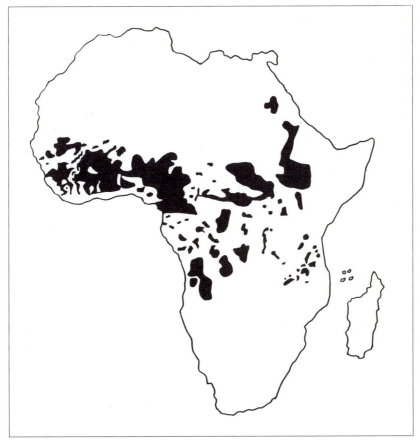

Figure 9.7. *Geographical distribution of onchocerciasis.*

cultivation begins, however, the natural vegetation is cleared away, the sources of organic materials are lost, and the fertility of the soil is depleted after only a few years of crop cultivation. Therefore, the farmers are forced to develop a shifting pattern of cultivation with a long fallow period in order to restore soil fertility. As long as the land is big enough to absorb a certain size of population, the farmers can practice this type of farming, restoring soil fertility by recycling during the fallow period.

As a result of their increases in population, many African countries have felt the threat of population pressure. Even in areas with favorable rainfall, forests are disappearing, resulting in damage in soil fertility, loss of water retention capacity, erosion of thin surface soil, and irreversible desertification.

The severity of the ecological conditions necessitates the system of shifting cultivation with a long fallow period to recover the fertility of the soil. But the increasing population pressure has meant that the fallow period has been shortened, with the result that there is insufficient time for the ecologically fragile marginal land to recover its fertility. It is now known that if the population density per square km exceeds twenty-five the natural ecosystem is under stress, and if it reaches thirty-five per square km, the agricultural system is in danger of desertification. Several countries in dry areas of Africa have already reached this dangerous level.

At present the Sudan-Sahel region is already overburdened with cattle far beyond the level of recycling of biomass production. The overgrazing of animals effectively destroys the vegetative layer, not only because animals devour the foliage of the trees and the grass, but also because they trample heavily on the ground, resulting in its compaction. The area becomes a desert. Recent experience suggests that a cycle of two years of cultivation followed by a three-year fallow period will allow the soil to recover its fertility—if the farmer does not burn grass or graze animals during this period. It is suggested that with the use of specially chosen plants, which can be green manure, the fallow period can be reduced by one year. If this were successfully implemented, the pressure of land shortage would be alleviated.

The practice of cutting trees for fuel wood also accelerates the desertification in certain areas.

Farming practices in Zambia illustrate some of these issues in an ecologically fragile arid area. In Zambia, people tend to plant cash crops. Apart from a relatively small number of maize farmers, cultivation in Zambia is still carried out by shifting cultivation using traditional slash-and-burn techniques called "Chitemene." The country's basic food crops—cassava, millet, sorghum, groundnuts, pumpkins, sweet potatoes and beans—grow well in poor forest soils with variable rainfall. The Chitemene system needs a large area to sustain it. (This system is used by a million people in the north and west of Zambia.) Cultivated areas remain fertile for about six years, when additional land must be cleared to allow the original soil a fallow period of five to twenty years.

To clear new land, or to re-clear land which has had sufficient fallow period, men climb trees up to twelve meters high and axe all the branches. Once the branches fall to the ground, the women and children heap them, using a sophisticated stacking system. The burning products a nutrient-rich ash which is then spread evenly over a proportion of the clearing.

Maize, now growing in popularity, was never the principal subsistence crop of Zambians. But the first colonial administrators, then foreign advisers, encouraged maize farming. They ignored women farmers and placed control of the crops in the hands of men.

Women perform all the tasks involved in the cultivation and processing (grinding, shelling, drying) of food. The rural depopulation is now serious, and there are not enough hands for harvesting.

One-third of Zambia's rural households are headed by women. They do not produce any maize for sale, and many are not visited by the government's agricultural extension workers. At any rate, these extension workers often cannot offer women useful advice, because they have little knowledge of traditional crops and do not consider women real farmers.

The particular hybrid maize, SR52 (known as high-yielding hybrid), which has been introduced in Zambia requires a long growing season. It is more sensitive to smaller environmental fluctuations (in soil type, temperature, rainfall, fertilizer and weeding) than the traditional maize. By encouraging only SR52, the government has reduced the flexibility of farmers to respond to drought. The methods of agriculture traditionally used by women, the cultivation of a number of different crops, ensured that, whatever the weather, some crops would survive. It also ensured that fragile soils were not overworked.

The International Union for Conservation of Nature and Natural Resources (IUCN) has observed that present yields and hoped-for increases in production can only be sustained if essential ecological processes like soil regeneration and nutrient recycling are maintained. Future increases in production may also depend on preserving genetic diversity locally for breeding purposes. The Chitemene system may be the only way in which much of Zambia's thin forest soil can be made to produce an adequate living for its farmers.

Another example is the Sudan. The introduction of boreholes is creating a serious problem. In the 1960s the Sudanese Government launched an ambitious project called "freedom from thirst," drilling hundreds of boreholes in semi-arid areas. In turn, herdsmen were able to increase the size of their herds, which soon destroyed the local vegetation and facilitated the advance of the desert.

The tendency to allow political considerations to override economic and environmental considerations has been observed. The Jonglei Project, which intended to siphon water from the south to the drier lands of the north at a cost of millions of dollars, was never completed and was eventually abandoned.

Sudan is one of five countries out of the forty-one in sub-Saharan Africa whose food production exceeds consumption. It has great potential for further agricultural development and is expected to become a bread-basket for the Arab world. FAO predicts that this year's harvest will be 4.6 million tons, exceeding the national consumption of 3.4 million tons. Farmers in the Kassala area are obliged to feed their camels with harvested grain because nobody buys the surplus grain that is produced. On the other hand, the government and aid agencies must move the grain from the surplus area to the five million people in the dry Darfur, Kardofan and Red Sea Provinces before the rains begin and large areas become impassable. The World Food Programme has given U.S. $5.8 million to buy 20,000 tons of local grain and to make an unusual payment for domestic transport. This unusually favorable contribution, however, can only provide enough for less than half a million people to survive for three to four months. Therefore, relief agencies have appealed to the United States and other countries for an extra U.S. $16 million in order to purchase food and another U.S. $33 million for domestic transport. These efforts, however, do not always go entirely according to plan. The merchants in the Sudan are a big political power and have been known to raise food prices during relief operations. This makes the merchants richer and reduces the amount of food purchased for their poor countrymen.

What should be the remedial treatment for this sick agricultural giant? The history of Sudanese agriculture illustrates that the government, particularly the Niemeri Regime, gave priority to the development of big projects for cash crop production, with little attention to small farmers and food crops. The gigantic Kenana plant complex for sugar and the ambitious Jonglei Canal program have both failed, leaving costly lessons of experience. Projects aimed at maximizing quick cash returns should not be repeated. By contrast, the Blue Nile Project (BNP), the biggest single agricultural program in the world, is still operating. It consists of large scale irrigation and small plats tenant farming. The BNP produces 85 percent of the national agricultural output and earns 65 percent of foreign currencies, in spite of the drastic fall of the price of cotton in the 1985 international market. The BNP is considered to be the foundation of the Sudanese economy. The present vulnerability to fluctuation in prices of cash crops is destroying the national agriculture budget, which should be available for remedial action against hunger. The new government's strategy for agriculture is sincerely awaited.

In the Sudan, in the area north of 14° N, the annual rain precipitation is less than 400 mm, and hence farming without irrigation is impossible. In the area of 14° N–9° N, the rain-fed cultivation of millet and sorghum is possible without irrigation. In the White Nile flood plain, south of 9° N, rain-fed cultivation of sorghum and millet is possible and the combined cultivation of roots and tubers will enable extensive cattle farming. In the area north of 14° N, the BNP type scheme will be the most appropriate form of agriculture and can serve as a model for other countries with arid conditions.

The British left behind an extensive railway network (5,500 km, although single-track) which links almost all the major urban centers. However, miserable weaknesses in its capacity and reliability were exposed during the recent national and international hunger relief efforts, when the poor maintenance of the railway, the difficulty in obtaining spare parts and the excessive power of the workers' union became evident. The rehabilitation and strengthening of this national railway, with financial and technical cooperation and international, multilateral and bilateral assistance, must be a key element of relief activities against hunger.

The country's storehouse facilities network needs to be strengthened. Localized hunger problems could be alleviated by using the national budget to purchase and store surplus harvests and to establish a short term credit system for farmers.

Suggestions for the Future

As Figure 9.8 and Table 9.1 illustrate, Africa needs to increase crop production by agricultural development.

In the areas of high rainfall, the application of more appropriate technology, the placement of higher priority on food crops than on cash crops, and the control of impeding endemic diseases will certainly increase production considerably. Soil conservation must also be maintained carefully. The size of the area with favorable rainfall is limited, however, as indicated in Figure 9.2, and the development of this humid area will soon reach full capacity.

Concurrently, most African countries are showing very high rates of population growth. The time to expand the arable land to the dry areas has arrived; this is the only possible choice. The construction of dams, elevation of water levels, the creation of artificial lakes and ponds for water reservoirs, and the eventual establishment of large and small scale irrigation schemes are necessary conditions for the development of agriculture.

In humid areas, water-associated endemic diseases are well recognized as impediments to socioeconomic development. However, the problem of water-associated endemic diseases is often forgotten or overlooked in areas where irrigation schemes have been undertaken for agricultural development. These areas were originally too dry to breed vectors of these diseases, were altogether free from these diseases, or were of such low endemicity that they were not considered a serious public health problem. Irrigation schemes, however, increased disease problems in these areas. The BNP's irrigation scheme is an excellent example. The area irrigated was originally a desert, with no schistosomiasis and a very

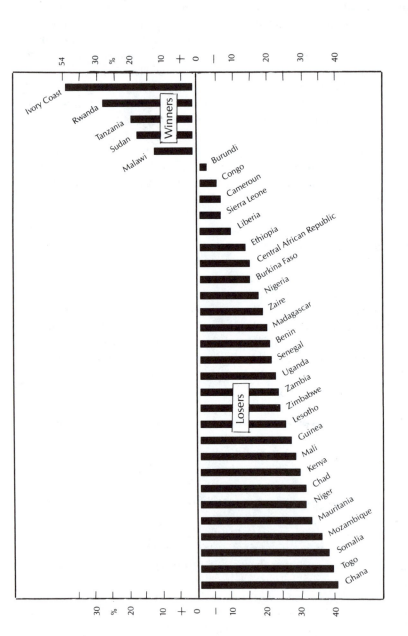
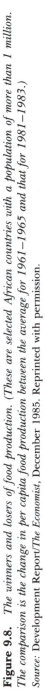

Figure 9.8. *The winners and losers of food production. (These are selected African countries with a population of more than 1 million. The comparison is the change in per capita food production between the average for 1961–1965 and that for 1981–1983.)*
Source: Development Report/*The Economist*, December 1985. Reprinted with permission.

low incidence of seasonal malaria occurring only in the rainy season. Both were insignificant public health concerns. However, the water surfaces created by the irrigation network became favorable breeding sites of vector anophelines and snails. During the harvest season of 1978–1979, holoendemic malaria and a high incidence of schistosomiasis paralyzed the workforce, causing a loss of millions of dollars. All formerly dry and safe areas which are irrigated risk becoming areas of manmade malaria and/or manmade schistosomiasis. Control measures should be included in the design stages, as prevention is the cheapest means of control.

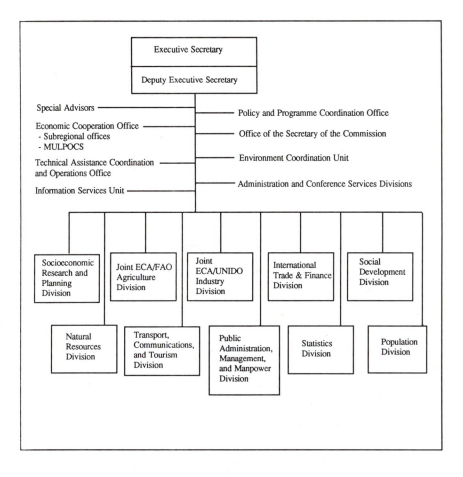

Figure 9.9. *Organization chart of the Economic Commission for Africa.*

African Regional Center for Research and Development of Coarse Grains, Pulses, Roots and Tuber Crops

Up to now the available data and information on coarse grains, pulses, roots and tuber crops in Africa have been scarce and scattered. Given the serious problems of chronic food shortages and malnutrition in this continent, it is highly recommended that an "African Regional Center for Research and Development of Coarse Grains, Pulses, Roots and Tuber Crops" be established in order to develop solutions for these problems. The Center should be established in conjunction with the United Nations Economic Commission for Africa (ECA) and with the political support of the Organization of African Unity (OAU).

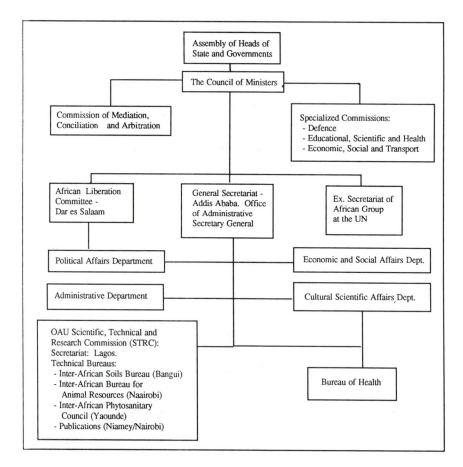

Figure 9.10. *Organization of African Unity.*

The Center should improve and develop high-yielding and dryness-tolerant varieties of maize, sorghum, millet, groundnut, pigeonpea, chickpea, blackgram, soyabean, greengram, cassava, enset (pseudo-banana), sweet potato, arrowroot, yam and Taro. The production, stock and distribution of seeds of such improved varieties, the application of fertilizer and the chemical and biological control of pests for each crop should be the main services of the Center. An outline for the statute of the Center has been drafted.

The Center and its network of the ECA would unify the research, development, information exchange and monitoring efforts at the regional and sub-regional levels, supplementing the national efforts of the Member States rather than competing with them. The activities would include the preparation of inventories of known technology,

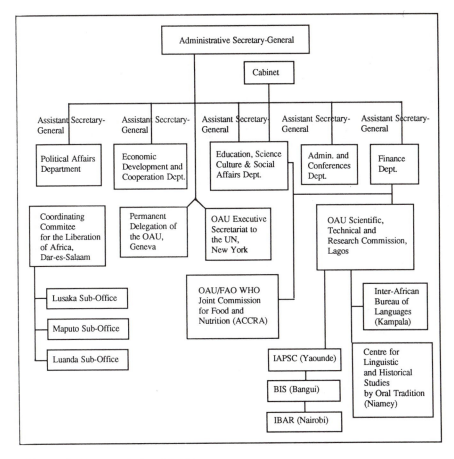

Figure 9.11. *Secretariat of OAU.*

followed by field tests, transfer and adoption, through a Technical Cooperation among Developing Countries (TCDC) approach. The socioeconomic component would be handled by ECA. ECA has Multinational Programming and Operational Centers (MULPOCs). Documentation would be carried out through the network of ECA (Figure 9.9). (The structure of the OAU is shown in Figures 9.10 and 9.11.)

10

Towards Basic Human Needs in Relation to Public Health and Nutrition

Yukio Kaneko and Koh'ichi Nidaira

Notwithstanding the impressive world economic development that has been achieved over the past quarter of a century, some 800 million people remain in absolute poverty, malnutrition, disease, high infant mortality, and low life expectancy. Their poverty has tended to cut them off from economic progress—they have remained outside the benefits of development.

To reduce absolute poverty it is critical to provide essential public services, particularly improved primary health care, clean water, and better nutrition. Domestic economic growth, of course, is needed to achieve this. But economic growth alone may not suffice; it often does not go as far towards helping the poor in the underdeveloped world as it does in the developed world.

In this situation the goal for governments in underdeveloped countries is to meet so-called basic human needs. Since the end of the 1970s the World Bank has conducted the following types of studies in this area (Burki and ul Haq, 1980):

General studies to explore the concept of basic human needs

Country and cross-country studies to determine the dimensions of basic needs and to review a range of policy interventions to improve the situation

*The authors would like to thank the editor of the symposium for his many helpful comments on the earlier version of the paper.

Sector studies to analyze the implications of meeting basic human needs in key sectors, such as nutrition, education, health, shelter and water supply, and sanitation

The conclusions obtained by these World Bank studies can be summarized as follows:

The only way that absolute poverty can be eliminated is by increasing the productivity of the poor.

To increase economic productivity, the contribution of such public goods as education, health care, and water supply are essential.

Expansion and redistribution of public goods are essential if basic human needs are to be met.

It may take a long time to increase the productivity of the absolute poor to a minimum level of satisfaction of their basic human needs.

In this paper we would like to discuss the present situation with regard to economic and social development, the interrelationship between these two areas, and the background and significance of the new international development strategy of Basic Human Needs (BHN) in relation to public health and nutrition in the underdeveloped world.

Economic and Social Indicators

Although the actual goods and services that would meet basic human needs differ from one country to another, it is commonly recognized that they should include nutrition, education, health, water and sanitation, and shelter. To clarify the present situation of social development in underdeveloped and developing countries, Khan and Zerby (1983), used the Wroclaw Taxonomic Method that was developed in the early fifties by a group of Polish mathematicians,[1] as well as quantitative economic indicators, to formulate quantitative social indicators representing six social categories: demography, health and nutrition, education, housing, culture, and political stability. They proposed a single index Measure of Development (MD), which they defined so that its values range between zero and one. According to their definition, the closer the value of MD is to zero, the more developed the country, and the closer to one, the less developed the country.

Using rankings of economic and social indicators that they calculated among ninety-seven countries for the year 1974–1975 and plotting a graph showing social indicators on the horizontal axis and economic indicators on the vertical axis, the position of development of these ninety-seven countries can be shown (See Figure 10.1).

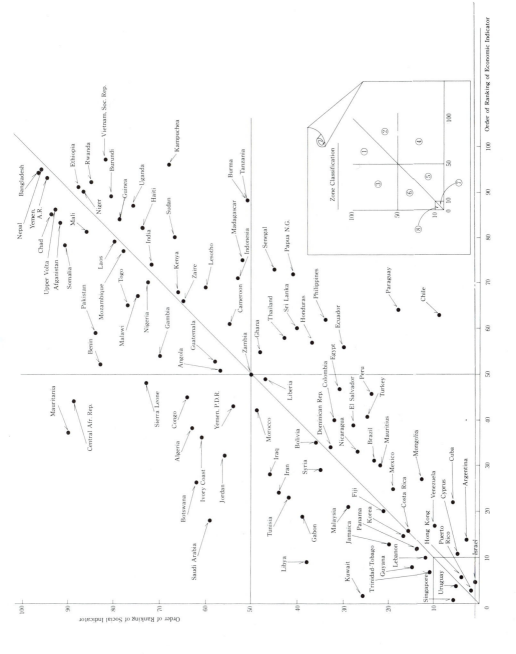

Figure 10.1. *Position of social and economic development.*
Based on Khan and Zerby, 1983.

These countries can be classified into eight groups, according to their present situation of social and economic development, as is shown in "Zone classification" in Figure 10.1.

Namely,

Group 1. Socio: seriously less developed; economic: less developed

Africa (11): Chad, Mali, Upper Volta, Somalia, Mozambique, Benin, Togo, Malawi, Nigeria, Gambia, Angola

Asia (5): Bangladesh, Nepal, Afghanistan, Pakistan, Laos

Middle East (1): Yemen Arab Republic

Caribbean (1): Guatemala

Group 2. Socio: less developed; economic: seriously less developed

Africa (13): Ethiopia, Rwanda, Niger, Burundi, Guinea, Uganda, Sudan, Kenya, Zaire, Lesotho, Madagascar, Tanzania, Cameroon

Asia (5): Vietnam Socialist Republic, Kampuchea, India, Burma, Indonesia

Caribbean (1): Haiti

Group 3. Socio: less developed; economic: developing

Africa (7): Mauritania, Central Afr. Rep., Sierra Leone, Congo, Algeria, Botswana, Ivory Coast.

Middle East (3): Saudi Arabia, Jordan, Yemen P.D.R.

Group 4. Socio: developing; economic: less development

Africa (2): Ghana, Senegal

Asia and Pacific (4): Thailand, Sri Lanka, Philippines, Papua N.G.

Latin America and Caribbean (4): Paraguay, Chile, Ecuador, Honduras

Group 5. Socio: developing; economic: less developing

Africa (4): Zambia, Liberia, Mauritius, Egypt

Middle East (1): Turkey

Asia (2): Cyprus, Mongolia

Latin America & Caribbean (11): Colombia, Peru, Brazil, Mexico, Costa Rica, Dominican Rep., Nicaragua, El Salvador, Venezuela, Argentina, Cuba

Group 6. Socio: less developed; economic: developing

Africa (4): Morocco, Tunisia, Libya, Gabon

Middle East (5): Iraq, Iran, Syria, Kuwait, Lebanon

Asia and Pacific (3): Malaysia, Korea, Fiji

Latin America & Caribbean (5): Bolivia, Jamaica, Panama, Trinidad-Tobago, Guyana

Group 7. Socio: developing; economic: moderate development

Asia (1): Hong Kong

Middle East (1): Israel

Latin America (1): Puerto Rico

Group 8. Socio: moderate development; economic: developing

Asia (1): Singapore

Latin America (1): Uruguay

Table 10.1 presents the number of countries which belongs to each development group by major regional area.

As shown in Table 10.1, thirty-one countries among forty-one in Africa, i.e., 76 percent of African countries, belong to Groups 1, 2 and 3. In the countries in these groups, the condition of life is poor: malnutrition, low life expectancy and high infant mortality are the consequence of a lack of supplies of public goods and services to meet basic human needs. The absolute poor have been cut off from the economic progress that has taken place elsewhere in their countries. Having remained outside successful development efforts, they have not been able to contribute much to it or to benefit fairly from it.

On the other hand, eighteen of twenty-four countries in Latin America—75 percent of Latin American countries—and seven of twenty-one countries in Asia and Pacific—33 percent of Asian and Pacific countries—belong to groups 5, 6, 7 and 8. These countries have made impressive progress in their levels of economic performance and fulfillment of social needs by benefitting from the recent economic recoveries in the United States and Japan and the beginning of recovery elsewhere in the industrial world.

Table 10.1
Taxonomy of the Current Levels of Development,
by Major Regional Areas

Development Group	Africa	Latin America and Caribbean	Asia and the Pacific	Middle East	Total
Group 1	11	1	5	1	18
Group 2	13	1	5	0	19
Group 3	7	0	0	3	10
Group 4	2	4	4	0	10
Group 5	4	11	2	1	18
Group 6	4	5	3	5	17
Group 7	0	1	1	1	3
Group 8	0	1	1	0	2
Total	41	24	21	11	

Source: Figure 10.1 (p. 241).

Economic Development Versus Public Health

The studies carried out under the auspices of the World Bank program on basic human needs in Sri Lanka, Brazil, Indonesia, Egypt, Mali, The Gambia and Somalia have been useful in highlighting the dimensions of unmet basic human needs in these countries and, thereby, in raising the consciousness of national policy makers. These studies have told us that, rather than global targets, individual social indices are needed (Burki and ul Haq, 1980). Table 10.2 summarizes data on development indicators of selected countries. In many United Nations conferences in recent years, an attempt has been made to set a time-specific target in the fields of education, health, water supply, nutrition and shelter. It would be useful now to clarify the broad dimensions of the problem in each area to determine its urgency.

In this section we would like to consider several aspects of basic human needs and public health and to clarify the relation between public health and economic development.

Infant Mortality and Population per Physician

A recognition of the linkages among and complementary nature of various basic human needs is necessary to improve the quality of life in underdeveloped and developing countries. For example, the increase of per capita gross national product (GNP), the decrease of population per physician, the appropriate level of nutrition, and the availability of water supply and sanitation would all improve the infant mortality rate.

Displaying per capita GNP as a comprehensive economic indicator on the horizontal axis and infant mortality rate on the vertical axis, the comparative positions in 1983 of forty countries, including developed countries, are plotted in Figure 10.2.

Each economic development group shows a rather distinct pattern in the relationships between infant mortality rate and per capita GNP. Among underdeveloped countries, such as Malawi, Nepal, Uganda, Tanzania, and Kenya, there is a much greater diversity in the fundamental condition of infant mortality relative to the differences in per capita GNP. In the early stage of the development process, therefore, more attention should be given to improving infant mortality rates rather than to substantially increasing economic activities. We have no evidence that economic activities could lower infant mortality, especially in underdeveloped countries.

Figure 10.2 depicts a turning point to a second stage of advancement. Infant mortality rates begin to decline more slowly around the level of such developing countries as Greece, Spain, Israel, Hong Kong, and

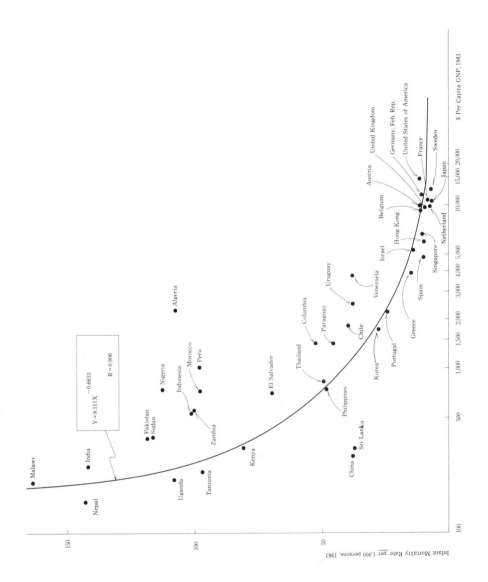

Figure 10.2. *The relation between infant mortality and per capita GNP.*
Source: Table 10.2.

Table 10.2

Summary of Development Indicators of Selected Countries

	Popula-tion per Physician 1980	Popula-tion per Nursing Person 1980	Daily Calorie Supply per Capita 1982	Infant Mortality Rate (Aged under 1) 1983	Life Expec-tancy at Birth (Male) 1983	Life Expec-tancy at Birth (Female) 1983
I. Low Income Economies						
Nepal	30,060	33,420	2,018	143	47	45
Malawi	41,460	3,840	2,242	164	43	45
Uganda	26,810	4,180	1,807	108	48	50
Tanzania	17,740	3,010	2,331	97	49	52
India	3,690	5,460	2,047	142	43	46
China	1,740	1,710	2,562	38	65	69
Kenya	7,890	550	2,056	81	55	59
Sri Lanka	7,170	1,340	2,393	37	67	71
Pakistan	3,480	5,820	2,277	119	51	49
Sudan	8,930	1,430	2,250	117	47	49
II. Lower Middle Income Economics						
Indonesia	11,530	2,300	2,393	101	52	55
Zambia	7,670	1,730	2,054	100	49	52
El Salvador	3,220	910	2,060	70	62	66
Morocco	10,750	1,830	2,671	98	51	54
Philippines	7,970	6,000	2,393	49	63	66
Nigeria	12,550	3,010	2,443	113	47	50
Thailand	7,100	2,400	2,296	50	61	65
Peru	1,390	970	2,114	98	57	60
Paraguay	1,310	1,100	2,820	45	63	67
Colombia	1,710	800	2,551	53	62	66
III. Upper Middle Income Economics						
Chile	1,930	450	2,669	40	68	72
Korea	1,440	350	2,936	29	64	71
Portugal	540	660	3,176	25	68	74
Algeria	2,630	740	2,639	107	55	59
Uruguay	540	590	2,754	38	71	75
Venezuela	990	380	2,557	38	65	71
Greece	430	600	3,554	15	73	77
Israel	370	130	3,059	14	72	76
Hong Kong	1,210	790	2,774	10	74	78
Singapore	1,150	320	2,954	11	70	75
IV. Industrial Market Economics						
Spain	450	330	3,341	10	70	78
Belgium	400	120	3,743	11	70	77
United Kingdom	650	140	3,232	10	71	77
Austria	400	230	3,524	12	70	77
Netherlands	540	130	3,563	8	73	80
Japan	780	240	2,891	7	74	79
France	580	120	3,572	9	72	79
Germany, Fed. Rep.	450	170	3,382	11	72	78
Sweden	490	60	3,224	8	75	80
U.S.A.	520	140	3,616	11	72	79

Sources: The World Bank, World Development Report 1985, Oxford University Press, 1985; The United Nations, Department of International Economic and Social Affairs, Demographic Yearbook, 1985; *Infant Mortality*, Population Bulletin of the United Nations, No. 14, 1982; World Health Organization, World Health Statistics Annual, 1985.

GNP per Capita US$ 1983	Food Aid in Cereals (1000t) 1983	Energy Consumption per Capita (kg of oil equivalent) 1983	External Public Debt Outstanding and Disbursed (Million $) 1983	Debt Service as % of Exports of Goods and Services 1983	Official Development Assistance (Million $) 1983	Population 1983	Average Annual Rate of Growth of GDP (1973–83)
160	44	13	346	3.0	0	15.7	3.0
210	3	45	719	20.3	0	6.6	4.2
220	14	23	623	—	0	13.9	−2.1
240	171	38	2,584	—	0	20.8	3.6
260	282	182	21,277	10.3	0	733.2	4.0
300	45	455	—	—	0	1,019.1	6.0
340	165	109	2,384	20.6	0	18.9	4.6
330	369	143	2,205	11.9	0	15.4	5.2
390	369	197	9,755	28.1	0	89.7	5.6
400	330	66	5,726	11.2	0	20.8	6.3
155	44	204	21,685	12.8	0	155.7	7.0
580	83	432	2,638	12.6	0	6.3	0.2
710	211	190	1,065	6.4	0	5.2	−0.1
760	142	258	9,445	38.2	0	20.8	4.7
760	49	252	10,385	15.4	0	52.1	5.4
770	0	150	11,757	18.6	0	93.6	1.2
820	9	269	7,060	11.3	0	49.2	6.9
1,040	111	550	7,932	19.6	0	17.9	1.8
1,410	1	187	1,161	14.9	0	3.2	8.2
1,430	1	786	6,899	21.3	0	27.5	3.9
1,870	2	755	6,827	18.3	0	11.7	2.9
2,010	53	1,168	21,472	12.3	0	40.0	7.3
2,230	0	1,194	9,951	26.7	0	10.1	4.4
2,320	2	982	24,593	33.1	0	20.6	6.5
2,490	0	776	2,523	19.8	0	3.0	2.5
3,840	0	2,295	12,911	15.0	0	17.3	2.5
3,920	0	1,790	8,193	18.3	0	9.8	3.0
5,370	0	1,932	15,149	19.6	0	4.1	3.2
6,000	0	1,647	224	—	0	5.3	9.3
6,620	0	4,757	1,244	1.3	0	2.5	8.2
4,870	0	1,858	0	0	0	38.2	1.8
9,150	0	4,401	0	0	480	9.9	1.8
9,200	0	3,461	0	0	1,605	56.3	1.1
9,250	0	3,083	0	0	158	7.5	2.8
9,890	0	5,397	0	0	1,195	14.4	1.5
10,120	0	2,929	0	0	3,761	119.3	4.3
10,500	0	3,429	0	0	3,815	54.7	2.5
11,430	0	4,156	0	0	3,176	61.4	2.1
12,470	0	5,821	0	0	754	8.3	1.3
14,110	0	7,030	0	0	7,992	234.5	2.3

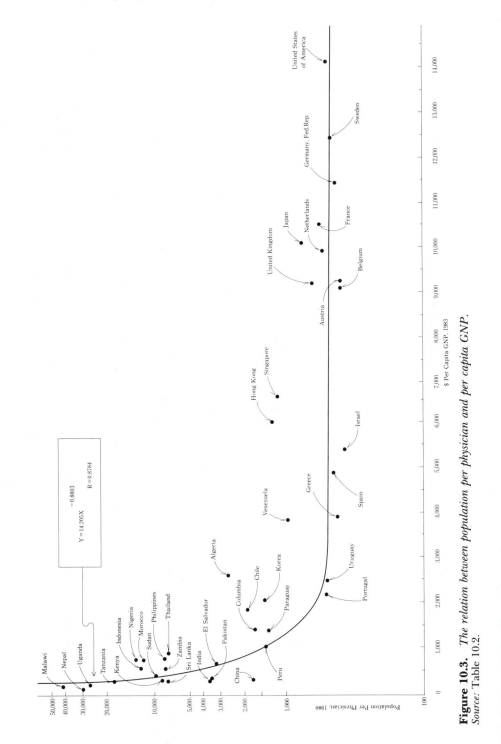

Figure 10.3. *The relation between population per physician and per capita GNP.*
Source: Table 10.2.

Singapore, whose per capita GNPs are equivalent to more than 4,000 U.S. dollars. Beyond this threshold, the infant mortality rate appears to lose its significance. On the other hand, population per physician varies in relation to per capita GNP as shown in Figure 10.3.

Regression curves in Figures 10.2 and 10.3 which show the relationship between the infant mortality rate and per capita GNP in Figure 10.2 and population per physician and per capita GNP in Figure 10.3 reveal the same relational patterns. And these also show that increase in per capita GNP tended to decrease both population per physician and infant mortality rate in underdeveloped countries whose per capita GNP ranged from 400 U.S. dollars to 2,000 U.S. dollars. It should be noted, however, that these causal relations are not exclusive and that other factors such as public health care, nutrition and decreasing rates of birth might influence infant mortality.

In developing countries and developed countries whose per capita GNPs were more than 5,000 U.S. dollars, both infant mortality rate and population per physician reached a level sufficient for sustaining human health.

On the other hand, we can see the positive non-linear correlation between population per physician and infant mortality rate in the following regression equation:

$$Y = 1.1481X^{0.6157}, \qquad R = 0.8410, \text{ sample size} = 40$$

Y: infant mortality rate
X: population per physician
R: correlation coefficient

This equation, which is derived from cross-section data of forty countries shown in Figure 10.2, indicates that a 10 percent decline of the population per physician reduced the infant mortality rate by about 6.16 percent.

Life Expectancy and Nutrition

The number of people in underdeveloped countries who received less than the minimum required level of nutrition increased from 368 million in the period 1967–71 to 424 million in the period 1974–76, according to a study report of the Food and Agriculture Organization of the United Nations. The greatest numbers of the undernourished people live in the poor countries of South Asia and sub-Saharan Africa, and a significant proportion of them are children below the age of fifteen years (Burki and ul Haq, 1980).

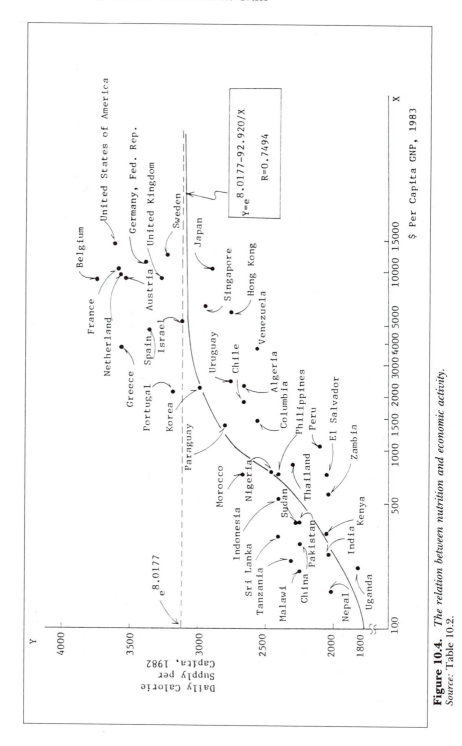

Figure 10.4. *The relation between nutrition and economic activity.*
Source: Table 10.2.

Figure 10.4 shows that the improvement of daily calorie supply per capita was not significantly related to the increase in per capita GNP in underdeveloped countries whose per capita GNPs were under 700 U.S. dollars, such as Nepal, Uganda, Malawi, Tanzania, etc. In these countries, increasing per capita GNP through rural development would not necessarily decrease the levels of malnutrition. Because improving malnutrition is such an urgent task, other means such as foreign food assistance should be considered as soon as possible in these seriously less developed countries.

There is no definite positive correlation between life expectancy and per capita GNP or between nutrition and per capita GNP, especially in the underdeveloped countries, as seen in Figures 10.4 and 10.5. These countries show wide ranges in nutritional intake, from around 2,000 to 3,500 calories, and in life expectancy, from around forty-five to seventy-five years old.

Let us examine the relationship between nutrition and life expectancy rate. The result of a regression using data on the forty countries was as follows:

$$Y = -1.3779X^{0.6957}, \qquad R = 0.7754, \text{ sample size} = 40$$

Y: Life expectancy
X: Nutrition (calorie supply)

It can be seen that the elasticity of nutrition to life expectancy is 0.6957, that is, a 10 percent increase in nutrition raises life expectancy by 6.957 percent.

On the other hand, using data on only the ten underdeveloped countries whose per capita GNPs are less than 400 U.S. dollars, we get a somewhat different regression. Namely,

$$Y = 2.697X^{0.8618}, \qquad R = 0.5601, \text{ sample size} = 10$$

Y: Life expectancy
X: Nutrition

It is interesting that the elasticity became greater in the latter case than in the former. We might conclude from this that nutrition has greater effect on the improvement of life expectancy in less developed countries than in the more advanced developing countries. However, we cannot conclude this with certainty because the correlation coefficients are insignificantly low.

Malnutrition has been viewed as a recent development problem in less underdeveloped countries. Considering the causes of malnutrition,

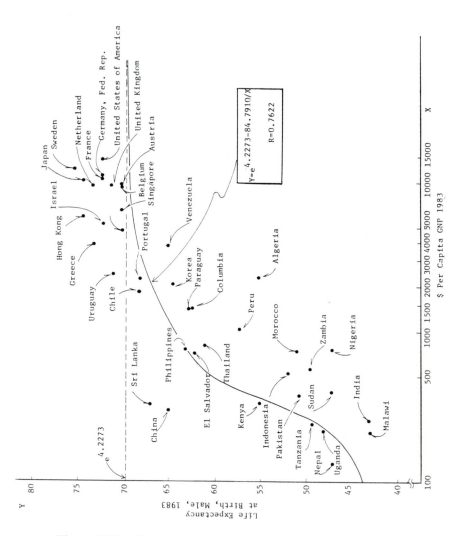

Figure 10.5. *The relation between life expectancy and per capita GNP.*
Source: Table 10.2.

Reutlinger and Selowsky (1976) demonstrated that one could not assert the root of malnutrition and policy palliatives without explicitly considering the distribution of food among different groups in the population. The malnutrition problem may not be solved simply by solving the aggregate food problem.

Nutrition is one of the main determinants of health, and health is regarded as a desirable end in itself. Health and nutrition interventions not only have an impact on human capital formation but also have implications for future earnings of individuals and the potential growth in GNP.

Economic Development Versus Starvation

The daily consumption of calories per capita is now 3,000–4,000 in advanced countries, but only approximately 2,000 in underdeveloped countries, as Figure 10.5 shows. Two-thirds of the population in the Third World takes in only the minimum calories necessary for health, or less, and they suffer from malnutrition.

Developed countries can increase food production when necessary because they have a highly developed agricultural infrastructure. But underdeveloped countries cannot be expected to accomplish a marked production increase per capita, because of the backwardness of their agricultural infrastructure, their high rate of population growth, and unstable crops.

The International Food Policy Research Institute predicted in 1984 that, over the long term, there will be increasing food surpluses in the North and increasing shortages in the South. At present, food shortages amount to 100 million tons and 800 million people suffer from malnutrition in underdeveloped countries, except for several newly industrializing countries. These newly industrializing countries have raised their nutrition levels in recent years, owing to their domestic agricultural policies and their successful economic growth strategies, as well as the use of imported food to supplement domestic crops. In these newly industrializing countries, nutrition levels have well exceeded those necessary for health both in quality and in quantity. The other nations in the Association of Southeast Asian Nations (ASEAN) have raised their levels of nutrition almost as favorably. On the contrary, however, the nutrition levels in most underdeveloped countries in Africa have remained less than the minimum. And not only the gaps between the North and the South, but also the gaps among the different nations of the South, have tended to widen. An effective development strategy and international economic cooperation will be required in order for these nations to improve their situation in the 1980s.

In underdeveloped countries whose levels of crop production are much less than their potentials, the malnutrition problem could be solved by increased production of food. But this cannot be accomplished without an institutional improvement. Land resources are distributed unevenly—in many underdeveloped countries the landlord class is only a small percentage of the population but owns 70–80 percent of the total farmland. Because of the concentration of landownership and economic clout, food resources often flow to the overseas market. Domestic demands remain unfilled because the poor and malnourished lack purchasing power.

The concentration of landownership has also contributed to a history of farmland being allotted for exportable cash crops. Although foreign currency is necessary for economic progress in all underdeveloped and developing countries, it cannot contribute to the improvement of living when income distribution is uneven. Under these circumstances, the percentage of the population that is malnourished would increase even while food and agricultural production were increasing.

The food problem cannot be settled unless every aspect is considered. Especially in underdeveloped countries, the institutional factors, such as farm land ownership systems, have reached a deadlock. Moreover, neither agricultural production nor industrialization will make any progress unless an increase occurs in the income of general farmers, because they shoulder the future demand of domestic industrial products.

We might say that international and domestic inequalities have come into being at the same time. A growth-oriented economic development strategy has been followed in both underdeveloped and developing countries since the 1960s but has never achieved brilliant success (Streeten, 1977; Streeten and Burki, 1978). Large sums have been invested in the agricultural and industrial sectors to increase production and to improve the infrastructure, and gradual improvements have been made in the production and distribution systems. However, this type of strategy has ultimately failed because it has not addressed needed institutional changes. This failure has reinforced both kinds of inequalities. The income gap between developed and underdeveloped countries has actually widened. And within the underdeveloped countries, the poor and needy have not received adequate income and food and poor farmers remain shut off from the benefits of innovation. The malnutrition problem has not been solved in underdeveloped countries, except for the newly industrialized countries (NICs), which have achieved a performance beyond their initial goals.

From Maximizing Income to Minimizing Poverty

Strains caused by the execution of the growth-oriented development strategy have left substantial numbers of people unemployed or poor. It was natural that in the face of the extreme poverty, the severe shortages of resources, and the high rates of population growth that occurred in the 1970s, alternate strategies were conceived. We will describe two of these alternate strategies for social and economic development that have been followed in underdeveloped countries.

The first strategy was to establish a New International Economic Order (NIEO) in place of the older order. The NIEO was a new concept that gained popularity in underdeveloped and developing countries in 1974, with adoption of the "Declaration and action program on the new international economic order" in the 6th United Nations Special General Assembly and the "Charter of economic right and responsibility among nations" in the 29th United Nations General Assembly of the same year. Most underdeveloped and developing countries claimed as their goal autonomous economic growth under the new international economic order; they insisted that the cause of their difficulties was the defects of the current international order (including the IMF and the General Agreement on Tariffs and Trade), under which free trade and market efficiency were promoted to the detriment of poorer countries. Instead, the NIEO sought a distributional equality between the North and the South, even if this meant that economic efficiency of the market was ignored to some extent. The NIEO strategy aimed at international fairness, equality of national sovereignty, sovereignty over natural resources, a reform of the international trade and monetary system, an increase in financial and technological assistance and independence, etc., in order to promote the economic and social development of underdeveloped countries.

We might say that the purpose of the NIEO is to settle economic conflicts, especially differences between the North and the South. Yet it has no explicit, concrete plan to solve domestic inequalities such as increases in unemployment and underemployment and severe poverty.

NIEO seems to assume, however, that the reform of the international economic system and the expansion of assistance to developing countries can lead to high rates of economic growth, with the consequence that low-income groups would attain more income and more welfare. This assumption is very similar to that behind the growth-oriented strategy— the traditional idea that only high rates of economic growth can eliminate both international income differentials and domestic poverty.

Another development strategy, called the Basic Human Needs (BHN) strategy, has been advocated by the International Labor Organization, the World Bank, and member nations of OECD's Development Assistance Committee. This strategy pays considerable attention to the elimination of absolute poverty by increasing the productivity of the poor; its main aim is to put an end to absolute poverty and malnutrition.

The BHN approach shifts our interest from maximizing income to minimizing poverty. A preliminary set of BHN indicators is as follows:

1. Food: Caloric supply per head, or calorie supply as a percentage of requirement; protein
2. Education: Literacy rates; primary enrollment
3. Health: Life expectancy at birth
4. Sanitation: Infant mortality; percentage of the population with access to sanitation facilities
5. Water Supply: Infant mortality; percentage of the population with access to potable water (Hicks and Streeten, 1979).

An important aim has been to meet such basic needs, on the assumption that serious poverty, malnutrition, and the other economic difficulties have been left unsolved by the growth-oriented strategy, which has intensified distrust of economic growth.[2]

A high rate of economic growth is a necessary condition for an increase in the income of the poor and needy, but it is not sufficient. Only when the socioeconomic structure is not a dual structure and when the development strategy emphasizes human-resources, will the relative income ratio of the poor and needy rise (Haq, 1978).

There are several reasons why economic growth has not made a definite dent in absolute poverty in underdeveloped countries. First, economic growth has supported a certain structure of production in these countries. A change has occurred from production for domestic consumption to cash crop for export. As a result, the countries have become less self-sufficient. That alone would not be important as long as they could get sufficient food from other countries. Since recent trends toward commercialization[3] in agriculture have required more intermediate inputs—such as feedgrains and agricultural facilities—the supply of food has been unstable. Thus, the absolute poverty in rural areas has not improved in underdeveloped countries.

Further, the minimum income alone would not relieve the poor and needy in underdeveloped countries. A variety of conditions must be met to achieve a standard of subsistence. Health and nutrition problems would be scarcely affected simply by supplying a certain quantity of food. While health depends on food supply, malnutrition is indirectly caused by inappropriate food or drink and diseases like diarrhea. Today's disease is the cause of tomorrow's hunger.

In underdeveloped countries, especially in the most underdeveloped countries of Asia and Africa, 15 million children die from malnutrition and infectious diseases every year, and it is said that 100 million children suffer from hunger and bad health. We cannot improve their lives without careful attention to the real state of these countries. Moreover, it should be noted that the weak are present in every society: the sick, the elderly, the handicapped, as well as children. The traditional growth-oriented development strategies have tended to ignore the welfare of the weak and therefore have not allowed them to enjoy the benefits of economic growth in most underdeveloped countries.

Fundamental Features of the BHN Strategy

The goal of the BHN strategy is to eliminate poverty and malnutrition by increasing the productivity and improving the health conditions of the low-income population.[4] We may not be able to rely on a government's welfare policy. Most underdeveloped countries cannot afford welfare policies such as those of some developed countries—which might include employment through public sector activities. Because the traditional growth-oriented development policy does not do enough to eliminate poverty, the BHN strategy aims to expand employment in the low-income bracket and thus yield a rise in productivity. This employment can be called poverty-oriented productive employment.

To raise productivity and increase the employment of poor producers and laborers, we need not only to create employment opportunities but to improve the circumstances of production and labor. These circumstances range from direct areas such as education and job training to indirect ones such as health, sanitation, and nutrition.

After considering everything, the BHN strategy emphasizes labor-intensive technology, small-scale enterprise, and agricultural and informal sectors instead of the traditional program of capital-intensive technology, large-scale enterprise, and manufacturing and modern sectors.

The BHN strategy also recognizes that public health depends on nutrition, education, water and sanitation, and shelter in the social sector. For example, the World Bank adopted an explicit policy of creating and developing institutions in education, health, water supply and other social sectors that will in time make good use of sector loans. This policy is one of the influential steps toward the BHN strategy.

The BHN strategy places more emphasis on agriculture and rural development, and the concrete policies are as follows.

Progress in agriculture will require an increased production of traditional crops through improvements in fertilizer, irrigation facilities and agricultural machines and implements, as well as a conversion to high value-added crops such as sugar, vegetables, and fruit. Considering the numbers of poor consumers in these countries, it would be advisable to produce more food staples for domestic consumption and fewer cash crops for export.

Rural development means improvement of the agricultural infrastructure and includes the following points.

1. Medicine and health, general education and nutrition among poor peasants
2. Technical development and professional training suitable for poor peasants
3. Enrichment of production-related activities, such as sale and repair of agricultural machinery, in farm villages, and establishment of distributional channels
4. Extension of a low-interest finance system for investment of small farmers
5. Security of employment for tenant farmers; land reform

These means toward agricultural production and rural development aim at an increase in income and the fulfillment of basic human needs of large numbers of poor peasants.

In this way the BHN strategy, as domestic policy, covers a variety of fields such as macroeconomic policy, employment policy, agricultural sector policy, technological policy, public health and social policy, educational policy, and institutional reform. As international policy it covers such areas as trade, development assistance, technical innovation, and multinational enterprise.

The BHN strategy is an innovation because of its special nature. It is quite selective in focusing attention on a specific population with unfilled basic human needs and in investing specific resources in them. Basic human needs are specified not by income, or by goods and services, but by property (for example, quantity of calories and protein). The BHN strategy provides resources to all people that are considered to be short of basic human needs—it does not concentrate on a specific area and sector.

Compared with the traditional growth-oriented development policy, which aims at the trickling down of economic growth, the BHN strategy is direct: it intends to assure a standard of subsistence and to increase welfare through the fulfillment of basic human needs.

We suggest, in principle, that the BHN strategy should be taken as a package. The BHN strategy as a comprehensive policy aims at stable economic and social development in underdeveloped countries. Individual steps in the BHN strategy do increase welfare and assure a standard of subsistence. But separate policy itself could not make underdeveloped countries stand on their own feet in the long run. Therefore, the appropriate policy package should be taken depending on the situation in each country. The strategy must not be standardized. Even if nutrition and public health would be the important problems to be settled first in many less developed countries, these countries might have a different order of priority in other aspects.

Notes

1. See Z. Hellwig, "Procedure of Evaluating High Level Manpower Data and Typology of Countries by Means of Taxonomic Method," in Z. Gostkowski, ed., *Towards a System of Human Resource Indicators for Less Developed Countries* (Poland: Ossolineum, 1972).
2. Adelman and Morris (1973) concluded that the economic growth of the 1960s was accompanied by a fall in the average income of the poor and needy (40 percent from the bottom) rather than a rise. Adelman (1975) formulated the relationship between economic growth and income distribution of the developing nations. According to Adelman, the relative income ratio of the poor and needy (40 percent from the bottom) had fallen in these countries where the real rates of economic growth per capita were below 3.5 percent. Under the present rate of population growth in developing countries, at least 5.5 percent rates of real growth would be required.

   On the other hand, Ahluwalia (1975) pointed out the relationship between rate of economic growth and share of low income bracket. The rate of income growth of the low income bracket has exceeded the rate of economic growth in those countries where a very high rate of growth has been achieved. The share of the low income bracket would be increased. But the results vary according to the country, even if all countries have attained the same rate of economic growth.
3. The less developed countries have large external public debts, and their governments need to earn enough foreign currency to cover interest payments. To do this they are often forced to export commercial food crops. Thus they must use official development aid (ODA) mostly to help develop cash crops and can only use a small portion of ODA for domestic welfare.
4. In this section, the authors use the works of: Burki and Haq (1980); Coombs (1980); J. ul Haq (1980); M. ul Haq (1980); Hicks (1974); Ilo (1976a, 1976b, 1977); Leipsiger (1981); McHale and McHale (1977); and Streeten (1977, 1978, 1979, 1980).

References

Adelman, I. "Growth, Income Distribution and Equity-oriented Development Strategies," *World Development* 3 (1975).

Adelman, I. and C. T. Morris. *Economic Growth and Social Equity in Developing Countries*. Stanford: Stanford University Press, 1973.

Ahluwalia, M. S. "Income Inequality: Some Dimensions of the Problem," in Chenery, H. B. et al., *Distribution with Growth* Oxford. Oxford University Press, 1975.

Berg, A. *Nutrition*. Washington, D.C.: The World Bank, Poverty and Basic Needs Series, 1980.

———. "A Strategy to Reduce Malnutrition," in The World Bank, *Poverty and Basic Needs*. Washington, D.C., 1980.

Burki, S. "Sectoral Priorities for Meeting Basic Needs," *Finance & Development* 7:1 (1980).

Burki, S., and M. ul Haq. *Meeting Basic Needs: An Overview*. The World Bank, 1980.

Chenery, H. B. "Poverty and Progress-Choices for the Developing World," *Finance & Development*, 17:2 (1980).

Coombs, P. H., ed. *Meeting the Basic Needs of the Rural Poor: The Integrated Community-Based Approach*. Pergamon Policy Studies, Washington, D.C.: World Bank, 1980.

Cruz, H. S. "The Three Tiers of "Basic Needs" for Rural Development," *Finance and Development* 16:2 (1979).

Dell, S. "Basic Needs or Comprehensive Development: Should the UNDP Have a Development Strategy," *World Development* 7 (1979).

Haq., J. ul. "An International Perspective on Basic Needs," *Finance and Development* 17:3 (1980).

Haq., M. ul. "Basic Needs and New International Economic Order," in Haq., K. ed., *Dialogue for a New Order*. New York: Pergamon Press, 1980.

Haq., M. ul. "Changing Emphasis of the Bank's Lending Policies," *Finance & Development* 15:2 (1978).

Hicks, N. L., and P. Streeten. "Indicators of Development: the Search for a Basic Needs Yardstick," *World Development* 7 (1979).

Hicks, N. L. "Is There a Trade off between Growth and Basic Needs?," *Finance and Development* 17:2 (1980).

———. "Growth vs Basic Needs: Is There a Trade-Off," *World Development* 2 (1974).

International Labor Organization. *Employment Growth and Basic Needs: A One-World Problem*. Geneva, 1976a.

———. *Background Papers: Vol. 1 Basic Needs and National Employment Strategies; Vol. 2 International Strategies for Employment*. Geneva: ILO, 1976b.

———. *Meeting Basic Needs: Strategies for Eradicating Mass Poverty and Unemployment*. Geneva: ILO, 1977.

Iseman, P. "Basic Needs: The Case of Sri Lanka," *World Development* 6 (1980).

Khan, M. H. *Socio-Economic Data Bank*. Sydney: The University of New South Wales Libraries, microfiche, 1978.

———. "A Comparative Study of Socioeconomic Development: Asia," *Asian Profile* 9:4 (1981).

Khan, M. H. *Socio-Economic Data Bank*. Sydney: The University of New South Wales Libraries, microfiche, 1978.

———. "A Comparative Study of Socioeconomic Development: Asia," *Asian Profile* 9:4 (1981).

Khan, M. H., and J. A. Zerby. "The Socioeconomic Position of Indonesia in the Third World," *Ekonomi dan Keuangan Indonesia* 31:1 (1983).

Leipziger, D. M. ed. *Basic Needs and Development*. Cambridge, MA: Oelgeschlager, Gunn & Hain, 1981.

Lisk, F. "Conventional Development Strategies and Basic-Needs Fulfilment: A Reassessment of Objectives and Policies," *International Labour Review* (March-April 1977).

McGranahan, D. V., et al. *Contents and Measurement of Socioeconomic Development*. New York: Praeger Publishers, 1972.

McHale, J., and M. C. McHale, *Basic Human Needs: A Framework for Action*. Houston: Center for Integrative Studies, University of Houston, April 1977.

Reutlinger, S., and M. Selowsky. *Malnutrition and Poverty*. The World Bank, 1976.

Sheehan, G., and M. Hopkins. "Meeting Basic Needs: An Examination of the World Situation in 1970," *International Labour Review* (September-October 1978).

Singh, A. "The 'Basic Needs' Approach to Development vs the New International Economic Order: The Significance of Third World Industrialization," *World Development* 7 (1979).

Srinivasan, T. N. "Development, Poverty and Basic Human Needs: Some Issues," *Food Research Institute Studies* 16:2 (1977).

Streeten, P. "The Distinctive Features of a Basic Needs Approach to Development," *International Development Review* 19:3 (1977).

———. "Basic Needs: Premises and Promises," *Journal of Policy Modeling* 1 (1979).

———. "From Growth to Basic Needs," *Finance & Development* 16:3 (1979).

———. "Basic Needs and Human Rights," *World Development* 8 (1980).

———, and S. J. Burki. "Basic Needs: Some Issues," *World Development* 6 (1978).

Szal, R. J. "Operationalizing the Concept of Basic Needs," *Pakistan Development Review* (Autumn 1980).

Tévoédjrè, A. "Employment, Human Needs, and the NIEO," in J. A. Lozoya, ed., *Social and Cultural Issues of the New International Economic Order*. New York: Pergamon, 1981.

11

A Public Health Approach to the "Food-Malnutrition-Economic Recession" Complex

Leonardo Mata

The authors in this volume disagree as to whether the current economic world recession and its accompanying adjustment policies affect nutrition and health. Based on the data presented throughout this volume and the discussions at the Takemi Symposium, I am not convinced that current world economic conditions have significantly changed the nutritional state and survival of children in less developed countries—except in certain regions of Africa. This is not to say that such an effect does not exist—economic adjustments made by nations at the macro level and by families at the household level might have acted as a buffer.

Any serious attempt to correlate economic phenomena with nutrition and health must take into account certain fundamental variables not immediately obvious to economists and policymakers. Discussions of this topic, for example, may suffer from problems in data collection which are particular to the field of public health. In addition, if the concept of malnutrition is to be used in a discussion of economics, it must be precisely defined in biological terms, and what we know of its causes must be understood and considered. Health factors, including illness, and other sociological factors which cause malnutrition need to be described. To understand these variables we must step outside the

*I want to thank Drs. John Wyon, Samuel Preston and David Bell for valuable comments on this chapter.

realm of policymaking and the discipline of economics. This chapter discusses some of these variables and their effects on analyses of health, nutrition and economic policy.

Causality of Malnutrition

First I will attempt to summarize, in simple terms, how malnutrition originates in most traditional and transitional nations (Mata, 1978). This knowledge is pivotal to hypotheses of possible interactions between changes in the macroeconomy and health.

The Role of Infectious Disease

Longitudinal monitoring of pregnancy, childbirth, growth, and survival in poor ecosystems is the best way to understand how children become malnourished (Mata, 1978, 1985). Figure 11.1 presents the growth chart of a typical child from a village in the Guatemalan highlands. Like 40 percent of village infants, this one had low birth weight due to intra-uterine growth retardation. Although many people assume that a deficient diet during pregnancy accounts for low birth weight, the etiology is much more complex. Factors include low maternal education, poverty and negative influences dating back to the mother's own childhood and adolescence (Guyer et al., 1985–86; Mata et al., 1976). Scientists are continuing to explore other plausible causal factors such as infection with *Mycoplasma* and other microorganisms during pregnancy, physical exertion, pollution, and deficient or insufficient prenatal care (Guyer et al., 1985–86; Mata et al., 1976; Braun et al., 1971; Tafari, 1981). However, the etiology and correction of some intrauterine growth retardation still puzzles physicians the world over.

The weight gain of the child shown in Figure 11.1 was adequate during exclusive breastfeeding, despite his low birth weight. With commencement of weaning—a process extending for one to three years in this village—the child underwent progressive malnutrition resulting primarily from recurrent infections. Most people working in hospitals or health centers or conducting nutrition surveys would classify a child like this as malnourished if seen at any point after weaning began. Little or nothing would be known about his past, even if the mother is interviewed, as language and other cultural barriers will frustrate interpretation. The cause of the child's malnutrition will probably be accepted as "lack of food."

Lack of food indeed helped cause this child's malnutrition, but not because food was not available. In fact, the child did not eat, or ate

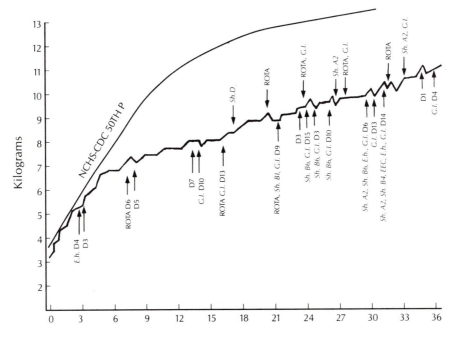

Figure 11.1. *Growth (weight in kilograms) of a typical child from Santa Maria Cauque, observed prospectively from birth to age three years. The growth curve is compared with the 50th percentile of the NCHS curve, to show that the child grew at adequate velocity during the first five to six months (while exclusively at the breast), and then began losing weight in connection with recurrent diarrheal disease episodes of various causes. By twelve months of age the child was evidently malnourished and remained so throughout. Deficits in weight (wastage) are generally accompanied also by deficits in height (stunting). Many episodes of diarrhea (and other infectious diseases not shown in the figure) are associated with fever, vomiting, anorexia, and metabolic alterations leading to malnutrition. Even if food was available, children may not be able to eat the required amount to compensate for successive losses due to infections.*

Key:

D = diarrhea. Numbers indicate duration in days.

ROTA = rotavirus

Sh.A. = Shigella dysenteriae

Sh.B. = S. flexnerii

Sh.D. = S. sonnei. Numbers indicate serotype.

EEC = enteropathogenic E. coli

E.h. = Entamoeba histolytica

G.l. = Giardia lamblia

poorly, as a result of frequent and recurrent infectious diseases often accompanied by anorexia. Actually, the longitudinal study showed that most children experience chronic recurrent diarrhea and other illnesses during one-third or more of their first three years of life (Mata, 1978, 1985).

The effect of diarrhea and other infectious diseases is multiple: anorexia, vomiting, impaired digestion, impaired absorption, metabolic alterations and increased nutrient needs and wastage (Mata, 1985; Mata et al., 1977; Tomkins et al., 1983). To illustrate one aspect of the impact of infection on the nutritional state, I will refer to negative effects of two hormonal substances—*Interleukin 1* and *cachectin* (tumor necrosis factor)—both released by body monocytes under the stimulus of infections or other stressful factors (Dinarello, 1983; Ceramy, 1983). These hormones account for formidable actions: in the brain, the beginning of fever and anorexia; in muscle, the breakdown of proteins and loss of tissue mass; in liver, the synthesis of abnormal macroglobulin; etc. These phenomena represent a host defense against infection—at a high nutritional cost. Even with mild infections, the body loses cells, plasma, electrolytes, amino acids and vitamins. Infected children may not accept food, even of the best quality. The paradox of "hungry children who cannot eat" actually exists. Lack of appetite in children is a common complaint of mothers throughout the world.

The problem described likely cannot be corrected by dumping food. The provision of food at the individual level would be effective if anorexia is resolved first, if recuperation from illness is achieved and if the child is removed or protected—at least temporarily—from his contaminated environment. However, nutritional recuperation is required in special cases, for instance, for malnourished children and for those at high risk, that is, when they are wasted (Waterlow and Rutishauser, 1974). Wasting is defined as a deficit of weight for height greater than 20 percent. Thus, energy-protein malnutrition will persist or even recur with greater severity after dumping food unless the basal social and biological conditions leading to growth retardation are corrected. Unfortunately, few long-term investigations have been conducted on the natural history of malnutrition, and most of them have not included the extensive studies on the microbiology and infectious diseases which are needed to document the staggering force of infection. Even worse is the fact that many people still have not heard or understood the significance of high rates of infection for the conditioning of malnutrition throughout the world.

The Role of Maternal Technology

Lack of food cannot be entirely ruled out in the causality of malnutrition inasmuch as there is evidence of some food deprivation with the commencement of weaning. During exclusive breastfeeding—at about six months of age—human milk generally provides the calories and nutrients needed for optimal growth. Thereafter, food supplements should be given in adequate composition and amount to support growth. Many people do know enough about feeding mixes of sufficient nutriture and caloric density for good nutrition and growth. But this situation is complicated by frequent infections and episodes of anorexia, vomiting and fever. Thus, nutritional deprivation frequently relates to deficient "maternal technology" (meaning family technology).

Good maternal technology (Table 11.1) consists of: (a) adequate knowledge and technique for preparation and administration of weaning foods; (b) appropriate handling of human and animal feces; (c) knowledge about signs and symptoms of dehydration and other life-threatening conditions; (d) acceptance of immunizations and other elements of modern medicine; (e) basic nutrition and health education; and (f) proclivity towards family planning (Mata, 1979). Mothers are not entirely responsible for inadequacies in maternal technology, inasmuch as they are trapped in ecosystems and societies that have not permitted them to acquire an understanding and knowledge of the ubiquitous fecal contamination of food and environment and other threats to child nutrition and survival. On the other hand, many women in villages and city slums possess effective maternal technologies, and their children thrive well despite the odds and hardships.

Table 11.1
Maternal (Family) Technology

1. Adequate technique to store and handle water for drinking and cooking

2. Correct handling and disposal of human and animal feces

3. Hand-washing and use of soap or ashes before handling children and preparing food; sufficient hand-washing after handling feces

4. Successful breastfeeding and adequate food supplementation during weaning, and during illness and convalescence; knowledge about adequate mixing of traditional foods and child-feeding technique

5. Capacity to recognize dangerous signs and symptoms of disease, and seek prompt treatment

6. Knowledge of oral rehydration therapy and other resources to treat diarrheal and respiratory diseases

7. Acceptance and demand of health care: prenatal care, immunization, antibiotic treatment

8. Acceptance of family planning and adequate reproductive behavior

9. Proclivity for community participation

The control of infection and the promotion of maternal technologies are the base of the strategy of Health for All by the Year 2000. The GOBI approach (of growth monitoring, oral rehydration therapy, breastfeeding, and immunization) fundamentally addresses the control and prevention of infectious diseases and their consequences as means to improve the nutritional status.

Structure of Infant Mortality

The evidence advanced to show an effect of the current economic recession on health (Jolly and Cornia, 1984; Grant, 1986) actually does not show the expected impact on sensitive health indicators like infant mortality or prevalence of malnutrition (Preston, 1986; Behrman, 1986). This may imply that the crisis has not been severe enough to affect the indicators or that adjustments have cushioned its negative influence. Furthermore, it is puzzling that infant mortality has declined, or at worst remained stable, in countries such as Costa Rica and Chile that were seriously affected economically while certain socialist countries, where full employment and other measures are always in effect, are facing a rise in mortality of children and older individuals (Klinger, 1982; Anderson and Silver, 1986).

I want to address now the question of causes of death in childhood, which is neglected in other discussions here. When infant mortality is above 50 per 1000 live births (as in most less developed countries), the main causes of death are diarrhea, acute respiratory infections, tuberculosis, childhood diseases (measles and pertussis), and tropical diseases (e.g., malaria). One study in India showed a significant relationship between intake of supplementary solid food and survival (Wyon and Gordon, 1970), but this was an area where many children were kept at the breast *without supplements* for long periods extending into the second year of life, that is, they were "starved at the breast."

In countries with an infant mortality below 30 per 1000 (Malaysia, Chile, Costa Rica, Panama, Trinidad-Tobago and Cuba) the infant mortality profile is similar to that of industrial nations, with neonatal deaths being as many as or in excess of post-neonatal deaths. To illustrate, the structure of neonatal mortality for Costa Rica in 1982 is shown in Table 11.2 next to that of Massachusetts in 1984. The overall rates were low in both places. Dominant causes of death in these populations were congenital defects (especially of the heart), and respiratory infection of the newborn. Most of the mortality is not preventable, and some of it is related to premature pregnancy, fetal immaturity and deficiencies in prenatal care and delivery procedure; still more mortality suggests inadequacies in the conduction of childbirth, reflecting excessive obstetric

Table 11.2
Structure of Neonatal Mortality in Massachusetts (1984) and Costa Rica (1982)

Massachusetts, 79,700 births			Costa Rica, 72,000 births		
Rank	*Cause(s)*	*Rate**	*Rank*	*Cause(s)*	*Rate**
1	Congenital defects	3.91	1	Congenital defects and complications in pregnancy	5.3
2	Respiratory infections	1.56	2	Ill defined conditions	2.1
3	SIDS**	0.92	3	Respiratory infections	1.5
4	Ill defined conditions	0.88	4	Diarrhea	1.0
5	Maternal conditions	0.75	5	Other conditions	0.6
6	Immaturity	0.75	6	Immaturity	0.5
	Total	8.77		Total	11.0

* Rate per 1000 live births; data for Massachusetts provided by Dr. S. Franklin, Massachusetts Department of Public Health, Boston.
** Sudden Infant Death Syndrome.

intervention. No evidence is found that malnutrition is an important cause of death in either place. The rate of low birth weight infants was about the same in both populations, about 8 percent.

The similarity of neonatal mortalities in Costa Rica and Massachusetts is interesting in that total fertility rate in Costa Rica in 1980 (3.7) was twice that in Massachusetts at about the same time (1.8). The slightly lower neonatal mortality in Massachusetts likely is accounted for by its lower fertility and by greater medical intervention that averts death among the very small babies. No data were found on the resulting associated quality of life. Rates of malnutrition (defined as weight for age or height below the fifth percentile of the National Center for Health Statistics growth curves) in Massachusetts were similar to those for Costa Rica around 1982 (Mata, 1985; Guyer et al., 1985–6).

Economic Recession and Adjustments

The preceding discussion on causality of malnutrition and structure of infant mortality casts doubt on a possible effect of economic recession of the current magnitude on nutrition, health and survival of children, at least in the countries discussed in the Symposium. Nevertheless, economic recession might have induced changes in behavior and life styles, which might have led to unwanted pregnancy, stress during pregnancy, family disruption, deficient prenatal care, dehumanized childbirth and child neglect and abandonment. If such changes occurred, their effects might take considerable time to become manifest. On the other hand, diminished food supply cannot be proposed to explain the current level of infant mortality in Costa Rica and similar countries, despite the fact that poverty is significantly greater and more obvious in them than, for instance, in Massachusetts.

It seems logical that economic recession may have an impact by inducing the following alterations: (a) deterioration of water supplies and sanitation; (b) attrition in programs for primary health care and delivery of medical services; (c) psychosocial disruption resulting in family and community instability and other manifestations of social distress; or (d) two or all of the above. Obviously, such changes will favor the occurrence of infectious diseases (Mohs, 1982) and/or child neglect (Mata, 1985) and hence will result in more malnutrition and death of children.

The crisis might also alter maternal behavior to induce child abuse and neglect. However, this is not likely to occur in traditional and transitional countries, as was the case throughout Latin America during the energy crisis of 1973, or more recently in countries stricken by the crisis of the 1980s. It should be mentioned here that malnutrition is not a primary killer, except in famine situations, and in isolated cases of severe edematous malnutrition (often called kwashiorkor), now in clear disappearance from developing countries. Malnutrition must be severe enough to render the host susceptible to die of other causes, primarily infections, but there is still a need for good data relating food intake, nutritional status and changes in immunity. On the other hand, infectious diseases are known to kill individuals of all sorts, including those who are wealthy and well nourished.

The lack of impact of economic recession might be related to socioeconomic adjustments in the household, or at the local and national levels, where some order of priorities is established. For instance, Costa Rica illustrates the impact of foreign aid in cushioning the adverse effects of the crisis.

Much could be done to ameliorate problems internally, however, if governments would decrease the emphasis in costly "paternalistic" programs of doubtful impact which cannot solve the basic social malady. Thus, it is apparent that economic strategies aiming at improving food availability will hardly have an effect on the nutritional status. Conceivably, an excess of food supplied to households might eventually be sold, and the money destined to satisfy other needs. This actually has been documented for a very small proportion of people that sell food obtained from national and international programs. Likely, the added income would alleviate intra-household tension and distress. I believe this and similar topics merit attention by economists and health professionals, as they might bear more on causality of malnutrition than on low food availability itself.

Does this analysis apply to all nutritional situations in the world? The answer clearly is no. To elaborate, in countries periodically stricken by natural or manmade disasters, food shortage may reach levels incompatible with survival, demanding relief action. Also, deprived rural and urban populations, and individual families, may suffer from shortage of food, and in these cases food must be provided until a dignifying solution is found. In such situations, however, food programs are only a palliative measure, perpetuating the status quo (Mata, 1978). Even after alleviation of famine, there is prompt return to underdevelopment with its mounting population problem (Watkins and Menken, 1985).

The Danger of Misconception

My final remarks are to stress the danger of equating malnutrition with lack of food, or the converse, good nutrition with adequate supply of food. Good nutrition and health result from a constellation of interacting factors, one of which is food availability. Evidence indicates that households throughout the world generally have enough food to satisfy the needs of most people (Johnson, 1984), particularly the highly vulnerable infants and toddlers; furthermore, many mothers know how to make good use of what is available (Mata, 1978; Mata, 1979). However, many factors interfere with proper food consumption and utilization, for instance, infections and inadequate family or maternal technologies. If malnutrition is equated with lack of food, the likely outcome is the prescription of food as the solution. Food intervention programs have not had a resounding effect on curtailing diarrhea and malnutrition (Mata, 1985; Beaton and Ghassemi, 1982; Feachem, 1986), because they leave causal factors undisturbed, namely, deficient maternal behavior, poor education, unsanitary environment, and deficient primary health. On the other hand, there is growing evidence to show that the cultural and technological endowment (maternal technologies) and the application of scientific knowledge on disease prevention and control (development of sanitary infrastructure and medical services), are more relevant than socioeconomic factors in explaining the dramatic improvement in health and survival throughout the world in recent decades (Mohs, 1982; Rosero-Bixby, 1986; Mata and Rosero, 1987; Halstead et al., 1985; Preston, 1985; Mensch et al., 1985).

It is essential to continue exploring relationships of economic recession and its ensuing adjustments with other determinants of nutritional status and health. For instance, it would appear logical to investigate possible influences of economic recession on the quality and quantity of primary health care, availability of transport and curative services. Also, the effects on the behavior and wellbeing of the family, as it relates to pregnant women, infants and young children, should be considered.

Conceptual models should be engineered for the determinants of nutritional status and health in marginal societies—the chief interest of the Takemi Symposium—during the pre-recession period and during economic recession itself. The latter, in turn, should be clearly defined and described. On the basis of a model of this kind, it would be possible to discern the kinds of data which should be gathered for a pre-recession period, specifically those which one expects will show significant changes during economic recession in nutrition and other indices of social malady.

References

Anderson, B. A., and B. D. Silver. "Infant Mortality in the Soviet Union: Regional Differences and Measurement Issues," Research Report 86–93. University of Michigan, Population Study Center, 1986, pp. 1–35.

Beaton, G. H., and H. Ghassemi. "Supplementary Feeding Programs for Young Children in Developing Countries," *American Journal of Clinical Nutrition* 35 (1982; supp.): 863–916.

Behrman, J. R. "The Impact of Economic Adjustment Programs," Chapter 5 of this volume.

Braun, P., et al. "Birth Weight and Genital Mycoplasmas in Pregnancy," *New England Journal of Medicine* 284 (1971): 167–171.

Ceramy, A. "Materials which Promote and Inhibit Biosynthesis of Cachectin. A Macrophage Protein which Induces Catabolic State: A Review," in Thomas P. Singer et al., eds., *Mechanism of Drug Action.* Orlando: Academic Press, 1983, pp. 175–186.

Dinarello, C. A. "Interleukin-1 and the Pathogenesis of the Acute-Phase Response," *New England Journal of Medicine* 311 (1983): 1413–1418.

Feachem, R. G. "Preventing Diarrhoea: What are the Policy Options?" *Health Policy Planning* 1 (1986): 109–117.

Grant, J. P. *The State of the World's Children 1986.* Oxford: Oxford University Press, 1986.

Guyer, B., et al. "Anthropometric Evidence of Malnutrition Among Low-Income Children in Massachusetts in 1983," *Massachusetts Journal of Community Health* 2 (1985–1986): 3–9.

Halstead, S. B., J. A. Walsh, and K. S. Warren. *Good Health at Low Cost.* New York: The Rockefeller Foundation, 1985.

Johnson, D. G. "World Food and Agriculture," in J. L. Simon, H. Khan, eds., *The Resourceful Earth: A Response to Global 2000.* Oxford: Basil Blackwell, 1984, pp. 67–112.

Jolly, R., and G. A. Cornia. *The Impact of World Recession on Children.* New York: Pergamon, 1984.

Klinger, A. *Infant Mortality in Eastern Europe, 1950–1980.* Budapest: Statistical Publishing House, 1982.

Mata, L. J. *The Children of Santa Maria Cauque: A Prospective Field Study of Health and Growth.* Cambridge, MA: MIT Press, 1978.

———. "Environmental Factors Affecting Nutrition and Growth," in M. Gracey and F. Falkner, eds., *Nutritional Needs and Assessment of Normal Growth*, Nestle Nutrition. Vevey: Raven Press, 1985, pp. 165–182.

———. "Malnutrition-Infection Complex and its Environment Factors," *Proceedings of the Nutrition Society* 38 (1979): 29–40.

———. "The Nature of the Nutrition Problem," in L. Joy, ed., *Nutrition Planning: The State of the Art.* New York: IPI Sci Tech, 1978, pp. 154–264.

Mata, L., R. A. Kronmal, J. J. Urrutia, and B. Garcia. "Antenatal Events and Postnatal Growth and Survival of Children in a Rural Guatemalan Village," *Annals of Human Biology* 3 (1976): 303–315.

———. "Effect of Infection on Food Intake and the Nutritional State: Perspectives as Viewed from the Village," *American Journal of Clinical Nutrition* 30 (1977): 1215–1217.

Mata, L., and L. Rosero. *Health and Social Development in Costa Rica: Intersectoral Action.* Washington, D.C.: Pan American Health Organization, 1987.

Mensch, B., H. Lentzner, and S. H. Preston. *Socio-Economic Differentials in Child Mortality in Developing Countries.* New York: United Nations, ST/ESSA/SER.A/97, 1985.

Mohs, E. "Infectious Diseases and Health in Costa Rica: The Development of a New Paradigm," *Pediatric Infectious Diseases* 1 (1982): 212–216.

Preston, S. H. "Resources, Knowledge, and Child Mortality: Comparison of the U.S. in the Late Nineteenth Century and Developing Countries Today." *IUSSP International Population Conference.* Florence, June 5–12, 1985, pp. 373–386.

———. "Review of Richard Jolly and Giovanni Andrea Cornia, editors, *The Impact of World Recession on Children*," *Journal of Development Economics*, 1986.

Rosero-Bixby, L. "Infant Mortality in Costa Rica: Explaining the Recent Decline," *Studies in Family Planning* 17 (1986): 57–65.

Tafari, N. "Low Birth Weight: An Overview." *Advances in International Maternal and Child Health.* New York: Oxford University Press, 1981, pp. 105–127.

Tomkins, A. M., et al. "The Combined Effects of Infection and Malnutrition on Protein Metabolism in Children." *Clinical Science* 65 (1983): 313–324.

Waterlow, J. C., and N. E. Rutishauser. "Malnutrition in Man," in Joaquín Cravioto et al., eds., *Early Malnutrition and Mental Development*, Symposium on Early Malnutrition and Mental Development. Stockholm: Almqvist & Wiksel, 1974.

Watkins, S. C., and J. Menken. "Famines in Historical Perspective," *Development Review* 11 (1985): 647–675.

Wyon, J. B., and J. E. Gordon. *The Khanna Study: Population Problems in the Rural Punjab.* Cambridge, MA: Harvard University Press, 1970.

PART III

APPROACHES TO HEALTH POLICY

12

Health Policy Responses: An Approach Derived from the the China and India Experiences

Lincoln C. Chen

There are several reasons why an assessment of health policy options in response to recent world economic crises is a daunting and perhaps insurmountable challenge. First, cause-and-effect linkages between the dynamics of the macroeconomy and the health of populations are multiple, difficult to pinpoint, and undoubtedly complex (Feinberg, 1982; Helleiner, 1985; Jolly, 1985; Killick, 1984; United Nations, 1986). One axiom of public health is the direct and consistent relationship between material well-being and health (Government of India, 1979; Halstead, 1985; McKeown and Record, 1962; Mosley and Chen, 1984). Thus, very marked economic fluctuations could be expected to generate corresponding changes in a population's health status. The relationship, however, is imprecise, and significant deviations—both positive and negative—are not unusual within and among societies (Caldwell, 1979; Halstead et al., 1985; Krishnan, 1976).

Another factor is the diversity of economic and health situations in the developing world. Retarded or negative economic growth, for example, has been concentrated in some countries of Latin America and sub-Saharan Africa, while some segments of Asia have been spared (Killick, 1984; United Nations, 1986; Williamson, 1983). The total international indebtedness of Third World countries was U.S. $900 billion in 1984; nearly half of this was owed by seven large borrowers in Latin America and Asia (Debt Crisis Network, 1985; Killick, 1984; Williamson, 1983).[1] Fifty smaller countries, many in Africa, may be equally or more

279

severely affected, but their population and debt sizes are more modest. Two giant Asian societies, China and India, have remained relatively immune from international economic turmoil.

Finally, there are limited empirical data from specific geocultural settings to document recent changes of health status that can be attributed indisputably to international economic forces. Considerable public controversy surrounds this subject (Debt Crisis Network, 1985; Jolly, 1985; Killick, 1984; United Nations, 1986).[2] Scientific agnosticism is perhaps an inevitable conclusion because of lack of empirical data and analysis (Helleiner, 1985; Williamson, 1983).[3] Also, many other momentous events have been taking place simultaneously. The acute health and nutritional crises in sub-Saharan Africa, for example, have multiple—not simply international economic—origins, including climatic and political instability (World Bank, 1984a). Inequitable patterns of health and development in some Latin American societies were already entrenched well before recent economic difficulties (Killick, 1984; Williamson, 1983).

Many hypotheses, nevertheless, could be advanced to link economic crises and austere macroeconomic adjustments with adverse impacts on health. Given the breadth and depth of economic adjustments in some countries, few aspects of these societies could be expected to remain unaffected. Developing countries are often primary product exporters, and promotion of exports could lead, for example, to further shifts away from subsistence food to cash crop production (Debt Crisis Network, 1985). Import restrictions are often accomplished through price increases to dampen domestic consumption demand (Williamson, 1983). Price increases along with wage freezes erode the purchasing power of the poor, labor, and the middle class (Marshall et al., 1983). Elimination of food subsidies and reductions of public welfare expenditures have obvious implications for the financing and the ultimate impact of public health and social welfare systems (Helleiner, 1985; Killick, 1984.) Most significantly, income and employment among the poor may deteriorate.[4] Even with data insufficiency, few would deny that recent economic adjustment experiences have invariably been associated with a further regression, or at best stability, of income distribution (Feinberg, 1982; Helleiner, 1985; Williamson, 1983).[5] We must conclude that, at least in the short run, the burden of slowed or negative economic growth and economic adjustment processes would be shouldered disproportionately by the poor, the disadvantaged, and women in particular (Jolly, 1985; United Nations, 1986).

Examination of health policy responses to international economic change could focus on whether adjustment policies exert an adverse impact on health and, if so, the mechanisms through which these presumed effects may operate. The former issue is complex and geoculturally specific and would make generalizations difficult; the latter would simply evoke many hypotheses without empirical support. A broader and more useful approach would be to address a set of fundamental, structural issues related to health policy in developing countries. What would be the basic components of health policy analysis? Are there common features and processes in the health sector across developing societies? If so, can a conceptual framework be developed? And finally, how would specific policy-relevant studies such as those in this volume on women, technology, drugs, and financing, relate to an overall approach? This chapter explores some of these questions. First it presents data on the health status and health systems in China and India, the world's two most populous countries. Such a comparison provides an empirical basis for a conceptual framework incorporating various health and nonmedical factors that determine the health of populations. The paper then concludes by highlighting selectively a set of generic issues fundamental to health policy analysis in developing countries.

India and China

The 1982 populations of India (733 million) and China (1,019 million) combined constitute nearly 40 percent of the world's population or 75 percent of people residing in low-income countries with per capita annual incomes below U.S. $400 (World Bank, 1984; World Bank, 1985). In addition to their demographic size, these two Asian societies share other features.[6] Both are ancient cultures which attained political independence about four decades ago. Both have low per capita income, modest levels of urbanization, and a predominance of agriculture in the economy (Table 12.1). Because both economies are continental in scale, they have been relatively protected from recent global economic fluctuations (World Bank, 1984b; World Bank, 1985).

Differences between these two giants are also noteworthy. Politically, China is a centrally controlled communist state, while India is a federated democracy operating a mixed economy. While the Chinese people are relatively homogeneous ethnically (93 percent Han), India's people are highly diverse—with fifteen major languages, many religions, and multiple caste, tribal, and cultural affiliations. The Chinese have achieved nearly universal literacy within a reasonably egalitarian social structure. In contrast, the vast majority of India's people remain illiterate and deeply imbedded in rigid social stratifications, as manifested by the Hindu caste system. Even so, both India and China may be classified as "superior health achievers" since their mortality levels are lower than

Table 12.1
Selected Development Indicators: India and China (1983)

	India	China
Demographic		
Population (millions)	733	1,019
Urbanization (%)	24	21
Labor force in agriculture (%)[a]	71	74
Economic		
GNP per capita (US$)	260	300
Absolute poverty (million)	300	100
Cereal availability per capita (gms/day)	414[b]	533[c]
Social		
Adult literacy[d] (%)	34	77
Enrollment primary school[e] (%)	79	100+

[a] 1981
[b] 1982
[c] 1979
[d] 1977
[e] 1982

Sources: D. T. Jamison, 1985; World Development Report 1985; C. Gopalan, 1985.

would be predicted by their respective national incomes (Caldwell, 1986; Halstead, 1985).

Health Status

Data in Table 12.2 show that India and China experience markedly different health situations. India has moderately high birth and death

Table 12.2
Health Indicators: India and China (1983)

	India	China
Crude Rates (per 1,000 population)		
Birth	34	19
Deaths	13	7
Natural increase	21	12
Fertility Rates		
Total fertility (per woman)	4.8	2.3
Mortality Rates		
Infant (per 1,000 livebirths)	93	38
Child 1–4 yrs (per 1,000 population)	11	2
Life expectancy (years)		
Male	56	65
Female	54	69

Source: World Development Report 1985.

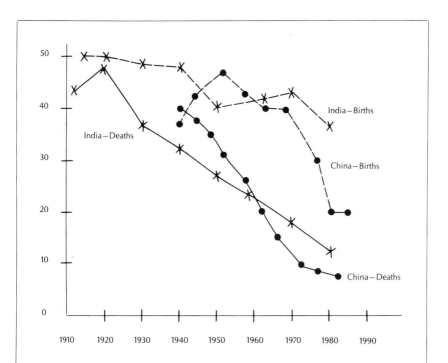

Figure 12.1. Crude birth and death rates in China (1940–1980) and India (1911–1981).

rates while China's are very close to those of economically advanced countries. China has achieved these dramatic health advances over the past three decades (Figure 12.1) (China Health Yearbook, 1983; Jamison et al., 1984).[7] Health in India has improved reasonably steadily throughout most of this century, but India's contemporary health situation continues to remain backward (Government of India, 1984; Vasaria and Vasaria, 1981).

A most interesting comparison between India and China is health disparities within societies. Despite its high overall life expectancy, China's health differentials are primarily geographic in character (Jamison, 1985). Infant mortality in rural China is 70 percent higher than urban levels, and the rate in backward Yangsu County is nearly three times that of the more advanced Shanghai County (Yu, 2985). Mortality rates in the minority regions of China may be considerably worse than generally reported. Health differentials are also marked in India. There the disparities are evident not only geographically but across many socioeconomic characteristics, as Table 12.3 shows (Government of

Table 12.3
Infant Mortality Rate (per 1,000 livebirths) in India According to Selected States, Literacy, Religion, and Child Sex (1979)

	Rural	*Urban*	*All*
All India	136	71	126
States			
Uttar Pradesh	184	168	172
Kerala	45	29	42
Literacy			
Illiterate	145	88	140
Literate	90	50	55
Religion			
Hindu	138	70	132
Muslim	126	76	104
Sex Child			
Female	131	71	121
Male	129	73	119

Source: Registrar-General of India, Survey on Infant and Child Mortality, 1979.

India, 1984; Jain, 1985; Vasaria and Vasaria, 1981). Indian rural infant mortality is nearly twice that of the level in urban areas, and the likelihood of infant death in the backward State of Uttar Pradesh is five-fold that of the socially advanced Kerala State (Government of India, 1979). Differentials are also pronounced between religious, caste, and class groups and socioeconomic characteristics such as literacy and mother's education (Bose and Desai, 1983; Jain, 1985; Vasaria and Vasaria, 1981). India is one of the few societies in the world where female life expectancy is briefer than male (Chen, 1982; Dyson and Moore, 1983).

Health Systems

Much has been written about China's remarkable success in improving the health of its people.[8] The advances are attributable to China's health system as well as to socioeconomic gains in the provision of basic needs—water, sanitation, and food (Gopalan, 1985; Halstead et al., 1985; Jamison, 1985; Panikar, 1986). China's health system prior to the 1980s has been marked by several innovations. Among the more significant have been mass mobilization of the people for preventive health efforts, including regular campaigns against the "four pests" (rats, flies, mosquitos, and bed bugs) and sexually transmitted diseases, mass vaccination, and control of the vectors responsible for the transmission of malaria and schistosomiasis. Another noteworthy feature has been the deprofessionalization of health care providers through the development of a mass cadre of barefoot doctors at the grassroots level. The mass application of paraprofessionals through a three-tier health care delivery system has helped extend the availability of basic services into remote regions. Third, China invests a relatively large proportion of its national resources in the health sector (Jamison, 1985; Panandikar, 1983). These investments have been both monetary and human, through contributions of unpaid labor. China's capacity to implement health care and other programs at the grassroots level has been the most outstanding feature of its success (Perkins and Yusef, 1984). Few countries can claim similar implementation capacity, including economically-advanced countries.

Organization. These favorable characteristics in China are only partially shared in India, which presents a far more complex picture. As a federated democracy, India's constitution assigns health and other social sectors to India's twenty-two states. The center may plan and fund health systems, but the ultimate responsibility for implementing them rests with diverse state governments (Government of India, 1980).

At the central union level, health is the responsibility of the Ministry of Health and Family Welfare (Banerji, 1985; Government of India, 1980). The Ministry has two operational departments—health and family welfare. The health department is responsible for health services, medical education, hospitals, and vertical disease control programs. The family welfare department is primarily responsible for family planning and secondarily for maternal-child health services. Other health-related fields are assigned to other ministries: nutrition to Social Welfare; water and sanitation to Housing and Public Works; and pharmaceuticals to Industries and Chemicals.

The organization of health departments at the state level mirrors the bifurcation of health and family planning at the center (Figure 12.2). Urban health services are provided through a network of state or municipal hospitals and dispensaries. The overwhelming bulk of India's people are in 576,000 rural villages, covered by a three-tier primary health care system (Table 12.4). At the district level (population about 1 million) are medical and family planning officers responsible for the entire district, including dispensaries and hospitals. At the block level (population about 100,000) are primary health centers. These, in turn, supervise and back up the work of subcenters, which optimally cover about 10,000 people through multipurpose workers. The bulk of basic services are provided by part-time community health workers based at the village level.

Personnel and Facilities. Table 12.5 shows that the pattern of health personnel in India and China are, at senior levels, rather similar (Gov-

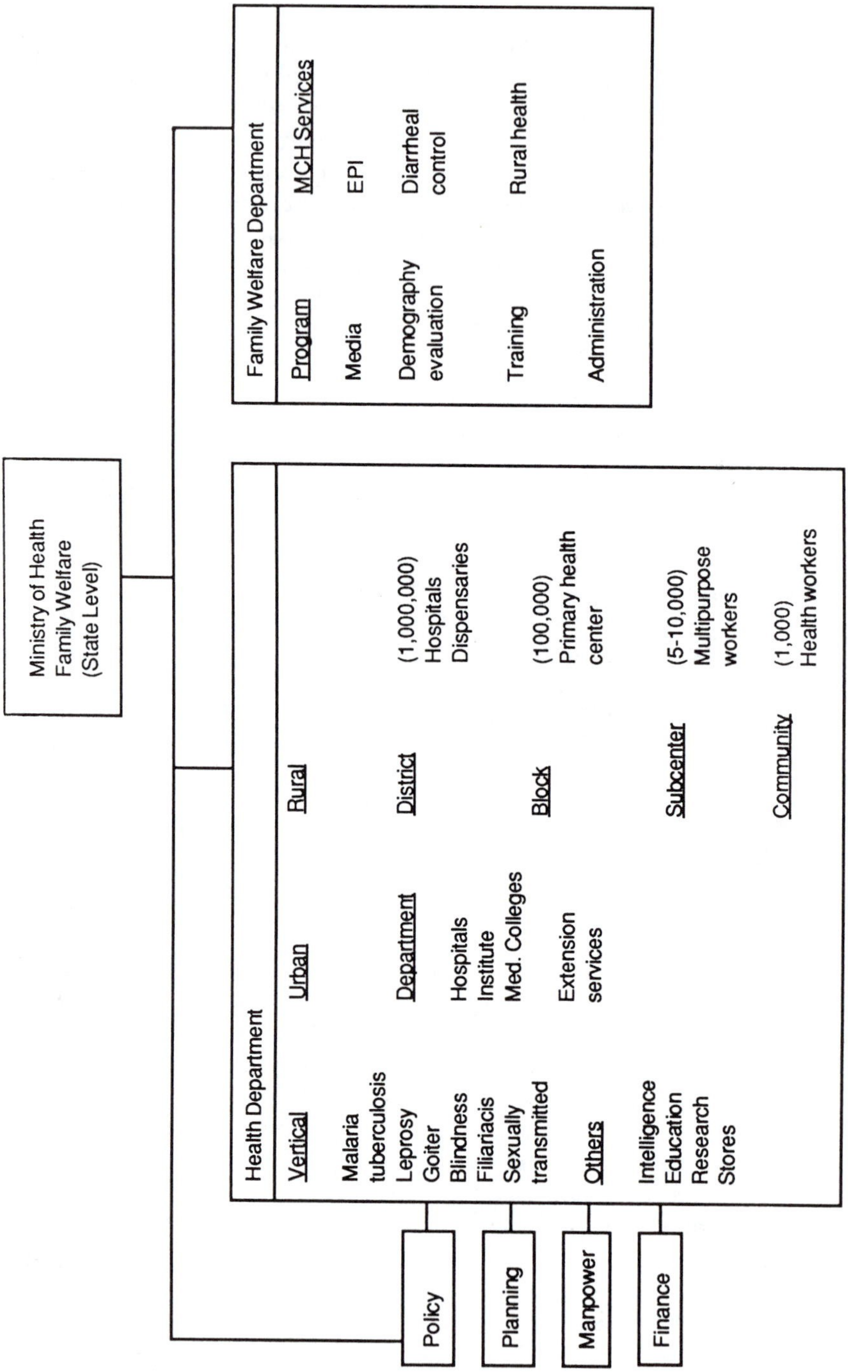

Figure 12.2. *Indian health system organization.*

Table 12.4
Structure of Rural Primary Health System in India

Level	Facilities	Staff	Village Serviced	Population Serviced
District	Hospital	Medical Officer	1,200–1,800	1,500,000
		Family Planning Officer		
Block	Primary	Medical Officer	80–100	80,000–120,000
	Health	Nurses		
	Centre	Pharmacist		
		Technicians		
	Subcenter	Health supervisors	25–40	30,000–40,000
	Subcenter	Health workers	8–10	10,000
Village	—	Community health worker	1	500–1,500

ernment of India, 1984; Jamison et al., 1984). Both have large numbers of western-trained allopathic doctors, and both have nurtured and subsidized traditional health practitioners.[9] At the middle and primary levels, differences become noticeable. The density of Chinese assistant doctors is similar to that of India's rural medical practitioners. There is considerable difference, however, between Chinese paraprofessionals—who have been trained and supervised as assistant doctors—and the unqualified, unregistered, commercially motivated rural medical practitioners one finds in India. At the grassroots level, China's health aides and barefoot doctors are four times more dense than India's village aides and community health workers. Moreover, in-depth observational studies in India have demonstrated high rates of absenteeism, diversion into private practice, and low work output among Indian health personnel (Banerji, 1985; Bose and Desai, 1983).

China's health facilities are also superior. China's hospital to population density is seven times that of India's, and it has four times the density of beds per population (Government of India, 1984; Jamison et al., 1984). China's bed availability for rural people, furthermore, is eight times that of India's. Much of India's primary health care infrastructure is still in the planning stage. In 1984, less than 30 percent of primary health centers were actually in operation, and less than half of the subcenters were staffed with trained multipurpose workers (Banerji, 1985).

Resource Mobilization and Allocation. Although their 1982 per capita GNPs are roughly similar (China, U.S. $265; India, U.S. $229), the share of national income invested in health differs (World Bank, 1985). India's per capita health investment is $2.70 or 1.2 percent of GNP

Table 12.5
Health Personnel and Facilities in India and China

	India		China	
	No.	Per 100,000	No.	Per 100,000
Personnel				
Senior				
Doctors (western)	271.6	37.	516.5	52
Doctors (traditional)	382.5	52	289.5	29
Pharmacist (all)	155.6	23	162.7	16
Middle				
Assist doc/Med practitioner	250.0	44	436.2	44
Nurses	160.9	22	525.3	53
Midwives	247.4	34	70.9	7
Primary				
Aides/Workers	140.8	19	769.5	78
Village Workers	313.2	42	1,839.6	185
Facilities				
Hospitals (all)	7.2	1	65.9	7
Beds (all)	500.6	67	2,017.0	203
Beds (Rural)	93.5	16	1,097.1	138

Sources: China: The Health Sector, World Bank, 1984; *Health Statistics of India*, Ministry Health Family Welfare, 1984.

(Banerji, 1985; Col and Roberts, 1984; Government of India, 1984; Gupta, 1984; Marshall et al., 1983; Pai Panandikar et al., 1983). This level is only one-third that of China's \$8.8 per capita or 3.3 percent of GNP (Jamison et al., 1985; World Bank, 1984; World Bank, 1985).[10]

Health sector resource mobilization patterns in India and China are compared in Figure 12.3.[11] Private sources constitute two-thirds of India's health finances; one-quarter is from government; and only 8 percent comes from insurance schemes. China, by contrast, has a tri-partite financing structure with about equal shares coming from state, private, and rural cooperative insurance sources.

The flow of resources through various health care delivery systems follows the patterns of financing. In India, two-thirds of the flow goes through the private commercial systems. Only one-quarter goes through government health services. Very small portions flow through private non-profit voluntary organizations and enterprise-related health systems. In China, the flow through rural collective systems predominates

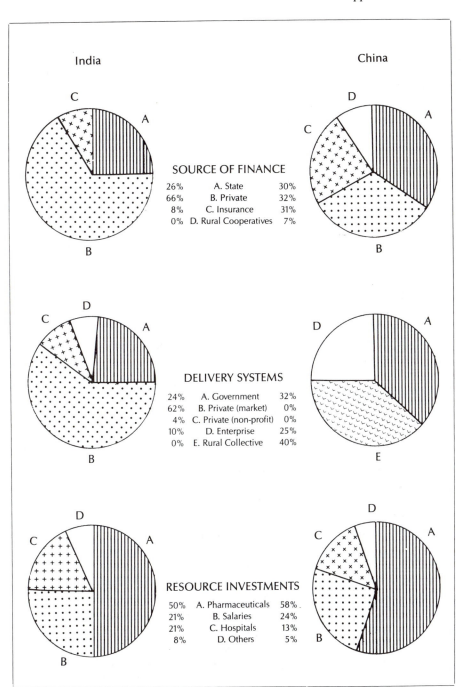

Figure 12.3. *Health resource mobilization and allocation: India and China.*
Source: China data from Jamison et al., 1984. India data compiled by author.

(40 percent), with smaller portions going through government and enterprise systems.

Resource allocations in health, however, are similar in China and India. In both cases, half or more of the resources are invested in pharmaceuticals, and nearly all of these expenditures are for modern, not traditional, drugs. About a quarter is allocated for personnel salaries. China's investment in hospitals is proportionately half that of India's.

Conceptual Framework

The comparison between China and India provides an empirical base for formulating a conceptual framework for health policy analysis. Such an approach begins with a focus on the health status of populations. A systematic approach to factors that determine the health of populations introduces considerations related to both the productivity of health care systems as well as the impact on health of social, economic, political, and environmental factors (Caldwell, 1986; Halstead et al., 1985; Mosley and Chen, 1984).

Figure 12.4 presents a schematic conceptual framework for the determinants of the health status of populations. In this approach, nonmedical factors include the quality of the physical environment, economic or material well being, nutritional status, reproductive patterns, and women/household capacity variables (Mosley and Chen, 1984). These nonmedical factors are the primary determinants of disease risk; they also condition preventive and therapeutic health responses. The quality of the environment (housing, water, sanitation, workplace) is a primary determinant of the risk of disease exposure and transmission. Nutritional status (agriculture, food) determines the biological capacity of the host to withstand disease onslaught and thus the severity and case-fatality of illness. Material well being (income, employment) determines the capacity of families to purchase an adequate environment and nutritional status. Economics also may shape client behavior, particularly the pattern of health service utilization (Khan and Prasad, 1984; Khan and Prasad, 1983). Patterns of reproduction (age, parity, spacing of births) determine the biosocial health risks of mothers and children.

Many studies have shown that even if environmental and economic variables are controlled, some families are consistently better, and others poorer, health achievers (Caldwell, 1986). Inadequately understood but powerfully significant is the capacity of families, particularly mothers, to manage health related investments and behavior within households. One measurable indicator of this capacity is maternal education (Caldwell, 1979; Ware, 1984). But the health capacity of a household

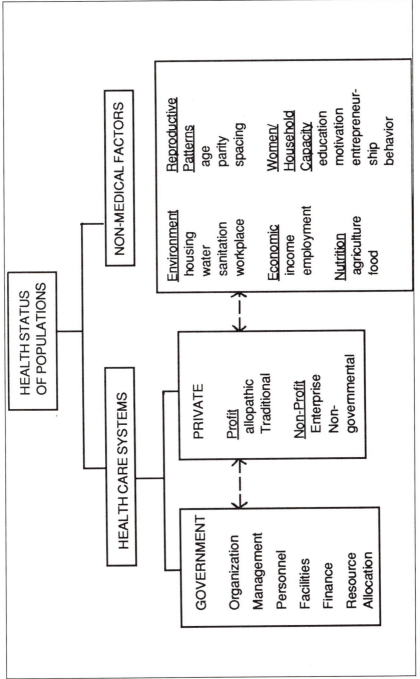

Figure 12.4. *Schematic framework on determinants of health status of populations.*

probably relates to a host of additional, poorly measured factors such as motivation, enterprise, and behavior (Ware, 1984). These probably exert their effects through both health care and nonmedical factors—such as disease prevention, improved nutrition, and more timely and effective prevention and management of illness.

The other major determinant of the health status of a population is the health system. One useful classification for health systems is public versus private. Such a dichotomy usefully classifies systems that are different in virtually all respects—objectives, organization, structure, personnel, financing, and client role. In developing countries, the better understood system is usually the public system. Subsidized by government budgets and usually directly operated by public extension bureaucracies, public sector health systems operate within reasonably well defined policy parameters.

The private systems are much more varied and difficult to map. Often multiple schools of health, both modern western (allopathic) and traditional, are involved. The commercially driven, for-profit private systems operate through fee-for-service payments, and health service providers may range from highly trained physicians to traditional practitioners to untrained providers including pharmacists. In some countries, nonprofit voluntary systems may also be significant, especially in societies with a history of religious or charitable movements.

Third party health insurance systems for employees in the formal labor sector could be either private, public, or some combination thereof. In most cases, these have multiple sources of funds—employee contributions, company funds, and public subsidy. Sometimes entirely separate health facilities have been established to service clients of third party or enterprise systems. The most common beneficiaries of these systems are government employees, industrial workers, social security recipients and pensioners. These systems are growing in rapidly modernizing societies but may be virtually absent in lowest income countries.

Overall, it should be noted that while the health system and nonmedical factors are depicted separately in Figure 12.4, they are in reality highly interactive and interdependent. In other words, non-medical factors can influence the shape and performance of health systems, and conversely, the performance of health systems can influence non-medical factors. The reduction of debilitating disease could facilitate the exploitation of previously inaccessible agricultural lands, and a reduction of malnutrition and morbidity could improve work performance. There may also be interactive processes between governmental and private sectors within the health system—such as the private production of pharmaceuticals for distribution in public systems or the part-time private practice of fulltime government-employed doctors. Thus, the processes and effects of health systems and non-medical factors are highly dynamic, interactive, and interdependent.

Health Sector Policy Analysis

A systematic policy approach to the health sector requires an understanding of the characteristics of the sector, its objectives, and institutional and financial structures and processes. Customary approaches to health policy include analyses of such issues as organization, management, personnel, facilities, technology, financing, and resource allocation (Baum and Talbert, 1985).

All of these elements are important, and policy analyses focusing on any of these individual elements can generate important policy-relevant insights. Considered separately, however, these individual components are incomplete and may be inadequate in several ways for effective policy implementation. First there are strong linkages and interactions between these components within the health system. Policy change in any single element could be frustrated by rigidities in other critical components. Further, topical approaches must be fortified by a broad and deep understanding of the health system in the context of the overall political economy. The historical, political, and economic forces in the political economy not only shape and condition the health sector—they also influence many non-medical factors. Finally, such approaches to the health sector may focus too heavily on "supply" issues—the delivery of technologies and services by the health system. Supply approaches may fail to incorporate adequately client demand issues (Caldwell, 1986; Khan and Prasad, 1983; Ware, 1984). Client preferences, health behavior, and the capacity of families themselves to generate health (with or without the health system per se) are critical in determining the efficiency and productivity of the health sector and ultimately the health status of populations.

Let us examine the China-India comparison to illustrate these propositions. At least on the surface, there are similarities between the Chinese and Indian health systems—in organization, management, facilities, personnel, and technology policy. Both China and India have developed three-tier horizontal health care systems which extend to the village level. These countries have invested heavily in modern hospitals and doctors while simultaneously subsidizing the traditional health systems. At the grassroots level, both have paraprofessionals providing basic services to the population. In both countries, about half of all health expenditures are for drugs. Hospitals and personnel salaries command most of the remaining resources.

Deeper analyses demonstrate critical differences, however. One comparison is the organizational controversy regarding the relative merits of vertical versus integrated program structures and the relative emphasis on preventive versus curative services. Curiously, prevention in both countries receives less than 10 percent of health resources (Jamison, 1984). Disease prevention in China, however, has achieved outstanding results through mass mobilization of peasants for health campaigns. These preventive health actions did not overtax the health budget in a poor society since monetary resources were supplemented by compulsory mobilization of surplus labor during slack agricultural seasons (Mosley and Chen, 1984; Panikar, 1986; Perkins and Yusef, 1984). China's success with vertical programs is probably unique to its sociopolitical conditions (Perkins and Yusef, 1984). Effective implementation depended upon China's strong political-administrative capacities at the grassroots level.

India, by contrast, has experienced mixed results with vertical programs. In the past 40 years, India has introduced many preventive campaigns—in family planning, malaria, filiriasis, leprosy, blindness, goitre, smallpox, tuberculosis, kala azar, Japanese encephalitis, and more recently an expanded program in immunization (EPI) and oral rehydration therapy (ORT) (Banerji, 1985). Of these health problems, only smallpox has been eradicated. The remaining have persisted and in some instances—such as malaria—resurged. India's health system is increasingly burdened by budgetary obligations and staff from defunct vertical programs in which permanently employed field staff have been left behind because of shifting priorities (Banerji, 1985; Bose and Desai, 1983).[12] India's vertical campaigns also depended entirely on a fulltime extension bureaucracy, not on unpaid labor, and pressures from the top could not generate indefinitely high productivity in the health sector. Policy realignment in India thus must also encompass organizational reform, particularly personnel policies. In India, personnel policies are uniformly applied throughout the civil service, not just in the health sector.

A similar contrast is noteworthy in policies related to personnel and facilities. China's barefoot doctors were a creation of the Chinese political-administrative system at the commune and brigade levels. The barefoot doctors fit into the local organizational structures of rural China; their functioning depends on these structures (Perkins and Yusef, 1984). The grassroots health worker in India operates in an administrative vacuum. The Indian community development movement, begun in the 1950s, is based upon an extension model originally transplanted from the United States. Parallel sectoral extension workers function within traditional village power configurations, which are hierarchical and socially stratified. India's extension approach has yet to overcome weaknesses in motivation, supervision, and training.[13]

In neither China nor India has there been broad recognition of and concern over the health consequences of drug use patterns and the large proportion of health resources invested in modern pharmaceuticals. In China, a state corporation produces the drugs, and there appears to be large-scale abuse of modern pharmaceuticals. In. India, public efforts have only recently been made to promote rationalization of drug production and consumption which are predominantly in the private sector (Baum and Talbert, 1985). The problem in India is grossly complicated by the fact that pharmaceuticals are not considered primarily within the domain of health. Rather, drug production and marketing are under the purview of the Ministry of Industries and Chemicals (Banerji, 1985; Bhagat, 1982).

Two common analytical approaches to these policy issues are technology cost-effectiveness and economic analyses. The application of cost-effectiveness techniques could theoretically contribute to more rational technology/drug selection. After all, cost-effectiveness introduces the concepts of priorities based upon disease prevalence, health impact, and feasibility of technological intervention as determined by efficacy and cost. Sophisticated technology analyses would also build in concern for client preferences, health behavior, and health service utilization. Economic analysis is a powerful tool for the mapping of the structure of the health system and for illuminating the system's actual (rather than articulated) priorities. Such financial techniques applied to China and India have demonstrated their power in generating insights about the structure of the health sector.

Taken to an extreme or isolated from the bureaucratic environment, these quantitative techniques may lose much of their relevance and usefulness. Assumptions built into cost-effectiveness analysis may overwhelm quantitative precision. Moreover, a narrow focus on cost-effectiveness may miss more fundamental constraints. India's selection of certain technologies and resource allocation patterns (hospitals and drugs) would appear inappropriate. The problem, however, stems not so much from inappropriate technology selection as from ineffective implementation by the extension bureaucracy. Policy change thus must deal with issues beyond technology cost-effectiveness. An example of the limitations of technology policy is tuberculosis control. According to cost-effectiveness analysis, tuberculosis is undoubtedly of high priority. It is highly prevalent, extracts a significant health toll, and has a low-cost, efficacious technological solution. But appropriate technology policies alone have failed to address the problem—80 percent of pulmonary tuberculosis patients that come to Indian clinics are turned away by physicians with only cough syrup (Banerji, 1985)!

Health system interdependencies can be seen clearly when proposed policy changes are rendered ineffective by a lack of corresponding shifts in budget allocations. In India, the recent priority given to primary health care and child survival has unfortunately not yet been reflected by budgetary reallocations. Instead of revamping health programs to reflect new priorities, policymakers in both India and China have tacked new "special programs" onto existing structures and made no organizational or budgetary shifts. Pure budgetary shifts would nevertheless be impossible without major realignments of organizational and personnel policies. In a dense bureaucratic and cautious political environment, fiscal policies to govern the role of the private sector, introduce user fees or develop risk-sharing arrangements are difficult to implement and often politically controversial. The Indian government does not charge for any public social service. The imposition of a user fee for health services, for example, would not only require entirely new bureaucratic procedures but could be perceived as violating the post-colonial state ideology of welfare socialism.

Political Economy of Health

While understanding of health sector policy options can be advanced through any specific lens (e.g. organization, technology, finances), such analyses are only useful to the extent that they are geoculturally specific and incorporate considerations of the broader context of the political economy. Historical, political, and economic forces operate on the health system both directly and indirectly (through nonmedical factors).

Health systems do not exist in a time vacuum—their histories both shape their present and constrain their future (Abel-Smith, 1984).[14] For China, the communist revolution has been a central determinant of China's performance in health. China's newly formed government, having no colonial past, was able to introduce a health care structure integrating local financing and implementation with its own unique political-administrative structures. In India, British colonialism introduced western medicine and medical structures well before the time of the peaceful transition to independence. The famous Indian Bhore Committee in 1946 recommended a national health strategy that contained all of the elements of what we today call primary health care (Government of India, 1946). A more recent report by the Indian Medical Research Council and the Indian Council for Social Science Research reaffirmed the Bhore recommendations (ICSSR-ICMR, 1981). Neither, however, has been able to overcome historical momentum or the constraints the political economy imposes.

In both China and India, the broader political context of health is important. China's communist government has consistently ranked health a high ideological—and thus budgetary—priority. However, China's repressive political system has also generated health problems. Political opposition is not tolerated and public information and debate are unheard of. Thus, 16–20 million Chinese died quietly of famine during the Great Leap Forward in 1959–1961 (Aird, 1982). By contrast, India is a highly socially stratified democracy with an open political process and a free press. India has recently achieved food self-sufficiency, but 40 percent of Indians still suffer from an inadequate diet. Lack of response by the Indian government to an acute famine would trigger public outcry and could perhaps bring down a government. But the Indian elite and political system are able to diffuse criticism of persistent mass hunger among nearly half of its people (Sen, 1983).

The linkage between politics and the health system is well illustrated by recent developments. The new Chinese "household responsibility system" has reintroduced the concept of economic incentives for individual productivity. Peasants and workers are now encouraged to produce privately for individual reward. This fundamental political change has had dramatic, perhaps unintentional, consequences for the Chinese health care system. With a population in pursuit of private gains, decision making has shifted from groups to families, previous operating structures have weakened, and health motivation can no longer be mandated but must be achieved through mass education.[15] The network of barefoot doctors has nearly collapsed, rural health care coverage has declined, county hospitals and rural clinics are in financial distress, and private medical practice has re-emerged. Well-to-do clients are now bypassing lower paramedical staff to present themselves directly at more advanced facilities (Hsaio, 1983; Krishnan, 1976). In India, recent policies liberalizing the economy may generate a similar trend towards capping of the public sector and stimulation of private enterprise (Government of India, 1980; Sen, 1986).[16]

History and politics are important, but health policy must also confront a fundamental question about economics. How binding are economic constraints on health in developing societies? Here we are not dealing with fiscal issues in the health sector but with the significance of economics as one of the non-medical factors determining the health of populations. At the simplest level, the relationship between per capita national product and life expectancy of populations is tight—more wealth, better health (Government of India, 1979; Halstead et al., 1985; World Bank, 1985). The role of socioeconomic development (versus medical technologies) in the historical decline of mortality in the now industrialized countries has never gained full scientific consensus (Caldwell, 1986; Grey, 1974; McKeown and Record, 1962). Moreover, there are many contemporary exceptions to the direct income-health relationship. Some countries (such as China, India, Sri Lanka, and Costa Rica) have achieved health standards clearly superior to those predicted by their income levels, while others (such as Saudi Arabia, Iran, Libya, Iraq, and Algeria) are clearly inferior health achievers (Caldwell, 1986; Halstead et al., 1985). The explanation for these cases of positive and negative deviance from economic prediction is not entirely clear.[17]

Economic binds are also imperfect at the household level. Some poor families are able to bear and rear healthy children, and conversely some well-to-do households cope poorly. In-depth field investigations have delineated some of the factors responsible, including female education, family entrepreneurship, and health behavior. Female education appears to be a powerful indicator of improved family health, even when income levels are controlled (Caldwell, 1979; Ware, 1984). Many hypotheses have been advanced to explain the power of women-related or household capacity factors. Some have argued that education imparts knowledge regarding the scientific basis of disease transmission (germ theory), while others have proposed that educated women are more likely to make effective use of preventive and curative health services (Caldwell, 1986). Others argue that it is not the knowledge imparted by education, but the socialization which promotes the adoption of an entire set of modern values and practices. Enhanced status of women in the family, some propose, shifts the distribution of power in the family and thus the distribution of intra-household resources towards women and children, the subgroups at highest health risk (Ware, 1984).

The significant conclusion here is that the family is the central production unit for health. Economic constraints may be important, but they are not insurmountable. Educational, behavioral, entrepreneurial, and other factors clearly play critical roles in the production of health. Effective health policy analyses, therefore, must squarely address this potential. In a recent review, Caldwell boldly concluded that "good health is within the reach of all"—rich and poor nations alike (Caldwell, 1986). He concluded that health standards require high levels of government investment in the health sector,[18] broad societal consensus that health is a high political priority, and enhanced status, education, and autonomy of women. The issues were not so much technical or bureaucratic as they were ideological and cultural—in which people perceived health and social equality as fundamental rights.

Conclusion: Economic Crisis and Health

This paper takes a broad approach to the determinants of health status of populations. In response to economic crisis, traditional health sector policy approaches might narrow too early on purely financial or technology problems. Health care financing is important, but it is inextricably linked to issues of health sector organization, personnel, technology, and the broader political economy. For the health sector, a systematic approach necessarily requires first an empirical review of existing health system structures, their deviations from articulated objectives, and their efficiency and productivity in generating good health. The broad view recognizes that nonmedical factors may be as or more important in the production of good health as the health care system.

This viewpoint leads to the conclusion that changes wrought by economic crisis may affect both health care systems and nonmedical factors. It is possible that changes in nonmedical factors may have far greater health consequences than changes in the health system per se. Health policy responses, therefore, cannot be disassociated from policy changes in other sectors. Generally, health sector resource levels are linked to investment levels in antipoverty, education, and social welfare programs. An important signal of adjustment policies, therefore, is the direction of resource movements in these related sectors. If cutbacks of public expenditures are necessary, and this is not necessarily accepted, then cutbacks in the health sector may or may not be more protective of health than cutbacks in other social sectors, such as antipoverty programs, food subsidies, and education.[19]

Some have argued that times of fiscal austerity are also opportunities for innovation. Equitable food rationing by the British during World War II resulted in improved nutrition during a time of crisis (Jolly, 1985). Recently, there have been international efforts, notably by WHO and UNICEF, to advance a child survival and development revolution involving the mass dissemination of low-cost health technologies, such as growth monitoring, oral rehydration, breastfeeding, and immunizations, known collectively as GOBI (Jolly, 1985). The movement involves not only appropriate health technologies, but also innovative social organizational forms for improving people's access to health technologies. Such deinstitutionized delivery systems move beyond the traditional medical establishments (such as hospitals) to emphasize new organizational structures involving village volunteers, mass media, schools, and churches. Both on their own right and in parallel with adjustment policies in social sectors, these approaches may represent new opportunities to improve cost-effectiveness, managerial efficiency, and targeting of services to the most prevalent health problems among the disadvantaged in the developing world.

The launching of these child survival programs and the recent fluctuations of the global economy suggest that improved monitoring of health status in developing countries is absolutely essential (United Nations, 1986). Information is particularly needed on health status across population subgroups, time, and geography. Whose health is affected? Who is bearing the burden? Where are the poor located? Which policies are affecting them adversely? The answer to these questions is fundamental to effective health policy responses.

Lack of data is due to the recency of the crises and also in part to weak information systems in developing countries. Another contributor has been the lack of interest of international institutions, such as the International Monetary Fund and the private banks.[20] These organizations have explicitly excluded health and welfare concerns from their programs aimed at economic stabilization. The primary objectives of these adjustment policies have been the restoration of balance of payments, economic productivity, and inflation control (Killick, 1984; Williamson, 1983). Income distribution, employment, poverty, health, nutrition, and other social welfare concerns thus far have been excluded from the policy agenda (Feinberg, 1982; Helleiner, 1985; Jolly, 1985). The reason offered is that these are internal issues properly left to sovereign governments. The basic assumption is that short-term belt-tightening is a necessary precondition for long-term economic health.[21]

The problem with this approach is that the poor, and poor women and children in particular, do not have the reserve for short-term belt-tightening. Severe cutbacks in employment, income, and public services would inevitably threaten health, including survival itself. Any effective health policy response to recent economic crises, therefore, needs to ensure that health among the disadvantaged assumes a highly visible position in the policy agenda (United Nations, 1986). Perhaps the most significant function of health policy is to ensure that health and nutrition, in addition to economics, command the highest priority in development and economic adjustment policies.

Notes

1. The seven largest international debtors are Brazil, Mexico, Argentina, Venezuela, Korea, Philippines, and Indonesia (Debt Crisis Network, 1985).
2. The debate over the validity of the "trickle-down" theory of economic development, wherein overall economic growth is presumed to diffuse downwards to the poor, has assumed a new dimension. There is now a re-articulation of an "adverse trickle-down" theory, wherein slow or negative economic growth disproportionately affects the

poor. It could be argued that both rapid and slow growth "trickle-down" effects are legitimate or that only the latter (slow growth) trickles down because of power imbalances in a society.

3. The UN Economic and Social Council recently observed significant deterioration of health and nutrition in many developing countries. "The poverty and nutritional situation, already bad, appears to have deteriorated further in many countries, especially in Sub-Saharan Africa and Latin America, where per capita incomes have fallen and public expenditure on health, education, and other basic services have been sharply cut-back" (United Nations, 1986). However, no data are presented and no evidence is advanced that this deterioration is due to international economic forces.

4. A review of adjustment experiences in Argentina, Brazil, and Chile during the 1970s showed that real wages declined, unemployment increased, and income distribution became more regressive (Marshall et al., 1983; Williamson, 1983).

5. Feinberg of the Overseas Development Council concluded that in "no case has it been claimed that a Fund (adjustment) program actually improved the distribution of income" (Feinberg, 1982).

6. The population of China is relatively homogeneous in comparison to India. The noted British economist, Joan Robinson, once wrote that whatever is written about India, if the opposite is written, both may be true!

7. Because these data are five or ten year averages, the dramatic mortality peaks of the Great Bengal Famine (1943) in India and the Great Leap Forward (1959–61) in China are not depicted.

8. Major policy changes in the Chinese political economy were introduced in the early 1980s. These have exerted profound influences on the Chinese health care system. This section primarily describes the system prior to these recent policy changes. In a later section, recent changes of the Chinese health care system are discussed.

9. The Chinese traditional medical systems are Han, Mongol, Tibetan, Ugyour, and others. The Indian traditional systems include Ayurveda, Unani, Homeopathy, Siddha, Tibetan, and others.

10. Indian resource investments in nutrition, water, and sanitation are excluded from these financial analyses.

11. Health financing and resource allocation data for China were obtained from the World Bank (Jamison et al., 1984; Jamison, 1985). Data for India are extraordinarily difficult to compile and analyze. Considerable information was obtained from many disparate sources (Banerji, 1985; Bhagat, 1982; Bose and Desai, 1983; Col and Roberts, 1984; Gupta, 1984; ICSSR-ICMR, 1981: Khan and Prasad, 1985; Pai Panandikar et al., 1983). Government expenditure patterns are complex because Five Year Plan allocations relate only to central government allocations; yet approximately two-thirds of public health sector expenditures are from the diverse recurring budgets of state governments. Moreover, the available data are often broadly categorized, producing detailed analysis. The most difficult estimate relates to the size and pattern of India's vast and complex private sector. Isolated health care expenditure surveys are available, but these show expenditure patterns ranging from Rs.3 to Rs.108 per capita annually. Crude averages were estimated through validation of these scattered estimates with more reliable financial data on turnovers in the pharmaceutical industry (Bhagat, 1982).

12. Foreign donor resources often play stimulate the establishment of vertical programs in India. High priority problems are identified, Five Year Plan resources are targeted (usually involving foreign aid), and specialized vertical programs are launched. The cost of these special programs, after the start-up phase, must be absorbed by the recurring regular budgets of state governments.

13. Functional time allocation studies in India have found that community health workers spend 44 percent of their work time on family planning and less than 25 percent on health or maternal-child health services (Banerji, 1985).

14. Abel-Smith noted that Bismark developed the German employee/employer health insurance fund (Aird, 1982). While risk sharing was introduced, physician fees were determined by the market beyond government control. Ever since, the cost structure of the German health system has been locked into a high cost trajectory. The German system, moreover, was transferred to Austria, Belgium, Italy, and Japan. And Japan transplanted the system into Korea during Korea's colonial period. All of these systems today are plagued by problems of high physician costs. In contrast, Scandinavia earlier selected a system to pay physicians from government budgets, which today accounts in part for Scandinavia's relatively lower-cost health care system.

15. Verbal report of Professor Carl Taylor, UNICEF representative in Beijing, May 4, 1986.

16. During the two post-oil price hikes in the 1970s, economic adjustment policies in India protected budgetary levels for health, food subsidies, social welfare, and anti-poverty programs. These protective policies were adopted during a populist-dominated phase of the political environment.

17. Caldwell noted that common features among the superior health achieving countries were religion (Hinduism or Buddhism), history of British colonialism, women's autonomy and education, higher relative investments in health, education, and social services, and a political environment fostering egalitarianism and social justice (Caldwell, 1986).

18. There is often substantial covariation in government expenditures for health and other social services. Commonly, high levels of investments in the health sector are accompanied by high levels of investments in education, nutrition services, and other social welfare activities.

19. Recently, the Sub-Committee on Nutrition of the UN Administrative Coordination Committee recommended a specific set of policies to protect the poor and disadvantaged during times of economic crises (United Nations, 1986). Recommendations at the national level aim at giving higher priority to the basic needs of the poor, including protection of their nutritional status, promoting employment and income, avoiding adverse price increases, restructuring health, water and educational services, and improving administrative management capacities. The recommendations for the international level include a more supportive international environment to enable developing countries to adjust while protecting the basic needs of the poor (United Nations, 1986).

20. An IMF spokesperson noted that "distribution among various social groups and among various public expenditure categories (arms spending or social outlays, productive investments or current operations, direct or indirect taxes) is a question decided by the governments. An international institution such as the Fund cannot take upon itself the role of dictating social and political objectives to sovereign governments (Williamson, 1983).

21. One policy issue is the tradeoff between short-term versus long-term health effects of crisis and adjustment. While there is legitimacy to this distinction, this paper avoids this issue on the presumption that those below absolute poverty have no long-term future without short-term survival. It is also debatable whether the time-related effects are primarily economic, health-related, or both. The inter generational transfer of poor health is a well-documented biosocial phenomenon.

References

Abel-Smith, B. "Global Perspectives on Health Service Financing," paper presented at Fifth Annual Conference of the Indian Society of Health Administrators, "Financing of Health Services in India." New Delhi, 1984.

Aird, J. S. "Population Studies and Population Policy in China," *Population and Development Review* 8 (1982): 277–278.

Banerji, D. *Health and Family Planning Services in India: An Epidemiological, Sociocultural, and Political Analysis, and a Perspective.* New Delhi: Lok Paksh Publishers, 1985.

Baum, W. C., and S. M. Talbert. *Investing in Development: Lessons of World Bank Experiences.* Washington, D.C.: World Bank, 1985.

Bhagat, M. *Aspects of Drug Industry in India.* Bombay: Center for Education and Documentation, 1982.

Bose, A., and P. B. Desai. *Studies in Social Dynamics of Primary Health Care.* Delhi: Hindustan Publishing Corporation, 1983.

Caldwell, J. C. "Education as a Factor in Mortality Decline: An Examination of Nigerian Data," *Population Studies* 33 (1979): 395–413.

———. "The Conditions of Unusually Low Mortality: Optimum Paths to Health for All." Canberra: Australia National University, Department of Demography, mimeo, March 1986.

Chen, L. C. "Where Have the Women Gone? Insights from Bangladesh on the Low Sex Ration of India's Population," *Economic and Political Weekly* XVII (1982): 364–372.

China Health Yearbook 1983. Beijing: People's Health Publishers, 1983.

Col, N., and M. Roberts. "Allocating Health Resources in Gujarat State, India." Boston: Harvard School of Public Health, Pew Curriculum Development Center, mimeo, 1984.

Debt Crisis Network. *From Debt to Development: Alternatives to the International Debt Crisis.* Washington, D.C.: Institute for Policy Studies, 1985.

Dyson, T., and M. Moore. "On Kinship Structure, Female Autonomy and Demographic Behavior in India," *Population and Development Review* 9 (1983): 35–60.

Feinberg, R. E. "The International Monetary Fund and Basic Human Needs," in M. Graham, ed., *Human Rights and Basic Needs in the Americas.* Washington, D.C.: Georgetown University Press, 1982.

Gopalan, C. "Food Production and Nutrition Trends in India and China," *Bulletin of the Nutrition Foundation of India* 6:3. New Delhi, July 1985.

Government of India. *Sixth Five Year Plan 1980–85.* New Delhi: Planning Commission, 1980.

———. *Health Survey and Development Committee Report* (Bhore Committee). New Delhi: Manager of Publications, 1946.

———. *Survey of Infant and Child Mortality.* New Delhi: Office of Registrar-General of India, 1979.

————. *Health Statistics of India 1984*. New Delhi: Central Bureau of Health Intelligence, Directorate General of Health Services, Ministry of Health and Family Welfare, 1984.

Grey, R. H. "The Decline of Mortality in Ceylon and the Demographic Effects of Malaria Control," *Population Studies* 28 (1974): 205–229.

Gupta, J. P. "Current Position, Trends and Policy Issues in Health and Financing in India." New Delhi: National Institute of Health and Family Welfare, mimeo, 1984.

Halstead, S. B., J. A. Walsh, and K. S. Warren, eds. *Good Health at Low Cost*. New York: Rockefeller Foundation, 1985.

Health for All: An Alternative Strategy. Report of the Joint Study Group ICSSR-ICMR. Pune: Indian Institute of Education, 1981.

Helleiner, G. K. "Stabilization Policies and the Poor," Working Paper no. B.9. Toronto: University of Toronto, Department of Economics, April 1985.

Hsiao, W. C. "Transformation of Health Care for 800 Million." Boston: Harvard School of Public Health, Institute for Health Research, 1983.

Jain, A. K. "Determinants of Regional Variations in Infant Mortality in Rural India," *Population Studies* 39 (1985): 407–424.

Jamison, D. T., et al. *China: The Health Sector*. Washington, D.C.: World Bank, 1984.

Jamison, D. T. "China's Health Care System: Policies, Organization, Inputs, and Finance," in *Good Health at Low Cost*. New York: Rockefeller Foundation, 1985.

Jolly, R. "Adjustment with a Human Face." The Barbara Ward Lecture, Society for International Development, 1985.

Killick, T. *IMF Stabilization Programmes*. London: Overseas Development Institute, 1984.

Khan, M. E., and C. V. S. Prasad. "A Study of Health Seeking Behavior in Himachal Pradesh." Baroda: Operations Research Group, Monograph, 1984.

————. "Health Financing in India: A Case Study of Gujarat and Maharashtra." Baroda: Operations Research Group, Monograph, 1985.

————. "Utilization of Health Services in Rural India—A Comparative Study of Bihar, Gujarat, and Kerala." Baroda: Operations Research Group, Monograph, 1983.

Krishnan, T. N. "Demographic Transition in Kerala: Facts and Factors," *Economic and Political Weekly* XI (1976): 1203–1224.

Marshall, J. L., S. Mardones, and I. L. Marshall. "IMF Conditionality: The Experiences of Argentina, Brazil, and Chile," in J. Williamson, ed., *IMF Conditionality*. Washington, D.C.: Institute for International Economics, 1983.

McKeown, T., and R. G. Record. "Reasons for the Decline of Mortality in England and Wales During the Nineteenth Century," *Population Studies* 16 (1962): 94–122.

Mosley, W. H., and L. C. Chen, eds. *Child Survival: Strategies for Research*. Cambridge: Cambridge University Press, 1984.

Pai Panandikar, V. A., R. N. Bisnois, and O. P. Sharma. *Organizational Policy for Family Planning.* New Delhi: Uppal Publishing House, 1983.

Panikar, P. G. K. "Financing Health Care in China: Implications of Some Recent Developments," *Economic and Political Weekly* XXI:16 (April 1986): 706–710.

Perkins, D., and S. Yusef. *Rural Development in China.* Baltimore: Johns Hopkins University Press, 1984.

Sen, A. K. "How Is India Doing?" *New York Monthly Review of Books.* New York, 1983.

Sen, P. S. "Stabilization, Income Distributions and Poverty in India." New Delhi: Indian Council for Research on International Economic Relations, mimeo, 1986.

United Nations. *Economic Recession, Adjustment Policies and Nutrition.* New York: United Nations, Economic and Social Council, E/ICEF/1986/INF/9, April 16, 1986.

Vasaria, P., and L. Vasaria. "Indian Population Scene After 1981 Census: A Perspective," *Economic Political Weekly* XVI:44–46 (1981): 1727–1780.

Ware, H. "Effects of Maternal Education, Women's Roles, and Child Care on Child Mortality," in Mosley and Chen, eds., 1984.

Williamson, J. *IMF Conditionality.* Washington, D.C.: Institute for International Economics, 1983.

World Bank. *Toward Sustained Development in Sub-Saharan Africa: A Joint Program of Action.* Washington, D.C.: World Bank, 1984a.

———. *World Development Report 1984.* Washington, D.C.: World Bank, 1984b.

———. *World Development Report 1985.* Washington, D.C.: World Bank, 1985.

Yu Su-En. "Health Statistics of the People's Republic of China," in Halstead, Walsh, and Warren, eds., 1985.

13

Weathering Economic Crises: The Crucial Role of Women in Health

Joanne Leslie, Margaret Lycette, and Mayra Buvinic

It has been estimated that at least 75 percent of all health care takes place at the family or individual level (Levin et al., 1979, cited in Coeytaux, 1984). Within households it is women, particularly in their role as mothers, who have the greatest responsibility for promoting the family's health and nutrition. In this chapter we are concerned with three questions: What are women's multiple roles and how do these influence the health and nutrition of their families? To what extent have recent economic difficulties directly or indirectly influenced women's roles and thus their capacity to protect and promote family health? And in what ways can a better understanding of the realities of women's lives help planners to design more realistic and thus more effective health and nutrition policies and programs?

Although the health of women themselves is an important social concern, as it affects both women's capacity to lead satisfying, productive lives and their ability to bear and raise healthy children, this chapter does not focus on determinants of women's health. Two recent monographs (Hamilton, Popkin and Spicer, 1984; Stinson, 1986) provide insightful analyses of determinants of women's nutrition and health in developing countries. Similarly, consideration of the significant contribution that women make as providers of health care in their roles as traditional birth attendants, community health agents, nurses, and physicians is also outside the scope of this chapter.

The chapter begins with a review of the trend, over the past decade, towards more participatory health strategies, drawing particular attention to the extent to which such strategies depend in one way or another on women. The second section of the chapter describes the multiple roles of women in developing countries, highlighting the increasing participation of women in market production. The third section considers how recent economic crises and related adjustments may have influenced women's ability to promote family health and nutrition. In the final section we offer recommendations concerning how health and nutrition programs could be more realistically planned around the potential time and financial contributions of women and identify certain development efforts outside the health sector targeted to women that may have important health and nutrition benefits.

Participatory Strategies for Health

In the past decade several innovative strategies for the delivery of public health have been developed. First came the widespread endorsement of primary health care, followed by an increased emphasis on cost recovery in the health sector and the so-called child survival revolution, which rests primarily on the four GOBI "technologies"—growth monitoring, oral rehydration therapy, breastfeeding and improved weaning practices, and immunization. All three of these strategies—primary health care, the child survival revolution, and cost recovery—have gained acceptance at least in part in response to a realization that the alternative state-financed, hospital-based curative approach was too expensive, reached too few people, and placed too little emphasis on preventive health care. Although there are important differences among them, all three approaches can be thought of as more participatory, and the participation they rely upon is predominantly, although not exclusively, that of women.

Primary Health Care

A central element of the primary health care approach, although one that has proven difficult to achieve (Parlato and Favin, 1982), is the desirability of community participation. Community participation is understood to include a voice in establishing local health needs, provision of labor and local resources for construction of facilities, and implementation of a range of preventive and curative activities (World Health Organization, 1978). To a reasonable extent, primary health care requires no dramatic changes in community behavior and practices, since many of the eight essential elements of primary health care are simply tasks that women have always done as part of their traditional domestic and/or subsistence agriculture responsibilities. The eight components of primary health care are usually accepted to be:

- health education
- nutrition and food
- maternal and child health care (including family planning)
- water and sanitation
- immunization
- disease control and prevention
- essential drugs
- treatment of common diseases and injuries

It is clear that women have always had primary responsibility for processing and preparing (and often producing) food, hauling water, providing home treatment of common diseases and injuries, and passing on health and nutrition knowledge from one generation to the next. Thus women have been the central providers of much of primary health care long before it was labeled as such. The elements of primary health care that involve the introduction of new health technologies also depend heavily on women.

To the extent that the introduction of a primary health care program, or the primary health care approach, requires women to fetch more water and firewood to improve household hygiene, to prepare more frequent and varied meals to improve household nutrition, to spend additional time participating in health and nutrition education sessions and taking children to be weighed and vaccinated, or to take on unpaid work as community health agents, primary health care may simply add to women's burdens in a way that is damaging to their own health or prospects for economic progress. Alternatively, it may meet with a disappointing lack of response from women if it is not seen to be in their self-interest.

On the other hand, primary health care may serve to reduce the burdens on women if it introduces appropriate technology to allow women to meet their traditional responsibilities more efficiently (examples would be community wells, small scale grain mills or increased availability of more effective western pharmaceuticals); reduces the time spent on child bearing and child care through increased child spacing and decreased child morbidity; or mobilizes other community members to assist women in their traditional tasks in the interest of improved health and nutrition for the community.

The Child Survival Revolution

The selective primary health care approach embodied in the child survival revolution relies primarily on the introduction of new health technologies and practices. For this reason, it is even more critical to ask who within the communities must learn to use these new technologies, or to adopt these new practices. There can be little doubt that women are the primary target group. To quote from UNICEF's 1986 State of the World's Children report, "whether we are talking about breastfeeding or weaning, oral rehydration therapy or immunization, regular growth checking or frequent handwashing, it is obvious that the mother stands at the centre of the child survival revolution" (UNICEF, 1986).

Of the four central components of the GOBI strategy, the only one that calls for continuing a traditional practice is breastfeeding. Breastfeeding was felt to warrant promotion, however, precisely due to a concern that substantial numbers of mothers were breastfeeding less—to the detriment of their children's nutritional status and health. Unfortunately, in the last ten years considerably more effort has gone into establishing the undeniable health benefits of appropriate breastfeeding (both directly and indirectly by increasing birth intervals) and into documenting regional and urban/rural differences in rates of change in infant feeding practices, than into understanding women's reasons for choosing a particular pattern for feeding their infants, or into assessing the costs and benefits of different infant feeding patterns given different family and economic structures. By and large the evidence shows that women recognize and appreciate the benefits to their infants of breastfeeding. They also, however, recognize that breastfeeding has substantial time and energy costs; that it is incompatible with certain kinds of work—most formal sector jobs and often agricultural work during the peak season; and may in certain cases—when mothers have several preschool age children and no other means of economic support—be detrimental to the wellbeing of their other children (Van Esterik and Greiner, 1981).

The other basic elements of the GOBI strategy—oral rehydration therapy, immunizations, improved weaning practices (which is usually grouped with breastfeeding), and growth monitoring—all demand that women first understand and accept new knowledge about their children's health and then that they incorporate new activities into their schedules. As with breastfeeding, the attention of the public health community has been focused more on establishing the health and nutrition benefits of these new technologies than in assessing their costs, particularly the costs to the beneficiaries. Each of these technologies is potentially life saving, and is certainly health promoting. Making them available as widely as possible increases the range of options available to families in developing countries to produce child health and nutrition, and that is clearly desirable. However, utilization of the GOBI technologies also requires a contribution of time and money on the part of someone responsible for the target child, usually the child's mother. Thus women are faced with the question of whether the benefits outweigh the costs.

The monetary costs of the technologies are generally modest, but they are not inconsequential, particularly for the poorest families. Such costs may include ingredients for home prepared oral rehydration salts (ORS) and special weaning foods, transportation costs to get to the location where immunizations are being given or growth monitoring is being done, and sometimes payment for packaged ORS, immunizations, growth charts, or community prepared weaning foods.

The time cost of the technologies may be relatively greater. Averaged out in terms of minutes per day, neither ORT, immunization, nor growth monitoring would add much to a mother's work day. The time costs are not distributed in this way, however, but are bunched. When a child needs ORT, someone must be in attendance almost constantly. In order to take a child to be weighed or to be immunized a mother may have to forego up to an entire day of work depending on the distance to be traveled and the length of the wait.

In contrast to the periodic time costs of ORT, immunizations and growth monitoring, provision of appropriate weaning foods is a daily activity. Initial supplemental foods are not usually the same foods eaten by the rest of the family; weaning age children should eat more frequently than older children and adults; and avoiding bacterial contamination requires preparing small amounts at a time and carefully cleaning all utensils used. All of the above means that improving current weaning practices almost surely requires a substantial increase in the amount of time a mother and her helpers put into food preparation.

If we consider momentarily three other "technologies" that are frequently cited as important additional elements (beyond GOBI) of the child survival revolution—food, family planning and female education—we find that they appear to involve fewer utilization costs and more direct benefits to women than the more central GOBI technologies. For example, the small amount of extra food per day that should be eaten by pregnant and lactating women, which can make such a significant difference in their own and their infants' health, entails relatively less work for women than does supplementary food for weaning age children because it does not need to be especially prepared. Although it is undoubtedly desirable for pregnant and lactating women to eat more frequently than other adults and to consume foods that are more energy and protein dense, they will benefit greatly from simply eating an extra portion of the regular family fare at the usual meal times. Family planning and female education offer clear direct benefits to women aside from their indirect benefits for child survival and development. The reduction in maternal mortality and the reduced drain on women's time and energy that family planning makes possible (through increased child spacing) may make family planning the element of the child survival revolution that is most immediately valuable to women in the short term, although female education may be of even greater value in the long run, as is discussed at the end of this section.

Cost Recovery

Of the three participatory health strategies, the growing emphasis on cost recovery or fees for service is the one most clearly responding to increasingly constrained government and international funds for the health sector. Families have always made substantial investments in medicine and services to prevent or cure illness, although the burden of paying traditional healers or birth attendants may have been less in the instances where payment in kind (either goods or services) was accepted. On the other hand, to the extent that modern drugs and immunizations are more effective than traditional remedies, the total cost to families of using modern rather than traditional medicine may actually be less. Whether the cost of modern medicine is greater or less than that of traditional medicine, it increasingly requires cash payments, and in this context the role of women as earners of income may be as important to family health as are their home production roles. Women's ability to earn income makes an important contribution to the capacity of any poor household to purchase health services and other determinants of health, but it will be particularly crucial in households where the woman is the sole or primary source of economic support, or where men and women have separate areas of economic responsibility and health and nutrition fall into the woman's sphere.

Women's Education: The Catalyst

Although not a health strategy in and of itself, improvement in women's educational status has in the past ten years been increasingly appreciated for its central importance as a determinant of family health and nutrition. Research done in the late 1970s in developing countries found a surprisingly consistent positive effect of maternal education on infant and child mortality rates and on child nutritional status in all regions (Cochrane, Leslie and O'Hara, 1981; Caldwell and McDonald, 1982). More recent studies have isolated the effect of maternal education from other socioeconomic variables and explored the relative importance of the multiple pathways through which maternal education may influence child health (Ware, 1984; Cochrane, 1986). Although higher levels of maternal education are usually associated with both higher levels of paternal education and higher levels of household income, most research has found a positive effect of maternal education on child survival and health separate from its association with other socioeconomic variables.

Higher levels of female education are associated with lower fertility, and thus the positive effect of maternal education on child survival is first explained by increased child spacing—but child spacing does not account for all the variation (Hobcraft, McDonald and Rutstein, 1983; Cochrane, 1986). Beyond child spacing, the most frequently hypothesized links between maternal education and child health are through increased use of health services, more decisionmaking power within the family and the community, and greater earning power. Clearly these three factors are central to the successful adoption and utilization of the participatory health strategies described above.

Women's Multiple Roles

The health strategies discussed in the previous section depend heavily on women's time contributions and cash outlays for ingredients, medicines, and fees. There is some question, however, as to whether women can easily make these contributions and, if not, how implementation strategies can be revised to facilitate women's participation. As a basis for addressing these issues, women's critical roles in home and market production are reviewed below.

Home Production Roles

Home production activities make vital contributions to the household economy, especially among lower income groups in developing countries, and it is typically women and female children who are responsible for this work. However, the System of National Accounts (SNA) used in most countries excludes the value of time spent preparing food, cleaning, and caring for children. This failure to take account of the time and effort that goes into home production leads to serious misrepresentation of the contribution of women to total output and, typically, underestimation of women's time and work burdens. The labor required for gathering firewood, obtaining water, and preparing food without the benefit of modern appliances is strenuous and time intensive. For poor women who tend to have large families, the bearing and nurturing of children can add considerably to physical chores and physical stress over a lifetime. In Nigeria, for example, Harrington has found that over 60 percent of a sample of Yoruba women aged 25–34 years had spent more than half of their lives either pregnant or breastfeeding (Harrington, 1983). Overall it is estimated that at any given time, one woman in six, aged 15–49 years, is pregnant in developing countries (Sivard, 1985).

Recently economists have begun to focus more on the central role of home production, home management, and home technology. Several attempts have been made to estimate households' "full income" by adding the value of household production to market income. In the Philippines, King and Evenson have estimated full income to be more than twice as much as market income. And while women contributed, on average, only 20 percent of the household's market income, they contributed almost 40 percent of full income (children contributed 28 percent) (King and Evenson, 1983). In Malaysia, the value of housework as a share of personal income is 38.5 percent (Kusnic and DaVanzo); studies in the United States and Canada show the share to be from 41 to 53 percent (Birdsall and McGreevey, 1983). It is estimated that the unpaid labor of women in the household, if given economic value, would add one-third (or $4 trillion) to the world's annual economic production (Sivard, 1985).

Time use studies have been the main tool used in home production analyses and they reveal a striking picture of household members' contributions (see Table 13.1). In general, they indicate that women work longer hours than men, and the poorer the country the more hours women work. Women in the United States work at home and outside the home an average of six hours a day. In the Philippines women work ten hours a day. In parts of East Africa women work sixteen hours a day doing housework, caring for children, preparing food, and raising between 60 and 80 percent of the food for the family (Fagley, 1976). In Burkina Faso, women have only a little more than one hour a day of time in which to perform personal care, undertake community activities, and socialize (McSweeney, 1979). Rural Javanese women work eleven hours a day compared to eight and one-half hours for men (Nag, White and Peet, 1978). In rural Botswana women work six hours a day in agriculture even during the slack season (Mueller, 1984).

Women's time allocation patterns are less fixed than those of men. Men's use of time does not vary much during their adult working lives. In contrast, time allocation by women and children is flexible, changing with the number and ages of children in the household and the annual cycle of agriculture and schooling (when children go to school at all). As the demand for childrearing time and for cash income increases over the household's life cycle, the burden of meeting this demand falls primarily on the wife and on children as they grow older. In the rural Philippines, fathers' time spent in child care, food preparation, marketing, and other chores is one to two hours daily, whether there is one child or seven. The nonfarming man spends more time in household work than the farmer, but this time is still less than one and one-half hours. Filipino women spend about two and one-half hours per day in market production (wage employment, farming, fishing, and income-earning work at home)—more if they are farmers—and seven to eight hours in home production—slightly less if they are farmers. Women with infants spend about two hours in market production and about nine hours in home production. Women with seven or more children spend less time in child care and home production than those with fewer children, but they increase proportionally their time spent in market production. Older children often substitute for adults in home chores and care of siblings. When there are seven or more children, men actually reduce their child care time (to about ten minutes a day) and increase their leisure time; thus children reduce the work load of the father but not of the mother (King and Evenson, 1983). In rural Peru as well, it is mothers and children who substitute for each other in cooking, hauling water, and animal care (Deere, 1983).

Women's home production is important to family health through curative care in the home and utilization of health services, as well as through preventive health care such as food preparation, breastfeeding, and family hygiene. It is usually women who prepare special foods and herbal remedies for those who are sick, and it is almost always women who nurse the sick and injured at home. In addition, when a family member needs to be taken for treatment or hospitalized, it is usually women who take on this responsibility. In most developing countries, hospitals do not provide food for patients, so someone from the family must stay at the hospital or go every day to bring food; again, it is women who usually perform this task.

It is also women who utilize, on behalf of themselves and their children, the maternal and child health services that comprise such a large fraction of health services in developing countries. It is by definition women who go for prenatal visits, and women most often seek family planning services. It is usually mothers who attend health and nutrition education sessions and who take children to be immunized and weighed.

Table 13.1
Average Hours per Day Spent by Men and Women in LDC Households: Results from Time Use Studies

Region & Country	Reference		Home Production	Subsistence and Market Production	Child Care	Total Work Time	Leisure/Personal Time	N	Sampling Method
Latin America									
Peru									
Machiguenga (rural)	Johnson, 1975	F	3.52	3.62	.98	8.12	3.98	1159	I
		M	.85	4.01	.11	4.97	5.67	572	
Nicaragua (rural)	Gillespie, 1977	F	3.28	4.36	.36	8.0	1.3	NA	I
Middle South Asia									
Bangladesh									
Manikganj (rural)	Caldwell et al., 1980	F	5.8	4.17	.4	10.37	5.1	23	S
		M	.29	7.31	.05	7.65	5.3	Households	
Dacca (urban)	Caldwell et al., 1980	F	4.66	1.77	.74	7.17	8.3	22	S
		M	.64	4.20	.07	4.91	9.8	Households	
Rural area 1980	Cain	F	7.68	1.68	NA	9.36	NA	NA	NA
		M	.93	8.57	NA	9.50	NA		
Rural area	Von Harder, 1977	F	6.07	5.95	NA	12.02	NA	NA	NA
Char Gopalpur	Cain, Khanam and Nahar, 1979	F	5.88	1.61	.80	8.29	NA	174	I
		M	1.24	7.04	.05	8.33	NA	138	NA
Pakistan									
Lyallpur (rural)	Anwar & Bilquees, 1976	F	5.75	8.25	.50	14.5	1.0	NA	I
India									
Rural area	INCCU,* 1977	F	4.50	10.75	1.0	16.25[a]	.75	NA	NA
Allahabad (rural)	Bhatty, 1980	F	4.22[b]	6.89	—	11.11	NA	264	S
								Households	
Nepal									
Rural area	Nag, White and Peet, 1978	F	3.66	7.42	1.1	12.18	NA	171	I
		M	1.88	8.06	.22	10.16	NA	131	
Rural area	Acharya & Bennett, 1982	F	3.82	6.15	.85	9.97	NA	478	R
		M	1.59	6.33	.15	7.92	NA	443	

Location	Source	Sex						Sample size	
Eastern South Asia									
Philippines									
Laguna (rural)	King & Evenson, 1983	F	5.36	2.51	2.06[c]	9.93	13.99[a]	99	I
		M	.91	6.85	.39	8.15	13.67		
Rural area	Ho, 1979	F	6.75	2.01	1.58	10.34	NA	488	I
Laguna (rural)	Popkin, 1983	F	5.8	5.2	1.4	12.4	13.9[a]	573	R
Rural area	Folbre, 1983	M	.39	7.3	.64	8.23	16.3	Households	
		F	6.06	.89	1.44	8.39	NA	573	R
		M	.39	8.38	.10	8.87	NA	Households	
Indonesia									
Java (rural)	Hart, 1980	F	4.3[b]	5.5	—	9.8	NA	87 Households	S
Java	White, 1975	F	4.17	5.9	1.03	11.1	NA	20 Households	NA
		M	.43	7.90	.37	8.7	NA		
Java	Nag, White and Peet, 1978	F	3.92	5.88	.80	10.6	NA	33	I
		M	.36	7.80	.24	8.4	NA	31	I
Sub-Saharan Africa									
Botswana Rural area	Mueller, 1984	F	3.58	2.06[e]	.36	6.0	5.03	957 Households	I
		M	.98	3.68	.04	4.7	6.34		
Tanzania Rural area	Kamuzora, 1980	F	3.89	9.98	NA	13.87	2.78	105	R
		M	1.32	10.75	NA	12.07	4.69	Male-headed households	
Rural area	Tobisson, 1980	F	8.71	2.08	—	11.51	—	15	I
Central African Republic Rural area	FAO, 1983	F	3.64	4.3	NA	7.94	NA	NA	I
		M	.22	5.28	NA	5.50	NA		
Zambia Rural area	UNECA, 1974	F	6.5[b]	9.5	NA	16.0	NA	55	NA
Ivory Coast Rural area	FAO, 1983	F	5.02	1.78[e]	NA	6.80	7.45	720	I
		M	.75	3.18		3.93	10.18	Houawholsa	
Senegal Damga region (rural)	Fieloux, 1985	F	5.03[b]	4.0	—	9.3	2.6	NA	NA
Burkina Faso Kongoussi Zone (rural)	McSweeney and Freedman, 1980	F	5.16	4.31	.3	9.50	3.91	5	I
		M	.28	7.27	.0	7.55	6.45	5	

[a] Includes sleeping time
[b] Includes childcare time
[c] Includes breast- and bottle-feeding time

[a] Study conducted during peak season
[e] Study conducted during slack season
* Includes only employed women

NA = Not available
R = Random sampling
S = Stratified sampling
I = Intentional sampling

Market Production Roles

Much of women's work in the household underpins all productive activities of society and directly contributes to family health. Women also participate, however, in market production activities that indirectly affect their ability to promote health. In the past three decades the number of economically active women has risen from 344 million in 1950 to 675 million in 1985 (Sivard, 1985). In developing countries, 42 percent of women belong to the labor force and constitute one-third of the total labor force. The ILO reports a continuing and pronounced upward trend even in these "extremely conservative estimates" (UNFPA, n.d.).

These sharply increased levels of economic activity have occurred to some extent because of women's improved educational attainment and society's changing mores but in recent years have been much more directly the result of declining living standards. More women work now than ever before because more women are increasingly responsible for the economic well-being of their families. Women are, in fact, the sole breadwinners in one-fourth to one-third of the families in the world (Sivard, 1985). This pressure on women to earn an income is a result, in part, of increasing monetization of economies worldwide and growing urbanization. Machine-made goods and goods not produced locally have found a place even in subsistence economies. Machine-made cloth, bicycles, agricultural products such as pesticides and fertilizer, and many other items have by now become necessities even in poor households and add to the household's need for cash. In urban areas, women are for the most part unable to gather fuel, grow crops, or produce other necessities as they could in the countryside; at the same time, they face transportation costs, rent changes, and utility payments associated with urban life—all of which add to the household's cash requirements.

Agriculture. In spite of rapid urbanization, two-thirds of women workers in developing countries continue to work in the agricultural labor force and estimates based on censuses, national surveys, and United Nations data show that they provide most of the agricultural labor essential to both food and cash crop production in the developing world. The United Nations claims that women farmers grow at least 50 percent of the world's food, and as much as 80 percent in the rural areas of some African nations (Sivard, 1985). According to recent estimates based on ILO and FAO data, women constitute 38 percent of the agricultural labor force in developing countries—46 percent in sub-Saharan Africa, 45 percent in South and Southeast Asia, 31 percent in North Africa and the Middle East, and 18 percent in Central and South America (Dixon, 1982).

These figures are undoubtedly biased downward, however, since official estimates systematically undercount unpaid family labor and fail to record women's multiple and seasonal responsibilities in household and market production (Boulding, 1983; Dixon, 1982). Even surveys that question women directly about their economic activities may produce extremely biased results. Relying on the perceptions of women or men about women's contribution to agricultural production, instead of observation of actual participation rates, results in measurement errors, especially in more traditional societies where women feel that they are expected to work only at home or where a wife's idleness is a status symbol for men. In a survey of women in agriculture in Cajamarca in Peru, for example, only 4 percent of the women said their principal occupation was farming. Yet when asked about specific agricultural tasks, 46 percent of the women were found to be the primary or secondary person in charge of crop production, and through a detailed agricultural labor accounting system, 86 percent were found to participate in agricultural field labor (Deere and Leon, 1982).

Women active in agricultural production in developing countries can be categorized as farm owners or managers, farm partners, unpaid family workers, or agricultural wage laborers. The distinctions among these categories are based on the woman's decision-making power, time spent in farming, and agricultural tasks.

Women who are farm owners or managers are the principal decision-makers in agricultural production, devote a major portion of their labor to farming, and are responsible for most agricultural tasks. Women farmers in sub-Saharan Africa are the most likely to fall into this category. In Kenya, studies indicate that 36 to 40 percent of farms are managed by women (Staudt, 1978; Moock, 1976). In Botswana, an examination of household decisions concerning the time of plowing and type of seed planted showed that women made these decisions on their own in 31 percent and 57 percent of the cases respectively.

In other regions of the world, women also work as farm owners and managers. In Peru, for example, 21 percent of the peasant women in one study were farmers on their own account, with their husbands (who often migrated in search of work) deriving income from other sources (Deere and Leon, 1982). In Jamaica, women are typically responsible for their family's agricultural production until their husbands leave their jobs in the urban areas at about the age of forty. At that point, the wives and husbands assume joint management of the farm (Von Harder, 1981).

Women farm partners share the responsibility for agricultural production with another household member, usually their husbands. Decisions are made collaboratively, both partners devote a major portion of their labor to farming activities, and tasks, though often divided by the prevailing sexual division of labor, are considered essential and complementary to each other. A study of eight villages in Nepal showed that women make 42 percent of household agricultural decisions and decide jointly with adult males in another 12 percent of the cases (Acharya and Bennett, 1981). In Thailand, where women also participate widely in agriculture, one study found that decisions on whether to borrow money and how to dispose of the products of family labor are decided jointly in 40 and 50 percent of the cases, respectively (Whyte and Whyte, 1982).

Women farm workers have less responsibility for decisions about family farm production yet are active in agricultural work. Their husbands or other relatives make the major agricultural decisions. The women's tasks, though essential to production, are often limited to certain activities which vary by season. These women may be excluded from labor force statistics since their field work is seasonal and other tasks they perform may be considered housework and not even included under the heading of unpaid family labor (Beneria, 1982).

Women who work principally as agricultural wage laborers also constitute an important segment of the agricultural labor force. Due to the commercialization of agriculture and the current economic crises in the Third World, landlessness has increased, forcing both women and men farmers into temporary wage labor (Lassen, 1980). In Sri Lanka, 72 percent of the female agricultural labor force is salaried (though women receive only 66 to 75 percent of the male wage), and in India 50 percent of the tea plantation labor is female (Blumberg, 1981). In Honduras, women make up 40 percent of the wage laborers in tobacco and almost 90 percent in coffee (Buvinic, 1982).

Formal Sector Employment. In the non-agricultural sectors, which account for one-third of the female labor force, industry and services provide roughly equal shares of jobs for women. Within these sectors, however, women tend to be clustered in low-skill jobs with little potential for training or advancement.

In Tanzania, for example, almost 29 percent of urban women wage earners are found in clerical work while 16.5 percent are engaged in hotel/bar/porter jobs (Shields, 1980). By contrast, only 4.5 percent of male wage earners are found in those occupations. Moreover, a mere 1.6 percent of female earners are engaged in "skilled" occupations, compared to 10.4 percent of males.

In Latin America, as well, women show a marked concentration in the lower status occupational categories, mainly in the service sector. For example, in Brazil, Chile, and Peru over 50 percent of economically active urban women are engaged in the service sector (PREALC, 1978). A 1977 survey of households and workers in four major urban centers of Colombia showed that 68.5 percent of the female labor force is engaged in the service sector (Rey de Marulanda, 1981). Earnings distributions clearly show that this sector is associated with low wages and thus a large portion of the female labor force falls into the low-income category.

Other sectors offer only limited employment opportunities for women. While there is ample evidence of an expanding industrial sector in Latin America, industrial workers make up only 10 to 20 percent of the female labor force. Although women may be incorporated into factory work, especially in the textile and food processing industries, an increasing emphasis on heavy industry will undoubtedly lower the percentage of women engaged in industrial employment. In Brazil, for example, the proportion of female workers in the manufacturing sector dropped from 18.6 percent to 11 percent during the period 1950–1970. Moreover, studies in Venezuela and Brazil show that after twenty years of industrial growth, the incorporation of women into the modern formal sector is still centered around traditionally female occupations (Schmink, 1982). Women's share in the industrial labor force of developing countries rose from 21 percent in 1960 to 26.5 percent in 1980 but largely because women provide cheap labor to a competitive international market for export of manufactures (Joekes, 1985).

Informal Sector Employment. Unable to gain higher-level (and thus better paid) formal-sector employment, increasing numbers of women have turned to self-generated employment in the informal sector either as a supplement to formal sector earnings or as their sole source of support. In urban areas women take up occupations such as street vending and personal domestic services. In rural areas they process and market produce and local handicrafts. Earnings and mobility are low in these informal sector activities, but for most poor women access to this sector is easy compared to the problems they face in obtaining formal sector employment. In much of the Third World, the informal sector rivals formal employment as a source of jobs for both men and women. In Bombay and Jakarta, for example, as well as in many African cities, 50 to 60 percent of the labor force is employed in the informal sector, which is the fastest growing segment of the economy. In many Latin American cities over 50 percent of the labor force works in the informal sector.

Women are quite disproportionately represented in these urban informal occupations. In urban Tanzania, for example, about 80 percent of the total female labor force is self-employed and 53 percent of all informal sector workers are female (Shields, 1980). In Belo Horizonte, Brazil, 47.3 percent of female heads of household are employed in the informal sector, versus only 14.9 percent of male heads (Merrick, 1976). In Peru, even when domestics are excluded, 40 percent of the informal sector labor force and 61 percent of the self-employed are women, compared to only 18 percent of the formal sector labor force. About 50 percent of the informal labor force of Brazil is female, and in Ecuador half of all women employed in urban labor markets work in the informal sector (Mazumdar, 1976). In Botswana and Nepal, more than 80 percent of the total female labor force is self-employed in the informal sector (Sundar, n.d.).

Informal sector employment tends to be concentrated in marginal activities and is associated with relatively low productivity. This is reflected in the close association between informal employment and lower average earnings, particularly for women. In Brazil, for example, informal-sector earnings are only 55 percent of those in the formal sector for men with incomplete primary education, and just 47 percent for females. Completion of primary education raises these earnings by 60 percent for men, but improves informal earnings for women by only 6 percent (Merrick, 1976).

In Tanzania, 47 percent of self-employed urban women, versus only 4 percent of men, had incomes of less than 100 shillings per month in 1971. In Kenya, 41 percent of informally employed women had incomes of less than 199 shillings per month, compared to 13.8 percent of men (Shields, 1980). A study of the informal sector of Mexico City shows that 23.7 percent of the total labor force of the city work in marginal jobs that pay less than minimum wage (U.S. $100 per month); notably, however, these jobs account for 72.2 percent of the female labor force versus 53.9 percent of the male labor force (Arizpe, 1976). Finally, in urban Peru, studies show that women hold 46 percent of the informal sector jobs and earn an average income of U.S. $30 per month versus U.S. $70 per month for men (Mazumdar, 1976).

The Balancing Act

Women in developing countries hold low wage, low status occupations as a result of their lower educational attainment relative to men and of cultural biases that restrict their employment opportunities. An equally important factor, however, may be their attempts to balance home and market production responsibilities by holding jobs that, while not highly lucrative, allow flexible hours or permit them to bring children along (Birdsall and McGreevey, 1983). As poor women's economic responsibilities increase, the pattern is for them to work longer hours and to continue to engage in home production activities. They apparently do not trade off one activity for another, but instead forego recreational activities and dedicate fewer hours to sleep, rest and relaxation. Popkin has found a one-to-one correspondence between increases in mothers' work time and decreases in their leisure time (Popkin, 1983).

Clearly women continue to have major responsibility for household work even when they are heavily involved in market work. Thus, women have strong incentives to engage in market work that is compatible with home production responsibilities. In Malaysia, for example, less than 5 percent of all women work in the professions, management, or clerical occupations—jobs not compatible with child care. In nearly one-third of jobs in sales and production occupations (small scale retail trade, weaving, food processing) filled by women who have young children, women have their children with them while they are working. This is true in only 16 percent of agricultural jobs filled by women with young children, but women in agriculture work fewer hours on average than those in marketing, thus limiting time spent away from young children (DaVanzo and Lee, 1983).

In Peru, in-depth interviews of market women indicate that they choose their occupation for the specific reason that it is compatible with child care and home responsibilities. In their informal sector activities, women are able to have their children not only accompany them, but also assist them in important ways such as transporting goods from the wholesale market, working in the stall, and bringing lunch from home to their mothers (Bunster, 1983). The role of children in assisting their mothers in trading was also found to be important among Yoruba women in Nigeria (Karanja, 1980).

Women's tendency to choose jobs compatible with home responsibilities indicates how serious a constraint time can be for women with multiple responsibilities. It is equally important to note, however, that market production activities provide women and their families with crucial income that may be one of the most important determinants of the level of family health and nutrition.

Many studies have found a positive relationship between household income (or increases in household income) and child nutritional status (Smith, Paulsen, Fougere and Ritchey, 1983; Kumar, 1977; Nabarro, 1984). Popkins's study in the Philippines specifically identified a significant positive effect of mother's labor force participation on the food energy intake of children, along with a negative (although not significant) effect of the per capita income of other household members (Popkin, 1983). Similarly, in Ghana, Tripp found that "although certain indicators of farm resources and investment were positively correlated with above average nutritional status, the most significant differences were noted with respect to the trading activities of the parents. The group of children which exhibited the highest proportion above the median weight for age were those whose mothers had their own income from trading" (Tripp, 1981). On the other hand, a study from Nicaragua that investigated a range of socioeconomic determinants of child mortality, health and nutrition found little evidence of a substantial impact of either women's predicted earnings or income of other household members on nutritional status (Wolfe and Behrman, 1982).

There is some additional evidence that women's income is particularly important in improving family health. In sub-Saharan Africa, for example, men generally spend money on housing improvements, some clothing, and supplemental food when necessary; they also hire labor and pay for production inputs, such as seeds, fertilizer, hoes, plows, etc., for their own crops. Women are responsible for another set of expenditures, including home-produced food, school fees and books, cooking utensils, dowries for their daughters, and medicine for themselves and their children (Guyer, 1980). In the Sudan, women are responsible for spending their independently earned income on food, clothing, and health care (Fruzzetti, 1985). Women's income routinely covers medicine for children and female relatives; and women's savings are critical for medical emergencies. In Asia and Latin America, men are more likely to be responsible for routine household expenses. However, a study of households in southern India concludes that children profit nutritionally when women's rather than men's, monetary contribution to household income increases (Kumar, 1977).

Moreover, the positive income effect of women's employment on children's health and welfare has not been shown to be offset by negative effects of reduced child care time by working mothers or the substitution of older siblings in child care to nearly the extent that has been assumed. Most of the studies that have specifically looked at the relationship between women's market work and child health have started from the premise that women's work would have a detrimental effect on child health, at least where work meant work away from home and child meant infant or preschool age child. Most researchers have recognized that there was likely to be both a time effect and an income effect, but there seems to have been an implicit assumption, at least in the early research, that the negative time effect was likely to outweigh any positive income effect.

Leslie's recent review of the findings of 21 studies that looked at the relationship between women's work and infant feeding practices and of 22 others that related women's work to child nutritional status, found that the empirical evidence from the studies does not support the conclusion that women's work will have a negative effect on child nutrition (Leslie, 1985). The review found that while no overall generalizations about a positive or negative effect of women's market work on child nutrition were warranted, certain interesting patterns did begin to emerge.

As far as women's work and infant feeding practices are concerned, most of the reported effects were not on initiation of breastfeeding but on duration, particularly on duration of exclusive breastfeeding. Several studies found that the only significant difference between working and non-working mothers was that mothers who worked away from home began mixed (bottle and breast) feeding earlier (Popkin and Solon, 1976; Akin, Bilsborrow, Griffen, Guilkey and Popkin, 1984; Winikoff, 1986). Soekirman found that in Indonesia mothers who worked in factories breastfed less frequently during the day but with equal frequency at night (Soekirman, 1983).

Interestingly, some studies suggested that certain categories of working mothers actually were more likely to breastfeed or to breastfeed longer than nonworking mothers. There was some evidence of a higher prevalence of breastfeeding among women farmers than among non-working women or women who worked in other occupations (Knodel and Debavalyz, 1980; Butz, Habitcht and DaVanzo 1981; Pathmanathan, 1985) and of more breastfeeding among women who worked at home than among women who did not work or who worked away from home (Popkin and Solon, 1976; Akin et al., 1981). In a recent review of World Fertility Survey data, Balkaran and Smith found that self-employed women reported longer duration of breastfeeding than women who did not work, although women in other occupations reported a shorter duration (Balkaran and Smith, 1984). It seems quite reasonable that women who work at home or who are self-employed might be better able to breastfeed than women in other occupations; what is more intriguing is why they should be more inclined or better able to breastfeed than women who report no market work.

The pattern of findings from studies that consider the relationship between women's work and child nutritional status is also interesting. A number of such studies found significantly more malnutrition among children of mothers who work than among children of nonworking mothers. However, most studies that reported such a finding have been methodologically quite poor, using intentional samples and simple cross tabulations, and disaggregating the sample neither by type of work done by the mother nor by age of the child. Often, in fact, maternal work was not the focus of the study but was simply one of a series of socioeconomic variables being tested for their relationship with child nutritional status. In addition, they have presumed the direction of causality—that mother's work is the cause and child malnutrition is the effect—without considering the possibility that both are independent results of the household's poverty level or that mothers might actually seek work because they perceive that their children are malnourished.

More useful findings emerge from several relatively recent studies that have focused specifically on the relationship between women's work and child nutrition, using multivariate analysis and disaggregating both independent and dependent variables. Several of these have been particularly valuable in directly considering the income effect, the time effect, or the interaction between the two. Kumar's study from India found that at comparable levels of household income child nutrition was lower when their mothers were in the labor force than when they were not, but at the same time increments in household income from employment had a positive impact on child nutrition only when these increments were attributable to women's employment (Kumar, 1977). Adelman's study of data from Peru found that in order for the child of a full time working mother to achieve the height of one whose mother did not work, the household with the full time working mother needed to have almost twice as much income (Adelman, 1983). Soekirman found that the negative effect of mother's employment on child nutritional status is only significant if mothers work more than 40 hours a week and earn less than the minimum wage; if mothers work more than 40 hours but are better paid, there is no significant effect (Soekirman, 1983).

Among the most interesting findings are those from two studies that disaggregated results in terms of the age of the child. Using data from Haiti, Haggerty finds that time spent by the mother in child care during the first year of life is more important for satisfactory growth than is income whereas the opposite is true in the second year (Haggerty, 1977). Consistent with this is her finding that women who work at home (compared with factory or market workers) have the least malnourished children in the zero to eleven month age group and the most malnourished in the twelve to twenty-three month age group. Similar findings emerge from Engle's study of women in urbanizing Guatemala (Engle, 1985); in this study children of working mothers were more poorly nourished than children of nonworking mothers during the first year of their lives (primarily due to a negative effect of domestic work on child growth) whereas children of working mothers were better nourished than children of nonworking mothers during the second year of life (primarily due to a positive effect of formal and informal sector work).

Economic Crises and Adjustment Programs: Sharpening the Conflict?

Given women's household and market production obligations, and their central role as promoters of family health, it is important to examine the impact of economic crises and adjustment programs on their ability to continue to fulfill these multiple roles. There are several effects that we might expect to see:

First, to the extent that economic adversity encourages more market work for women because their contributions to household income become more critical, the competing demands on women's time for household and market production may increase to the point that their capacity or willingness to spend a large amount of time on health or nutrition related activities and service utilization will decline.

On the other hand, if economic conditions and/or adjustment programs diminish women's income earning opportunities in the short term, through contractions in employment or through shifting women's production time to less remunerative informal sector work, the positive impact of women's income on child health and nutritional status will decrease. If, however, women whose economic opportunities diminish spend more time in home production, there may be some compensating positive impact on child welfare.

Women's educational attainment, which is strongly linked to better family health, may also suffer during economic crises in two ways. First, women who are increasingly under pressure to work outside the home due to male unemployment and reduced household incomes may expect children, and especially daughters, to substitute for them in home production. Several studies show, for example, that girls' time spent in care of siblings, cleaning, food preparation, and carrying water increases significantly as mothers' hours in market production increase. As a result girls' enrollment in school may decline or their performance suffer. Second, the need for fiscal restraint may translate into decreased public expenditure on education. If school fees are applied or raised in order to compensate for diminished public expenditure, parents may choose to send male rather than female children to school.

Diminished public expenditures on health may also affect women's health related activities. Decreased expenditures may translate into longer waits at clinics that are understaffed, for example. Given other demands on their time, women may be less willing to bring their children regularly to clinics even if the services are offered without fee. The application of fees to compensate for reduced budgetary allocation to health services may of course directly reduce women's willingness to use health services.

Finally, increased costs for food high in nutritional value, as a result of lowered food subsidies or general economic adversity, may discourage women from purchasing such food items.

Given the limited information available so far, it is difficult to determine whether the effects mentioned above have occurred in developing countries; whether they may yet occur after some lag period; and whether, to the extent that they have occurred they are due to adverse economic conditions, the adjustment programs being implemented to combat such conditions, or both. We here offer some data that suggests the likelihood of these potential effects.

Labor Force Participation and Unemployment

In Latin America real per capita income for the region as a whole dropped between 1980 and 1983; in sub-Saharan Africa real per capita income has fallen since 1979 to levels below those attained in 1970. In both regions, open unemployment rates have increased (in Latin America, from an average of 7 percent before the recent economic crisis to 10 percent in 1983), and low-productivity informal sector employment has increased (PREALC, 1985a). In sub-Saharan Africa the informal sector provided 52 percent of employment in 1980 compared to 44 percent in 1974 (Gozo and Aboagye, 1985).

Several studies hypothesize that, as female primary school enrollment rates have more than doubled in sub-Saharan Africa since the 1960s, women have joined the labor force in growing numbers, and that given the current saturation of formal and informal labor markets, women's unemployment in the formal sector has risen along with their participation in the most marginal occupations in the informal sector (Green, 1986; Gozo and Aboagye, 1985). In addition, it is suggested that the depression in food crop prices and increasing food insecurity in sub-Saharan Africa have affected rural women's work in two ways: in some cases, depressed food prices have reduced women's incentives to produce surplus food for sale, thus diminishing their incomes; in other cases, poorer women farmers and near landless women have increased their work time to meet family economic needs through increasing production on more marginal lands or in low-productivity informal sector activities (Green, 1986).

The data from Latin America are somewhat more concrete. In 1982, the peak economic crisis year for Costa Rica, women's share of the labor force increased to 26.2 percent (from 24.8 percent in 1980) and leveled off at 25.4 percent in 1983, an economic recovery year. At the same time, women's open unemployment rate increased from 7.8 percent in 1980 to 11.4 percent in 1982, and then fell to 9.6 percent in 1983 (Ministerio de Cultura, Juventud y Deportes, 1985).

In Brazil, women's labor force participation rates rose from 37.91 percent to 39.81 percent during the economic crisis period 1983–84, while men's participation rates rose only slightly (from 71.3 percent to 71.5 percent) (PREALC, 1985b).

In Chile, despite a trend toward long term declines in women's labor force participation, women's activity rates in the lowest quintile of the household income distribution increased sharply, from 18 to 22.4 percent, during the economic crisis in 1974–75 (Rosales, 1979). In Uruguay, women's economic activity rates and open unemployment in Montevideo increased substantially during the 1975–79 period of worsening economic conditions, while men's activity rates increased only slightly and their open unemployment rates actually fell (Prates, 1983).

In Latin America, as is suggested for sub-Saharan Africa, adverse economic conditions seem to have been drawing women into the labor market where, unfortunately, they are faced with increasingly limited formal employment opportunities. Thus, increasing numbers of women are joining the informal economy. In Bolivia, for example, women's share of informal sector employment grew from 37 percent in 1976 to 48 percent in 1983 (Casanova, 1985).

When economic crises and adjustment bring women increasingly into market production, demands on their time increase, potentially limiting their ability to participate in time intensive health strategies. In addition, because they face limited formal employment opportunities, women are increasingly working in informal sector occupations that have low productivity and are poorly paid—thus limiting their ability to participate in alternative health strategies that are more costly but less time intensive.

Education

Data available so far indicate no major losses in girls' access to schooling, either in terms of decreased enrollment or increased dropout rates, during the recent economic crisis years. In Latin America, boys and girls have nearly equivalent access, and there are no signs that this is changing (Sivard, 1985). The gap between girls' and boys' access to education remains high in Africa, particularly at secondary levels. Increases in enrollments at the primary level for both boys and girls slowed down during the early 1980s, but there is no indication of actual declines in girls' enrollment rates. It is possible that some negative effects will be revealed when data from the mid-1980s becomes available. For now, however, even if economic crisis and adjustment policies are inducing women to work or work longer hours outside the home, it appears that girls' schooling is not being sacrificed to allow daughters to substitute for their mothers in home production activities.

Table 13.2
Change in Percentage of Total Government Expenditures for Education and Health Over a Ten Year Period in Selected Developing Countries

	Education		Health	
Country	1972	1982	1972	1982
Nepal	7.2	9.9	4.7	4.5
Malawi	15.8	14.3	5.5	5.2
Uganda	15.3	14.9	5.3	5.2
Tanzania	17.3	12.1	7.2	5.5
Ghana	20.1	18.7	6.2	5.8
Kenya	21.9	19.9	7.9	7.3
Sudan	9.3	6.1	5.4	1.3
Bolivia	30.6	13.6	8.6	2.0
Zambia	19.0	15.2	7.4	8.4
El Salvador	21.4	16.9	10.9	7.1
Morocco	19.2	16.2	4.8	2.8
Philippines	16.3	16.0	3.2	5.3
Thailand	19.9	20.7	3.7	5.0
Costa Rica	28.3	22.6	3.8	32.8
Turkey	18.2	16.8	3.3	2.1
Tunisia	30.5	14.2	7.4	6.7
Paraguay	12.1	12.0	3.5	3.7
Syrian Arab Republic	11.3	7.1	1.4	1.1
Malaysia	23.4	15.9	6.8	4.4
Chile	14.3	14.7	8.2	6.8
Brazil	6.8	4.6	6.4	7.8
Republic of Korea	15.9	19.5	1.2	1.4
Argentina	8.8	6.2	2.9	1.1
Mexico	16.6	13.1	5.1	1.3
Uruguay	9.5	7.7	1.6	3.3
Venezuela	18.6	15.7	11.7	7.6

Source: World Development Report 1985. Table 26: Central Government Expenditure. Oxford University Press, 1985.

If the data continue to support this scenario, it will be a particularly positive outcome in light of the reduced share of public expenditures devoted to education in many developing countries (see Table 13.2). In Africa, for example, the share of education expenditures in total public expenditures has declined in low-income sub-Saharan countries from 17.7 percent in 1970 to 14.8 percent in 1983, and from 16.7 percent in 1970 to 10.5 percent in 1983 for all sub-Saharan countries on average (see Table 13.3).

To the extent that a reduced share in expenditures translates into lower quality of schooling, or the imposition of school fees to maintain the education system, we might expect to see girls' enrollment rates decline as parents begin to perceive the costs of education (in terms of

Table 13.3
Selected Education Indicators for Sub-Saharan Africa

		1960		1970		1983	
		P	*S*	*P*	*S*	*P*	*S*
% girls enrolled in primary (*P*) and secondary (*S*) education in:							
low income economies	(L):	31	25	38	30	43	33
all countries	(A):	34	25	39	31	44	34

		1970	1980	1983
Total public expenditures in	L	17.7	15.3	14.8
education as % total government expenditures:	A	16.7	16.7	10.5
Capital expenditures as %	L	11.5	10.3	10.5
total educational exp.	A	11.3	15.5	10.5
Primary public recurrent	L	46.3	42.7	43.3
expenditures as % total ed. exp.	A	43.7	44.2	39.4
Secondary public recurrent	L	27.9	28.1	31.0
expenditures as % total	A	28.3	30.9	44.4

Source: World Bank and UNESCO data.

fees or loss of girls' time in home production) outweigh the benefits (especially if quality of education declines). This may in fact be occurring in the short term with the effect being masked by a longer term trend toward girls' increased participation in education. Alternatively, despite a reduced share in public expenditures, absolute expenditures in education may have been sufficient to maintain quality of education at levels existing prior to the recent economic crises and to avoid substantial increases in school fees. Even more optimistically, families' tendency to trade off girls' education in favor of their time in home production may have diminished significantly as a result of improved cultural attitudes towards women.

Health and Food Expenditures

There is no direct evidence that health service utilization has diminished during recent economic crises. However, it is clear that health expenditures as a proportion of total public expenditures have diminished in many developing countries. In only six out of twenty-six countries for which data is reported in the most recent World Development Report has the proportion increased, while reductions have been substantial in countries such as Tanzania, Bolivia, Sudan, Morocco, El Salvador, Syria, Malaysia, Argentina, Mexico, and Chile (see Table 13.2).

Our own field observations indicate that these reductions in the share of health expenditures have often translated into shortages of vehicles, fuel, or vehicle maintenance services which have severely limited the outreach capabilities of health and nutrition programs. Health workers are now frequently in the position of having to serve only those families who can make the trip to the nearest clinic or hospital, usually located in major towns or cities. For rural women, such trips can be inordinately costly, in terms of both time and money. Moreover, in many societies, it is considered inappropriate for women to travel long distances alone, so that women may be further discouraged from attempting to obtain health services.

Aside from the effects of reduced outreach, lowered health expenditures undoubtedly lead to reduced staffing of clinics and hospitals which in turn means that clients must wait for longer periods of time in order to receive services. Again, faced with competing demands on their time, women are likely to be discouraged from seeking health care for themselves and their children as these time costs of services rise.

Finally, economic crises and adjustment policies have likely provided further justification for the trend towards imposition of user fees as part of cost recovery strategies in health services. Again, there is no direct evidence of the effect of more widespread and higher service fees on women's utilization of health services. However, several studies show that women often spend large proportions of household income on medicines and immunization (UNICEF, 1986). User fees which would further raise the proportion of income devoted to health care may discourage women's use of health care services and induce them to utilize less effective traditional health services and homemade cures, at least when these are less costly or can be paid for in kind.

In a number of countries, such as Egypt, Colombia, and Sri Lanka, economic austerity has resulted in reductions in food subsidies as part of attempts to generally reduce public expenditures; moreover, the IMF has been advocating reduction or elimination of cheap food policies as part of recent proposed adjustment programs. Because food expenditures are a large proportion of the household expenditures among lower income groups, these reductions may have particularly adverse affects on the poor. Pinstrup-Andersen reports estimates of reductions in real income ranging from 5.5 to 9 percent among the lowest income groups as a result of a 10 percent increase in the price of food in Sri Lanka, Thailand, Egypt, India, and Nigeria (Pinstrup-Andersen, 1985a).

A considerable number of studies suggest that the income and price effects of reducing cheap food policies will lead to significant reductions in food expenditures, particularly among the poor (Pinstrup-Andersen, 1985b). However, the nutritional effect of reductions in food expenditures is not always clear. Many studies may overstate the effect of income on nutrition because they rely on expenditure data and do not take into account changes in the type of food purchased, such as an increase in purchases of semi processed foods. Behrman and Wolfe, for example, find relatively little effect of income when nutrients are used directly as the dependent variable (Behrman and Wolfe, 1984). In addition, reduction of cheap food policies may result in increased prices for food producers, although several studies indicate that the impact of improved prices for producers is not great for the rural poor because they do not earn a large share of their incomes from food production (Pinstrup-Anderson, 1985). While more research is needed on the effects of lowered food subsidies and rising food prices on nutrition and health, we might hypothesize that any negative effects will particularly apply to low income landless women and urban women who may be forced to reduce food expenditures, and possibly nutrient consumption, in response to higher food prices and reduced food subsidies.

Conclusions and Recommendations

The role of women as producers of health and nutrition is so central, and operates through so many different linkages, that it would be possible to assert that virtually any development activity that affects women will have an influence on family health. These various linkages are not equally important as determinants of health, however, nor are they equally open to influence by policy decisions or program design. Our recommendations, therefore, will focus first on three aspects of development programs outside the health sector that are particularly significant in terms of women's influence on health—reducing women's time conflicts, increasing women's incomes, and improving women's access to education and training. We then turn our attention to the health sector, and suggest how a recognition of the opportunity cost of women's time, the potential conflicts between home and market production, and the increasing access by women to cash income may have implications for the appropriate design of health programs and policies.

General Development Programs

Time, income, and education appear to be the three major, interrelated factors influencing women's ability to promote health and nutrition for themselves and their families. The time women invest in preparation of nutritious food, care of children, and visits to health providers is a critical aspect of the role women play as promoters of health and one that is typically associated with the daily home production activities of women.

Women's market production activities may make this time contribution particularly burdensome. As previously noted, women typically reduce leisure and personal care time in order to fulfill both market and home production roles. There is no doubt, however, of women's need to perform market production activities in order to contribute to the family's economic well being. Moreover, given the monetary costs of producing health, women's income earning roles are directly related to improved health and nutritional well being of the family.

Finally, women's education is directly linked to improved family health. Yet, ironically, girls' access to education may be limited when they are called upon to substitute in home production activities as mothers attempt to maintain home production outputs while fulfilling market production obligations. It is heartening, however, to note long term trends toward increasing enrollment rates for girls despite the potential opportunity costs of the time they spend in school.

Given the critical nature of these three factors, effectiveness of health strategies will be enhanced by development policies or programs that (1) reduce women's time conflicts (by improving their productivity in both home and market production); (2) increase women's incomes; and (3) improve women's education (both directly and through diminishing the opportunity costs of girls' time taken away from home production to attend school). We offer below a few suggestions as to how these goals might be achieved.

Reducing Time Conflicts. The introduction of appropriate technologies for use in home production activities is one of the most important ways in which women's time conflicts can be reduced. A significant amount of women's time spent in home production can be released through the introduction of light machinery for grinding grain, fuel efficient cookstoves to minimize firewood needs, reforestation of land near villages with fast growing trees to improve availability of fuelwood, and more abundant water supplies made available closer to where people live. In addition, women's time will also be freed through the development of improved crop drying techniques and more efficient and inexpensive food preparation utensils and equipment.

Increasing Women's Incomes. Given the extent of women's participation in agriculture and informal sector enterprise activities, the incomes and thus the ability to promote family health of a substantial fraction of the lowest income women can be improved through increasing productivity in these sectors. Improved productivity in income-earning activities will also reduce women's time conflicts in addition to increasing their incomes.

Agriculture:

- Promotion of agricultural extension through cooperatives (which are often male-dominated), tenants' groups, and land reform committees tends to bypass rural women. Women's access to agricultural extension and training can be significantly improved by utilizing promotion and information distribution systems that reach women such as existing women's production groups, and outreach at places where women typically meet.
- Training programs are important for improving women's agricultural productivity. Those that take place near women's homes, minimizing travel and time away from the household, will reach many more women farmers.
- Women farmers are more likely to be reached through agricultural extension systems that offer incentives for agents to work with small-holders, train agents in a farming systems approach, and target crops with which women are involved.
- Productivity is often related to agricultural credit. Women farmers, who seldom hold title to land or property, will more likely be eligible for credit when innovative collateral options such as crop liens and group guarantees are used.

Informal Sector Activities:

- Women can significantly improve their productivity if they are given technical assistance with record keeping, management, and marketing. Because of low educational attainment, many women lack knowledge of even the most simple record keeping systems.
- To ensure women's access to technical assistance and credit, promotion of such programs should be carried out through organizations to which women belong or through word of mouth in the marketplaces where women work.
- As with women farmers, minimal and flexible collateral requirements will improve the access to credit of women who work in the informal sector. Solidarity group lending and group guarantees are effective substitutes for traditional collateral requirements.
- Flexible repayment requirements in loan programs, such as those that allow borrowers the choice of repaying loans in very frequent, small amounts, improve women's access to credit and reduce their rates of default on loans.

- Deregulation of interest rates and other financial reforms that improve the availability of small loans and lower the transactions costs of borrowing will also improve women's access to credit.

Improving Education. The critical link between women's education and improved family health and nutrition is well established. Women's access to education and educational attainment can be encouraged through greater emphasis on outreach programs to publicize the economic and health benefits of women's education and through development of simple educational materials for literacy classes to reach women who are beyond the age for participating in formal education. Several specific approaches to improving women's access to education have been found to be effective:

- Increasing the numbers of schools in a given area (and in cases where education is segregated increasing the numbers of girls' schools) reduces the distance that girls must travel to school and seems to alleviate concerns about the safety and propriety of girls' school attendance.

- Flexible timing of both formal and informal education programs is important in encouraging girls' and women's attendance, especially during peak agricultural periods.

- Classes held for short periods of time on a daily basis, rather than those held for longer periods one or two days a week, are more likely to allow girls and women to maintain their home production activities and thus will encourage their attendance.

- The introduction of even small scholarships and/or stipends seems to encourage girls' school attendance despite the opportunity costs of their time away from home production activities. There is some evidence that these programs also have spillover benefits of encouraging school attendance after stipends are eventually reduced or eliminated.

Health Sector Programs

Operational level. Since women are the main consumers of health and nutrition services (on behalf of themselves and their children) and since inadequate coverage of health services is a major problem, it is important to modify health programs so as to increase their accessibility to and utilization by women. The World Bank's 1980 *Health Sector Policy Paper* cites inadequate coverage of health services as the major problem with the health sector in most developing countries (World Bank, 1980). This inadequate coverage is attributed to a range of issues that affect either the availability of services or their utilization or both, such as:

- Health facilities are not geographically accessible.
- Availability of services is erratic.
- Services are often of doubtful value.
- Economic barriers exclude many persons.
- Services provided are of low priority to the population.
- Health services are not based or focused in the community.
- Patients do not comply with the recommendations for treatment.

We suggest below a number of ways in which health programs could be modified to improve their accessibility to women and/or increase the likelihood of their utilization.

Delivery Issues.

- The timing of activities related to routine or preventive health care should take into consideration both the daily and seasonal dimensions of women's workloads. Immunization campaigns in rural areas, for example, should be scheduled for the slack not the peak agricultural season.
- Growth monitoring and health and nutrition education sessions should be scheduled for a time during the day when women are not normally fetching water or fuel or preparing the main meal of the day; usually this means afternoons. (Often health agents or their supervisors like to get their work taken care of in the morning; this leads to such sessions being scheduled for a time when large numbers of women are unable to participate.)
- Taking into consideration the competing demand for women's time, it may prove to be cost effective (even given the high cost of fuel and vehicle maintenance) to bring preventive services such as immunizations and growth monitoring to each community, and even to each household, through mobile teams or clinics. (Population densities and the condition of roads will also be important considerations in deciding on the efficiency of mobile health services.)
- Drugs, contraceptives, and curative services need to be made available at reasonable times and distances through such mechanisms as satellite health posts, flexible clinic hours and informal (sometimes private sector) distribution mechanisms in order to increase their utilization.

- Strategies such as ORT, home prepared weaning foods and growth monitoring can sometimes be implemented by mother substitutes. Therefore, it may prove more efficient in terms of mothers' time to promote the participation of siblings, grandparents, or even fathers in these activities.

Promotion Issues. Another way in which the utilization of health services or the adoption of more appropriate health and nutrition practices by women could be increased relates to the way that these are promoted. Mobilizing the necessary resources at the household level requires, to some extent, appealing to women's self-interest. It is clear that illness within the family has major time (and money) costs to women. One study in Kenya, for example, found that visits to clinics required at least half a day no matter how trivial the complaint and that the time lost by women due to medical visits ranged from one to two hours to a day per week (Hanger and Moris, 1973). Another study in Cameroon found that twelve percent of wage employed women reported having formally quit work at some time in their careers to care for a child who was ill for a prolonged period of time (DeLancy cited in Bryson, 1979). It seems reasonable, therefore, that underlining the potential time savings of reduced child morbidity could provide a strong incentive for preventive health care. If women are convinced that taking the time now to improve household hygiene or to get their child immunized will save them expenditures on medicine and/or loss of work time in the future, this could increase their motivation or provide them with a justification to present to other family members.

Another potential benefit of improved child health or nutrition that may motivate mothers or others in the household is better school performance. Many families in developing countries place a high value on education and make considerable efforts, even sacrifices, to allow their children to go to school. Reduced child morbidity or improved child nutrition may acquire considerably more value in the eyes of parents when seen as something that enhances the child's chances of succeeding in school.

The above proposals are not meant to suggest that families fail to value increased child survival and improved child development for their own sake, but simply that given the costs associated with adopting new and better health and nutrition practices (or maintaining beneficial traditional ones such as breastfeeding), benefits to the household as well as benefits to the child may need to be stressed.

Day care. Given women's increasing participation in work away from home, day care for children also contributes to health. It may be important that provision of or support of day care for children be accepted as a legitimate—even a priority—health activity. Day care increases women's employment options while offering a convenient location for the provision of health and nutrition care for children. In some cases day care even offers working mothers the chance to continue breastfeeding or to breastfeed more frequently.

While day care may sometimes mean a large, formal government- or business-supported center, many of the day care services that are most useful to and best accepted by mothers are small, informal and located in the communities where families live (WHO, 1981). To the extent that such informal, community day care centers involve modest facilities and payment of a local woman or even mothers taking turns being responsible for the children, they may also be much less expensive than centrally located or workplace day care. Provision of day care is often thought of as a luxury, something too expensive for poor countries or communities. But the costs may not be excessive compared to the benefits: day care offers women better employment opportunities and children better health, and perhaps even better school achievement. It is also worth noting that, after income generating opportunities, day care facilities are one of the needs most frequently cited by women in developing countries (WHO, 1981; de Souza, personal communication).

Policy Implications. Beyond the issues raised above concerning the design and promotion of health and nutrition services, it seems important at least to consider whether what we know about women's multiple roles and the effect of recent economic crises and adjustment policies on women has implications for how resources should be allocated more broadly within the health sector. Needless to day, there are other important issues to be addressed, but if priorities are to be assigned among the components of primary health care or the interventions that comprise the child survival revolution, the question of which health activities can most efficiently be used by women, or which ones will be most beneficial to women, undoubtedly deserves to be considered.

With the objective of improving the acceptance and impact of various health and nutrition interventions, it may be useful to consider two important questions. How time consuming is the utilization of each intervention? And perhaps more importantly, does the intervention offer significant future time savings for women? Of course, time costs and potential time savings will depend on a variety of factors, including whether the intervention is preventive or curative, the proximity of clinics, women's ease of access to transportation, waiting time at clinics, family size, etc. Although empirical data on the time costs and time savings of specific health and nutrition interventions is extremely limited, we offer the following distinctions as a basis for further discussion and research.

1. As long as they are made available at times and locations that are convenient for women, utilization of immunizations, family planning and appropriate curative medicines (such as antibiotics for acute respiratory infections) is relatively low cost in terms of time; even when there is a monetary cost, these seem to be services for which mothers, and other family members, are willing to pay. More importantly, these services offer significant savings of women's time.

- Immunizations can virtually eliminate several of the major causes of infant and child morbidity in the developing world and thus substantially reduce the amount of time women are forced to spend caring for sick children (as well as reducing the stress a mother experiences worrying about a severely ill child). It has also been suggested that immunizations can reduce child disability by approximately 30 percent (UNICEF, 1986). This will clearly avoid the time expenditure and the reduced employment options associated with caring for a disabled child.

- The increased birth intervals made possible through family planning give women more time to recover strength between pregnancies and may reduce or at least space out the particularly time consuming tasks associated with caring for a new infant.

- Finally, the use of antibiotics, when appropriate, for the treatment of child illness (particularly for ones that are quite prevalent such as acute respiratory infections) can dramatically reduce the length of time that a child is ill and thus, once again, contribute to easing the constraints on women's time.

2. Breastfeeding is somewhat intermediate in terms of its relative efficiency for women. Breastfeeding is time consuming and constraining on women's employment options, but it can also make a significant contribution to easing the competing demands on women's time. Compared with bottle feeding, breastfeeding reduces the number of illnesses during the first year of life and probably costs less money (even when the cost of the additional food needed by a lactating mother is taken into consideration). At the same time, to the extent that it increases birth intervals, breastfeeding offers the same family planning benefits to women as does contraceptive use.

3. Although they can have important benefits in terms of child survival and child development, the time costs of utilizing ORT, growth monitoring and improved weaning practices appear to be considerable while the potential time and money savings to women from these technologies seem to be quite limited. The main effect of ORT is to prevent death and perhaps to slightly reduce duration of disease, but there is no

evidence that ORT reduces the incidence of diarrhea, which is the leading cause of child morbidity among children over the age of one in a majority of developing countries. Similarly, growth monitoring and improved weaning practices offer significant potential for preventing child malnutrition and thus increasing child survival and achieving better child development, both physically and mentally. Nonetheless, evidence as to whether improved child nutrition has a significant effect on reducing child morbidity is mixed, and thus the potential for saving women time and money (through fewer child illnesses) would not seem to be as great as with other health interventions.

These distinctions are offered as food for thought, not as firm conclusions. We certainly do not wish to suggest that health practices and interventions fall neatly into two categories—those that are "good" for women and those that are not. However, a consideration of the relative costs and benefits of different health and nutrition interventions to women may suggest that some deserve a higher priority than others, or at least that some modifications may need to be made in the delivery or promotion of those that come with higher costs and relatively fewer obvious benefits.

References

Akin, John S., et al. "The Determinants of Breastfeeding in Sri Lanka," *Demography* 18 (August 1981): 287–307.

Anwar, Seemin, and Faiz Bilquees. "The Attitudes, Environment and Activities of Rural Women: A Case Study of Jhok Sayal," Research Report No. 98. Islamabad: Pakistan Institute of Development Economics, 1976.

Arizpe, Lourdes. "Women in the Informal Labour Sector in Mexico City: A Case of Unemployment or Voluntary Choice?" Paper presented at the Women and Development Conference, Wellesley, MA, June 2–6, 1976.

Balkaran, Sudat, and David P. Smith. "Socio-economic Differentials in Breastfeeding." *WFS Comparative Studies (Cross National Summaries): Additional Tables*. Presented at the 1984 World Fertility Survey Conference on Findings, London, 1984.

Behrman, Jere R., and Barbara L. Wolfe. "More Evidence on Nutrition Demand: Income Seems Overrated and Women's Schooling Underemphasized," *Journal of Development Economics* 14 (January-February 1984): 105–128.

Beneria, Lourdes, ed. *Women and Development: The Sexual Division of Labor in Rural Societies*. New York: Praeger, 1982.

Bhatty, Zarina. "Economic Role and Status of Women: A Case Study of Women in the Beedi Industry in Allahabad." ILO World Employment Programme Research Working Papers. Geneva: International Labor Organization, 1980.

Birdsall, Nancy, and William Paul McGreevey. "Women, Poverty and Development," in Mayra Buvinic, Margaret A. Lycette and William Paul McGreevey, eds., *Women and Poverty in the Third World*. Baltimore: Johns Hopkins University Press, 1983, pp. 3–13.

Blumberg, Rae Lesser. "Females, Farming and Food: Rural Development and Women's Participation in Agricultural Production Systems," in *Invisible Farmers: Women and the Crisis in Agriculture*. Washington, D.C.: Agency for International Development, Office of Women in Development, 1981, pp. 24–102.

Boulding, Elise. "Measures of Women's Work in the Third World: Problems and Suggestions," in Mayra Buvinic, Margaret A. Lycette, and William Paul McGreevey, eds., *Women and Poverty in the Third World*. Baltimore: Johns Hopkins University Press, 1983, pp. 286–300.

Bryson, Judy C. "Women and Economic Development in Cameroon." Washington, D.C.: United States Agency for International Development, mimeo, 1979.

Bunster, Ximena. "Market Sellers in Lima, Peru: Talking About Work," in Mayra Buvinic, Margaret A. Lycette, and William Paul McGreevey, eds., *Women and Poverty in the Third World*. Baltimore: Johns Hopkins University Press, 1983, pp. 92–103.

Butz, William P., Jean-Pierre Habitcht, and Julie DaVanzo. "Improving Infant Nutrition, Health, and Survival: Policy and Program Implications from the Malaysian Family Life Survey." Report prepared for the U.S. Agency for International Development. Santa Monica, CA: The Rand Corporation, 1981.

Buvinic, Mayra. "La Productora Invisible en el Agro Centroamericano: Un Estudio de Caso en Honduras," in Magdalena Leon, ed., *Las Trabajadoras del Agro*. Bogota, Colombia: Asociacion Colombiana para el Estudio de Poblacion, 1982, pp. 103–114.

Cain, Mead. "The Economic Activities of Children in a Village of Bangladesh," in Hans Binswanger et al., ed., *Rural Household Studies in Asia*.

Cain, Mead, S. R. Khanam, and S. Nahar. "Class, Patriarchy, and the Structure of Women's Work in Rural Bangladesh." Center for Policy Studies Working Paper No. 43. New York: Population Council, 1979.

Caldwell, J. C., et al. "The Control of Activity in Bangladesh." Australian National University Department of Demography, Working Papers in Demography, 12. Canberra: Australian National University, 1980.

Caldwell, John, and Peter McDonald. "Influence of Maternal Education on Infant and Child Mortality: Levels and Causes," *Health Policy and Education* 2 (1982).

Casanovas, Roberto. "Los trabajadores por cuenta propria en el mercado de trabajo: el caso de la ciudad de La Paz," in Carbonetto et al., *El Sector Informal Urbano en Los Paises Andinos*. Ecuador: Instituto Latinoamericano de Investigaciones Sociales and Centro de Formacion y Empleo para el Sector Informal Urbano, 1985.

Cochrane, Susan. "The Effect of Education on Fertility and Mortality." Education and Training Series Report Number EDT-26. Washington, D.C.: The World Bank, 1986.

Cochrane, Susan H., Joanne Leslie, and Donald J. O'Hara. "Parental Education and Child Health: Intracountry Evidence," *Health Policy and Education* 2 (1982): 213–250.

Coeytax, X. Francine. *The Role of the Family in Health: Appropriate Research Methods.* Geneva: World Health Organization, 1984.

DaVanzo, Julie, and Donald Lye Poh Lee. "The Compatibility of Child Care with Market and Nonmarket Activities: Preliminary Evidence from Malaysia," in Mayra Buvinic, Margaret A. Lycette, and William Paul McGreevey, eds., *Women and Poverty in the Third World.* Baltimore: Johns Hopkins University Press, 1983.

Deere, Carmen Diana. "The Allocation of Familial Labor and the Formation of Peasant Household Income in the Peruvian Sierra," in Mayra Buvinic, Margaret A. Lycette, and William Paul McGreevey, eds., *Women and Poverty in the Third World.* Baltimore: Johns Hopkins University Press, 1983.

———. "Rural Women and Agrarian Reform in Peru, Chile and Cuba." Paper presented to the Second Annual Women, Work and Public Policy Workshop, Harvard University, Cambridge, MA, April 1982.

Deere, Carmen Diana, and Magdalena Leon de Leal. *Women in Andean Agriculture: Peasant Production and Rural Wage Employment in Colombia and Peru.* Geneva: International Labour Organization, 1982.

Dey, Jennifer. "Women in African Rice Farming Systems." Paper presented to the Second Annual Women, Work and Public Policy Workshop, Harvard University, Cambridge, MA, April 1982.

Dwyer, Daisy. "Women and Income in the Third World: Implications for Policy." Working papers, no. 18. New York: The Population Council, 1983.

Engle, Patricia. "The Intersecting Needs of Working Women and Their Young Children: A Report to the Ford Foundation." Report prepared for the Ford Foundation, mimeo, 1980.

Fagley, R. M. "Easing the Burden of Women: A 16-hour Workday," *Assignment Children* 36 (1976): 9–28.

Fieloux, Michele. "Developpement, Emigration Masculine et Travail Feminin: Le Cas des Femmes Toucouleru de la Region du Damga (Moyenne Valee du Senegal)." Paper presented at the International Workshop on Women's Role in Food Self-Sufficiency and Food Strategies, Paris, January 14–19, 1985.

Folbre, Nancy. "Household Production in the Philippines: A Neo-Classical Approach," Michigan State University Working Paper No. 26. East Lansing: Michigan State University, 1983.

Fruzzetti, Lina. "Farm and Hearth: Rural Women in a Farming Community," in Haleh Afshar, ed., *Women, Work and Ideology in the Third World.* New York: Tavistock, 1985.

Gillespie, Vivian. "A Modified Time-Budget Methodology for Gathering Baseline Data on the Roles and Responsibilities of Rural Women in Nicaragua." Report prepared for Agency for International Development, Office of Women in Employment. Washington, D.C.: International Center for Research on Women, 1977.

Gozo, K. M., and A. A. Aboagye. "Impact of the Recession in African Countries: Effects on the Poor." Geneva: International Labor Organization, mimeo, 1985.

Green, Reginald Herbold. "Stabilization, Adjustment and Basic Needs in SSA: Annotated Jottings Toward An Agenda." Sussex, England: Institute for Development Studies, mimeo, 1986.

Guyer, Jane I. "Household Budgets and Women's Incomes." Working Papers, no. 28. Boston, MA: African Studies Center, Boston University, 1980.

Haggerty, Patricia Ann. "Women's Work and Child Nutrition in Haiti." Unpublished M.A. thesis. Cambridge: Massachusetts Institute of Technology, 1981.

Hamilton, Sahn, Barry Popkin, and Deborah Spicer. *Women and Nutrition in Third World Countries*. New York: Praeger, 1984.

Hanger, Jane, and Jon Moris. "Women and the Household Economy," in Robert Chambers and Jon Moris, eds., *Mwea: an Irrigated Rice Settlement in Kenya*. Munich: Welteorum Verlag, 1973.

Harrington, Judith. "Nutritional Stress and Economic Responsibility: A Study of Nigerian Women," in Mayra Buvinic, Margaret A. Lycette, and William Paul McGreevey, eds., *Women and Poverty in the Third World*. Baltimore: The Johns Hopkins University Press, 1983.

Hart, Gillian. "Patterns of Household Labor Allocation in a Javanese Village," in Hans Binswanger et al., eds., *Rural Household Studies in Asia*. Singapore: Singapore University Press, 1980.

Ho, Teresa. "Time Costs of Child Rearing in the Rural Philippines," *Population and Development Review* 5 (1979): 643–662.

Hobcraft, John, John McDonald, and Rutstein Shea. "Child Spacing Effect on Infant and Child Mortality," *Population Index* 49 (Winter 1983).

Indian National Commission for Cooperation with UNESCO, National Institute of Public Cooperation and Child Development. *Role of Working Mothers in Early Childhood Education*. Paris: UNESCO, 1977.

Joekes, Susan. *Women and the World Economy*. New York: Oxford University Press, for the U.N. International Research and Training Institute for the Advancement of Women, forthcoming.

Johnson, Allen. "Time Allocation in a Machiguenga Community," *Ethnology* 14:3 (1975): 301–310.

Kamuzora, C. Lwechnugura. "Constraints to Labour Time Availability in African Smallholder Agriculture: The Case of Bukoba District, Tanzania," *Development and Change* 11 (1980): 123–135.

Karanja, Wambui Wa. "Markets Women and Children in Nigeria: Some Notes from Lagos." Oxford: Oxford University, mimeo, 1980.

King, Elizabeth, and Robert Evenson. "Time Allocation and Home Production in Philippine Rural Households," in Mayra Buvinic, Margaret A. Lycette, and William Paul McGreevey, eds., *Women and Poverty in the Third World*. Baltimore: Johns Hopkins University Press, 1983.

Knodel, John, and Nibhon Debavalya. "Breastfeeding in Thailand: Trends and Differentials, 1969–1979," *Studies in Family Planning* 11 (December 1980): 335–377.

Knudson, Barbara, and Barbara A. Yates. *The Economic Role of Women in Small Scale Agriculture in the Eastern Caribbean: St. Lucia.* Barbados: University of the West Indies, 1981.

Kumar, Shubh. "Role of the Household Economy in Determining Child Nutrition at Low Income Levels: A Case Study in Kerala." Ithaca, New York, mimeo, 1977.

Lassen, Cheryl A. *Landlessness and Rural Poverty in Latin America: Conditions, Trends and Policies Affecting Income and Employment.* Cornell University Special Series on Landlessness and Near-Landlessness, No. 4. Ithaca: Cornell University, Rural Development Committee, 1980.

Leslie, Joanne. "Women's Work and Child Nutrition in the Third World." Washington, D.C.: International Center for Research on Women, 1985.

Lycette, Margaret A. "Improving Women's Access to Credit in the Third World: Policy and Project Recommendations." ICRW Occasional Papers, no. 1. Washington, D.C.: International Center for Research on Women, 1984.

Mather, Celia. "Rather than Make Trouble, It's Better Just to Leave: Behind the Lack of Industrial Strive in the Tangerang Region of West Java," in Haleh Afshar, ed., *Women, Work, and Ideology in the Third World.* New York: Tavistock, 1985.

Mazumdar, Dipak. "The Urban Informal Sector," *World Development* 4 (August 1976): 655–679.

McSweeney, B. G. "Collection and Analysis of Data on Rural Women's Time Use," *Studies in Family Planning* 10 (1979): 379–383.

McSweeney, B. G., and Marion Freedman. "Lack of Time as an Obstacle to Women's Education: The Case of Upper Volta," *Comparative Education Review* (June 1980): S124–S139.

Merrick, Thomas W. "Employment and Earnings in the Informal Sector in Brazil: The Case of Belo Horizonte," *Journal of Developing Areas* 10 (April 1976): 337–354.

Ministerio de Cultura, Juventud y Deportes. *Situacion de la Mujer en Costa Rica: Evaluacion del Decenio 1975–1985.* San Jose, Costa Rica: Ministerio de Cultura, Juventud y Deportes, Direccion General de Mujer y Familia, 1985.

Moock, Peter R. "The Efficiency of Women as Farm Managers: Kenya," *American Journal of Agricultural Economics* 58 (December 1976): 831–835.

Mueller, Eva. "The Value and Allocation of Time in Rural Botswana," *Journal of Development Economics* 15 (1984): 329–360.

Nabarro, David. "Social, Economic, Health, and Environmental Determinants of Nutritional Status," *Food and Nutrition Bulletin* 6 (March 1984): 18–32.

Nag, M., B. N. F. White, and R. C. Peet. "An Anthropological Approach to the Study of the Economic Value of Children in Java and Nepal," *Current Anthropology* 19 (1978): 293–306.

Parlato, Margaret, and Michael Favin. *Primary Health Care: Progress and Problems.* Washington, D.C.: American Public Health Association, 1982.

Pathmanathan, I. "Breastfeeding—A Study of 8750 Malaysian Infants," *Medical Journal of Malaysia* 33 (December 1978): 113–119.

Pinstrup-Andersen, Per. "Food Prices and the Poor in Developing Countries," *European Review of Agricultural Economics* 12 (1985a): 69–85.

————. "The Short-Term Impact of Macro-Economic Adjustment Policies on the Poor with Emphasis on the Nutrition Effects: the Need for Research." Washington, D.C.: International Food Policy Research Institute, mimeo, 1985b.

Popkin, Barry. "Rural Women, Work, and Child Welfare in the Philippines," in Mayra Buvinic, Margaret A. Lycette, and William Paul McGreevey, eds., *Women and Poverty in the Third World*. Baltimore: Johns Hopkins University Press, 1983.

Popkin, Barry M., and Florentino S. Solon. "Income, Time, the Working Mother and Child Nutrition." *Environment Child Health* (August 1976): 156–166.

Prates, Suzana. "El Trabajo de la mujer en una epoca de crisis (o cuando se pierde ganando)," in *La mujer en el Uruguay: Ayer y Hoy*. Montevideo, Uruguay: Grupo de Estudios sobre la Condicion de la Mujer en el Uruguay.

Programa Regional del Empleo para Latina America Latina y el Caribe (PREALC). *Mas Allá de la Crisis*. Summary paper. Santiago, Chile: Organizacion Internacional del Trabajo, 1985a.

————. *Mas Allá de la Crisis: Trabajos Presentados a la IV Conferencia del PREALC*. Santiago, Chile: Organización Internacional del Trabajo, 1985b.

————. *Participación Femenina en la Actividad Economica en America Latina (Analisis Estadístico)*. Santiago, Chile: Organización Internacional del Trabajo, 1978.

Rey de Marulanda, Nohra. *El Trabajo de la Mujer*. CEDE Documentos 063. Bogota, Colombia: Universidad de los Andes, Centro de Estudios sobre Desarollo Económico, 1981.

Reynolds, Dorene. "The Household Divided: Competition for Cash between Husbands and Wives in West Pokot, Kenya." Paper presented at the Annual Meetings of the American Anthropological Association, Washington, D.C., December 3–7, 1982.

Rosales, Osvaldo Villavicencio. "La Mujer Chilena en la Fuerza de Trabajo: Participación, Empleo, y Desempleo (1957–1977)." Santiago, Chile: Universidad de Chile, 1979.

Schmink, Marianne. "Women in the Urban Economy in Latin America." Working Paper No. 1. New York: The Population Council, 1982.

Shields, Nwanganga. *Women in the Urban Labor Markets of Africa: The Case of Tanzania*. World Bank Staff Working Paper no. 380. Washington, D.C.: The World Bank, 1980.

Sivard, Ruth Leger. *Women: A World Survey*. Washington, D.C.: World Priorities, 1985.

Smith, Meredith, et al. "Socioeconomic, Education, and Health Factors Influencing Growth of Rural Haitian Children," *Ecology of Food and Nutrition* 13 (1983): 99–108.

Soekirman. "The Effect of Maternal Unemployment on Nutritional Status of Infants from Low-Income Households in Central Java," unpublished PH.D. thesis. Cornell University, 1983.

Staudt, Kathleen A. "Administrative Resources, Political Patrons, and Redressing Sex Inequities: A Case from Western Kenya," *Journal of Developing Areas* (July 1978).

Stinson, Wayne, *Women and Health*. Geneva: World Federation of Public Health Associations, 1986.

Sundar, Pushpa. "Credit and Finance Needs of Women Workers." Mimeo, n.d.

Tobisson, Eva. "Women, Work, Food and Nutrition in Nyamwigura Village, Mara Region Tanzania." Tanzania Food and Nutrition Centre Report No. 548. Dar Es Salaam: Tanzania Food and Nutrition Centre, 1980.

Tripp, Robert B. "Farmers and Traders: Some Economic Determinants of Nutritional Status in Northern Ghana," *Journal of Tropical Pediatrics* 27 (February 1981): 15–21.

United Nations Children's Fund (UNICEF). *The State of the World's Children 1986*. New York: UNICEF, 1986.

United Nations Fund for Population Activities (UNFPA). "Labor and Population," *Population Profiles* 5. New York: UNFPA, n.d.

United Nations Economic Commission for Africa. "The Data Base of Discussion of the Interrelations between the Integration of Women in Development, Their Situation, and Population Factors in Africa." Addis Ababa: United Nations Economic Commission for Africa, 1974.

United Nations Food and Agricultural Organization. "Time Allocation Survey: A Tool for Anthropologists, Economists, and Nutritionists." Food Policy and Nutrition Division. Rome: Food and Agricultural Organization, 1983.

Van Esterik, Penny, and Ted Greiner. "Breastfeeding and Women's Work: Constraints and Opportunities," *Studies in Family Planning* 12 (April 1981): 184–197.

Von Harder, Martius. *Fraven in Landliechen Bangladesh: Eine Empirische Studie in Vier Dorfern im Comilla District*. Saarbrucken: Verlag der ssip-Scheiften Breitenback, 1977.

Ware, Helen. "Effects of Maternal Education, Women's Roles and Child Care on Child Mortality," in W. Henry Mosley and Lincoln C. Chen, eds., *Child Survival: Strategies for Research*. A Supplement to *Population and Development Review* 10. New York: The Population Council, 1984, pp. 191–214.

White, Benjamin. "The Economic Importance of Children in a Javanese Village," in M. Nag, ed., *Population and Social Organization*. The Hague: Mouton, 1975, pp. 127–140.

Whitehead, Ann. "'I'm Hungry Mum': The Politics of Domestic Budgeting," in Kate Young, Carol Walkowitz and Roslyn McCuyllagh, eds., *Of Marriage and the Market: Women's Subordination in International Perspective*. London: CSE Books, 1981.

World Health Organization. *A Report on Alternative Approaches to Day Care for Children*. Geneva: World Health Organization Maternal and Child Health, Division of Family Health, 1981.

———. *Primary Health Care*. Geneva: World Health Organization, 1978.

Whyte, Robert Orr, and Pauline Whyte. *The Women of Rural Asia*. Boulder, CO: Westview Press, 1982.

Winikoff, Beverly. "The Infant Feeding Study: Summary." Report prepared for U.S. Agency for International Development. New York: The Population Council, 1986.

Wolfe, Barbara L., and Jere R. Behrman. "Determinants of Child Mortality, Health and Nutrition in a Developing Country," *Journal of Development Economics* 11 (October 1982): 163–194.

World Bank. *Health Sector Policy Paper*. Washington, D.C.: The World Bank, 1980.

———. *World Development Report 1985*. Washington, D.C.: The World Bank, 1985.

14

Drug Supply and Use in Developing Countries: Problems and Policies

Adrian Griffiths

Drugs: The Position of Developing Countries

The Market

Modern health care is to a large extent synonymous with modern drugs. In developing countries, in the absence of the basic prerequisites of good health—adequate nutrition, safe drinking water, basic sanitation and environmental health measures—drugs play an even more decisive role as the first line of defense against disease. Despite their crucial importance, drugs are neither adequately supplied nor rationally used in developing countries. This paper reviews the key problems affecting drug supply and use, and the reactions of different countries to them.

The estimated pharmaceutical consumption of developing countries, including China, in 1982 was around $18.2 billion—somewhat more than a fifth of total world consumption. Among developing countries a small number accounted for a large proportion of consumption; for example, China alone accounted for almost a quarter of the total; Brazil accounted for well over a third of consumption of Latin America, and Nigeria and Egypt accounted for half the total consumption in Africa (IMS; U.N. Centre on Transnational Corporations, 1983).

*This chapter benefitted considerably from several discussions with Ms. S. Foster, economist, in the Action Programme on Essential Drugs at WHO, Geneva.

International trade in drugs increased at an estimated annual average of 9.6 percent at current prices from 1977 to 1982 to reach $14 billion ($8 billion in finished products and $6 billion in intermediates). Developing country imports rose from $2.5 billion in 1976 to $4.47 billion in 1982, i.e., 32 percent of world imports. However, they accounted for only 4.4 percent of world exports ($0.62 billion), leaving a negative net balance of $3.85 billion, of which roughly 70 percent was for finished products (Avramovic, 1985; Rigoni, Griffiths, Laing, 1985).

Manufacturing Capability

The stage of manufacturing capability of the pharmaceutical industry in developing countries varies widely. Broadly speaking, developing countries can be divided into three groups as far as drug manufacturing capability is concerned:

Group 1 countries (such as Costa Rica, Sierra Leone, Lesotho, and Malaysia) have little or no manufacturing capability and rely largely or completely on imports of finished drugs.

Group 2 countries (such as Colombia, Kenya, Togo, Zambia, Pakistan and Thailand) have some manufacturing capability, including in the more advanced cases, some production of simple bulk drugs from intermediates, but mainly formulation and packaging of finished products from imported bulk drugs.

Group 3 countries (such as Argentina, Brazil, Mexico, S. Korea, Egypt, and India) have acquired an advanced manufacturing capability, including some production of active substances (intermediates) and basic chemicals, and some product and process research and development.

Data are given in Table 14.1 for a sample of countries in each group. Group 1 countries are generally those which are too small, too poor, or both, to develop a viable drug manufacturing capability. However, as shown by the example of Malaysia, and more recently by much smaller, poorer countries such as the Comoro Islands and Burundi, limited local formulation and packaging are possible with appropriate outside help. While such ventures are rarely economically competitive against imports, they may help to save scarce foreign exchange and improve continuity of supply.

In Group 2 countries, while local production may reach very high shares of total consumption (e.g., 95 percent in Colombia and 75 percent in Thailand in 1980), imports of intermediates and semi-finished drugs by definition remain high (e.g., over three-quarters of consumption in

Table 14.1
The Pharmaceutical Industry in Selected Developing Countries, 1980

Country	Population, mid-1979 (million)	GNP per Capita $	Drug Spending per Capita $	Drug Production (million)[c] $	Drug Consumption (million) $	Production of Finished Drugs (percent of consumption)	Market Share of Foreign Firms (percent)[d]
Group 1:							
Costa Rica	2.2	1820[b]	13.3	21.0	28.0	75.0	82
Malaysia	13.1	1370	5.2	34.0	68.5	49.6	64
Sierra Leone	3.4	250	3.2	0.2	11.0	1.8	100
Group 2:							
Colombia	26.1	1010	20.8	532.0	560.0	95.0	88
Thailand[a]	45.5	590	7.3	250.0	335.0	74.6	na
Kenya[a]	15.3	380	2.1	8.0	32.5	24.6	90
Group 3:							
Argentina	27.3	2230	68.8	1900.0	1920.0	99.0	53
Brazil	116.5	1780	12.7	1301.5	1544.0	84.3	76
Mexico	65.5	1640	15.7	973.9	1100.0	88.5	72
Egypt	38.9	480	8.2	273.9	320.0	85.6	30
S. Korea	37.8	1480	16.6	950.0	630.0	150.8	16
India	659.2	190	1.3	1450.0	880.0	164.8	70

[a] Thailand 1979, Kenya 1978.
[b] Half the production was exporter.
[c] Brazil 1979, Costa Rica 1977, Malaysia 1978.
[d] Majority of wholly owned subsidiaries of foreign drug companies.
Source: United Nations Centre on Transnational Corporations, 1983.

Colombia and 75 percent in Thailand in 1980), imports of intermediates and semi-finished drugs by definition remain high (e.g., over three-quarters of consumption in Colombia and Thailand in 1980) since local capacities are still almost entirely confined to dosage formulation and packaging. As might be expected, foreign subsidiaries generally retain the bulk of the market in group 2 countries.

While it is much easier for the more developed countries to build an advanced drug manufacturing capability, the presence of Egypt and India in group 3 show that a high GNP per capita is not a prerequisite. What both these countries have in common is a relatively large home market, a pool of qualified technical personnel and a coherent drug sector policy.

For example, in Egypt the pharmaceutical industry grew out of the nationalization program in the early 1960s and the creation of three joint ventures with foreign companies, supported by the systematic development of an ancillary infrastructure in chemicals, research, and training. As a result, by 1980 the public sector produced 70 percent of consumption. The three joint ventures and one foreign subsidiary started in 1979 provided a further 13 percent; the remaining 17 percent were being met by imports. Patent and trademark market protection remain in force, but the local industry occupies a dominant position and has successfully negotiated favorable licensing and joint venture agreements. At the same time, local producers still depend on imports for a substantial proportion of chemical intermediates, and production plant. Incentives for local production include import protection, refusal of manufacturing licenses for competing products, and extensive fiscal concessions. However, over the last ten years more positive measures have been taken to develop joint ventures.

India adopted a more mixed strategy, regulating but not nationalizing foreign companies (which still had a 70 percent share of the market in 1980), while stimulating local production, both private and public, in all phases of manufacture. As a result, it now has the most vertically integrated drug industry in the developing world and was already producing almost two-thirds more than it consumed by 1980.

S. Korea, with the advantage of a much higher GNP per capita ($1480 compared to India's $190 in 1980—cf. Table 14.1) has also been highly successful. Production has increased from $0.99 million in 1971 to $1,150 million in 1981. Only fourteen of its 300 drug companies are foreign subsidiaries, and they have only 16 percent of the market, mainly because of the government's standing bar against majority owned foreign companies. However, the Foreign Capital Inducement Act and other more recent laws are designed to encourage and protect foreign investment and are reported to be effective.

Conclusions and Policy Implications

The decision to make rather than buy is often superficially attractive—self-sufficiency, local employment, export potential, and foreign exchange savings are among the advantages cited by advocates of local production. In practice, the local market is often too limited to be viable, exports are correspondingly unlikely, local employment is generally limited and qualified staff are scarce, so the end result can easily be dearer drugs of lower quality. The crucial requirement in developing local production is therefore an objective analysis of its technical and economic viability in the specific circumstances of the country concerned. Broader issues are involved in the more developed countries, for the question goes beyond the viability of individual plants to the interrelationship between different stages of manufacture and government policy for the whole sector within the overall development strategy.

Joint ventures with multinational companies can be an important advantage in terms of financing capacity and technical knowhow. However, many developing countries have experienced serious difficulties and disputes because of their failure to negotiate adequate agreements, particularly on key issues such as royalty payments, transfer of technology, and obligation to license unused patents, specification of export markets to which surplus local production may be sold, transfer prices, price and profit controls, investment protection, expatriation of profits, etc. The experience of countries like Egypt and S. Korea shows that mutually satisfactory agreements can be reached by competent negotiators working within a clear sector policy. In this context, more use could be made of technical cooperation between developing countries to exploit the positive experiences of the more successful countries and of the specialized resources of the World Bank and other regional development banks.

The Economic Recession and Drug Supply

The effects of the economic recession, triggered by sharp increases in oil prices, on developing countries, have already been extensively described and analyzed. The most important effects for our purposes have been the large and prolonged drop in exports, the deterioration of the terms of trade and exchange rates, and the swing from overliquidity and cheap credit to underliquidity and much dearer credit. By 1983–84 the average real GDP per capita was estimated to be down to its 1976 level in Latin America and below its 1970 level in sub-Saharan Africa. The result has been a massive increase in the foreign debt of the developing countries, from only $100 billion in 1971 to $600 billion in 1982, and around $970 billion at the end of 1985. Debt service costs doubled from $55 billion to $109 billion between 1978 and 1982 and, despite a large increase in rescheduling, were still at $103.4 billion in 1984.

The uncomfortably large number of countries which used foreign borrowing to finance public sector deficits and maintain consumption and those which plunged heavily into long-term infrastructure projects not directly productive, now face rigorous economic constraints on their development, many of them into the 1990s. This latter pattern has been frequent in the least developed countries such as those of sub-Saharan Africa. For example, half of the Congo's external debt was incurred for infrastructure investments, and in the Gabon a third went on the trans-Gabon highway alone. Indeed, in sub-Saharan Africa even industrial projects have not fared well for various reasons. A recent survey of 345 such projects found four-fifths of them performing inadequately (IMF, 1984; World Bank, 1985; Cline, 1983; Hugon, 1985; Institute de l'Enterprise, 1985).

Foreign aid and loan-funded developments during the early and mid-seventies generated new recurrent costs in the public sector. As the recession deepened, public revenues fell behind expenditures, loan funding of deficits became increasingly costly and difficult, and capital and recurrent spending had to be cut back. In the health services, staff costs are the largest single item of recurrent spending. Rational reductions therefore implied payroll cuts, i.e., reducing staff members or pay or both. However, government employees are a strong and vocal pressure group, and payroll cuts are strongly opposed both economically and politically. Reductions or less than inflation increases in recurrent budgets therefore tended to be focused on non-staff items. (Opportunities for reallocating capital to sustain current budgets were limited, for a large share of capital budgets generally come from non-transferable foreign aid and loans for specific projects.)

Among the non-staff items, drugs and medical supplies have almost invariably suffered. They are the largest recurrent budget items after staff; they commonly accounting for 20–40 percent of public health service recurrent budgets and therefore are the only major choice for cuts after staff. As noted, most developing countries, particularly the least developed ones, import a high proportion of their drugs—if not as finished products than as bulk intermediates for local formulation and packing. Drug budgets have therefore been strongly sensitive. The cuts in domestic budgets are compounded by the shortages of foreign exchange needed to pay for imports. Though public sector drug imports rarely exceed 1–2 percent of total imports, when debt service/exports ratios reach 30–60 percent or more, competition for foreign exchange becomes intense and drug imports are rarely the first preoccupations of hard-pressed Ministries of Finance.

In addition, the exchange rates of many developing countries have fallen, often dramatically, and local currency budgets have rarely been increased sufficiently to compensate for the drop in purchasing power. Finally, the foreign exchange allocated is often released late and irregularly so that planned purchases become impossible and crisis buying drives up prices still further.

The effects of the economic recession on private sector drug supplies have been mixed. On one hand, as overall purchasing power has stagnated or fallen, the demand for drugs has been dampened or at least has deviated to cheaper remedies, including traditional ones which can be paid for in kind. One the other hand, the failure of supplies in the public sector in many developing countries has driven patients to buy them from the private sector, thus leading to a tacit privatisation of drug supplies.

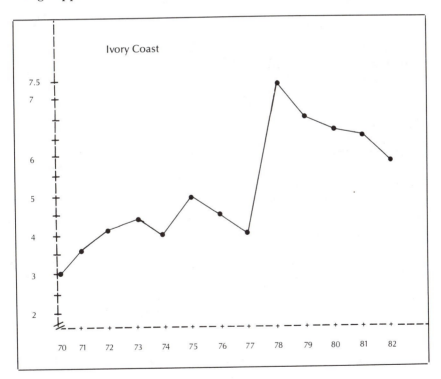

Figure 14.1. *Real drug imports per capita since 1970: Ivory Coast ($).*
Source: Data from Dunlop and Over, 1985.

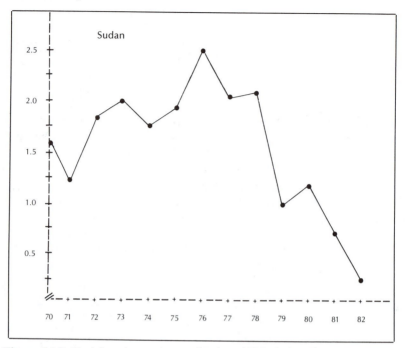

Figure 14.2. *Real drug imports per capita since 1970: Sudan ($).*
Source: Data from Dunlop and Over, 1985.

The Effects on Imports

Figures 14.1 through 14.3 illustrate the effect of the recession on real drug imports per capita in three sub-Saharan African countries: the Ivory Coast, the Sudan, and Tanzania. All three show a pattern which probably applies to most countries in the region: an upward trend until the late seventies, followed by a sharp downward trend since then. In the Ivory Coast, real per capita drug imports were 27 percent lower in 1982 than their peak level in 1978. In the Sudan, where external debt service reached seven times export earnings, real per capita drug imports in 1982 were barely a tenth of their 1976 peak and even lower than they were in the mid-sixties. In Tanzania, the upward trend ended with a sharp fall in 1976, followed by a temporary recovery in 1977 and 1978, then a sharp and uninterrupted fall to about the same level as the Sudan by 1984 (Dunlop and Over, 1985). These figures become even more dramatic when viewed against the massive decline in health caused by the regional drought which affected twenty-four countries in the region from 1982 to 1984. For example, UNICEF estimated that

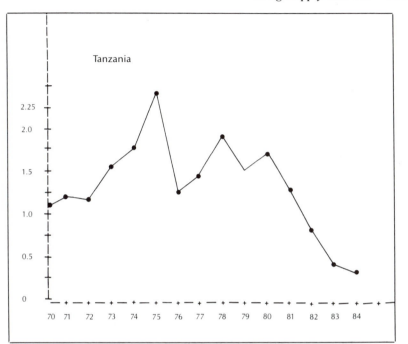

Figure 14.3. *Real drug imports per capita since 1970: Tanzania ($).*
Source: Data from Dunlop and Over, 1985.

the drought caused at least 1 million extra child deaths, i.e., about a quarter more than expected in 1984 (UNICEF, 1985).

Public Health Service Drug Budgets

The data in Figures 14.1–14.3 refer to total drug imports. A closer look at the experience of two other African countries, Togo and Zambia, shows the effect of the recession on public drug budgets. In Togo, the economy grew by an average of 7 percent a year in the decade to 1975 and was boosted further by the five-fold increase in the price of phosphate, the main export. The recession hit the economy in the middle of the third national plan, designed to achieve economic takeoff. Phosphate export earnings collapsed, followed by those of agricultural exports in the 1982–84 drought. The plan ended prematurely with an austerity budget, and the IMF assisted debt rescheduling and refinancing in 1979. In 1981, the fourth national plan was aborted, budgetary austerity increased, and a stabilization plan was introduced with the aid of the IMF and Paris Club creditors. Further structural adjustment plans have followed and are reported to be working well. Nevertheless, gross domestic product (GDP) per capita, at 1978 prices, fell by almost a quarter from 1979 to 1983, i.e., 37 percent per capita. Given the annual increase in population of 3.5 percent, it is not expected to regain its 1979 level until the late 1990s or the turn of the century.

The government budget (at constant 1978 prices), excluding public debt service, was cut by 22 percent between 1979 and 1983. The real per capita budget of the public health services fell by 40 percent from African Financial Community Franc (FCFA) 1722 to around 1025. Such a reduction was extremely serious in itself, but though a freeze on recruitment and pay was introduced in 1983, the share of the recurrent budget allocated to non-staff items, of which the largest component was drugs and medical supplies, fell from some 30 percent in 1978 to 18 percent in 1984, with actual disbursements still lower. Even in nominal terms the non-staff budget fell 29 percent. In real terms, allowing for the decline in the FCA franc and world inflation in drug prices, it fell by 60 percent or more, so that the real drug budget per capita in 1984 was less than a third of that of 1978 (IMF, 1984; WHO, Drug Action Programme, 1985).

The salient points of Zambia's economic situation may be summarized by a few key indicators. The price of copper, which represents 90 percent of merchandise exports and a third of GDP, fell by 57 percent in the decade to 1984, and real GDP per capita fell by a quarter. The terms of trade index fell by some 30 percent and the current account deficit rose from around 12 percent in the later seventies to a peak of 20 percent in the early eighties. By 1984, despite drawing down reserves and heavy foreign borrowing, imports had been forced down to below a third of their 1974 level in real terms. In addition, non-guaranteed imports were being charged price premiums of 70 percent or more to cover anticipated delays in payments. A sweeping program of economic adjustment is now well under way, but debt service is nevertheless expected to consume 50 percent of export income through to 1988. Unless extraordinary loans and further debt rescheduling and refinancing can be arranged, there will be a new outflow of capital for the rest of the decade. A series of devaluations, culminating with the introduction of foreign exchange auctions in late 1985, have brought the kwacha/dollar exchange rate down to less than a seventh of its 1981 level.

Despite these extremely difficult circumstances, public health expenditures were accorded high priority, their share of government budget increased from around 10.5 percent in 1981 to 14 percent in 1986. Total spending actually increased in real terms by around 10 percent, but this was mainly due to the large increase in the local currency value of committed foreign aid. Recurrent spending fell by some 4–5 percent, approaching 20 percent per capita. The share of the recurrent health budget allocated for drugs and medical supplies has remained at around a fifth since 1981, so other things being equal the per capita drug budget would also have fallen by 20 percent. However, allowing for the fact that three quarters of drug expenditures are in foreign exchange and are therefore affected by the dramatic fall in the exchange rate, the real per capita value of the 1986 drug budget is not more than a fifth to a quarter of what it was in 1981. This estimate coincides with estimates by physicians and others in Zambia, that the required drug budget may be four to five times the actual allocation (Zambia).

Conclusions and Policy Implications

Evidently ministries of health can do nothing about the overall economic constraints, but they could do more within these constraints.

First, they need to develop a concerted effort with ministries of finance to ensure that, whatever the budget accorded for drugs, including the required foreign exchange component, it is made available in a programmed fashion. This would allow drug purchases to be rationally planned to obtain maximum value for money, rather than being made on a crisis basis as and when budgets and foreign exchange are released.

Second, ministries of health need to make a much greater effort to quantify and price drug requirements so that they can make a coherent case for their minimum budget requirements and indicate the impact of shortfalls on the functioning of the health services.

Third, as indicated above, in many countries, the budgetary adjustments made under economic constraints have so distorted resource mixes that staff no longer have the material resources to do their work. Corrections to maintain the minimum balance of resources are therefore imperative.

Fourth, new sources of funding need to be urgently considered for health services in general and drugs in particular. Among the options worthy of serious examination are:

Prescription fees (for first prescriptions within an episode of treatment, so as not to penalize cases needing multiple prescriptions).

Consultation fees (per first consultation for an episode of illness).

Taxes on products harmful to health or which incur health service costs. Collection is administratively feasible and net yields are potentially significant for tobacco (particularly cigarettes), for alcohol (preferably an ad valorem tax), and for motor vehicle registrations or insurance, to cover the costs of road accidents.

Health insurance and provident fund schemes for workers earning above a minimum income (e.g., as now being considered in Botswana and Zambia).

Specific Drug Supply System Problems and Reactions

In addition to the above macro problems, which involve issues far beyond the health sector, there is a series of problems which are specific to drug supply systems. The main component activities of drug supply systems are:

Selection: deciding what drugs are needed

Quantification: calculating how much of each drug is needed

Procurement: selecting supplies, placing and monitoring orders, checking delivery and quality, and paying suppliers

Distribution: reception, storage, stock control, transportation, and record keeping for monitoring drug supply and use

Use: prescription, dispensing and patients' use of drugs (Management Sciences for Health, 1982).

The key problems encountered in each of these activities and reactions to them are reviewed in turn below.

Selection

Selection involves decisions about the drugs to be made available, their dosage form (e.g., tablet, syrup, injectable) strengths, and packaging. Logically, given that the need for drugs far exceeds the ability to pay for them in developing countries, it might be expected that only the most cost-effective drugs to cope with the morbidity patterns of each country would be selected. In practice, until the late seventies, drug selections in both the public and the private sectors were generally determined by a haphazard mixture of historical habit, individual clinical preferences, and marketing pressures.

The first step towards more rational choice of drugs came in 1975, when the World Health Assembly debated the experience of a few countries with essential drugs to meet basic health care needs. A working document produced by WHO consultants explained the concept and proposed both selection criteria and a preliminary list of drugs. This in turn led to the first expert committee on the selection of essential drugs and publication in 1977 of the first selection guidelines and a model list of essential drugs (EDL), from which each country could develop its own list. Since then, the EDL has been revised and updated every two years (WHO, 1977, 1979, 1983).

There was considerable opposition to EDLs at the outset, notably from the drug industry, pharmacists, and physicians, who argued that EDLs restricted access to drugs and the clinical freedom of physicians to prescribe the most appropriate drugs in each case (Pharmaceutical Manufacturers Association, 1979). The industry also argued that EDLs would discourage research. The argument concerning the effect on research had little credibility, since some nine-tenths of the drugs on WHO's EDLs were available as generics and so had already benefitted from the full period of patent protection during which their research and development costs are normally recouped. The arguments concerning restriction of access and choice were hard to sustain against the overwhelming evidence of inadequate and inappropriate drug supply and use in developing countries, and the manifest therapeutic and economic logic of the EDL selection criteria. These criteria are summarized as follows:

1. In each country, essential drugs should be selected by a *local committee*, including members competent in clinical medicine, pharmacology, and pharmacy and health workers of the types who will use drugs.

2. The international *generic name* of each drug should be used, if available.

3. Essential drugs should offer the widest possible *coverage* of the pattern of prevalent morbidity affecting the population for which they are intended.

4. The drugs selected should take account of the treatment *facilities* available; the availability, training and experience of *personnel; financial* resources and costs; and *demographic, generic,* and *environmental factors*.

5. Only drugs for which sound *scientific data* on efficacy and safety are available should be selected.

6. Each drug selected must be available in a form in which *quality, bioavailability* and *stability* can be assured under expected local conditions (including storage conditions and local diseases such as diarrhea or liver disease which may affect pharmokinetic patterns).

7. When two or more drugs seem similar in the above respects, the choice between them should be based on a careful evaluation of their relative *efficacy, safety, quality, price,* and *availability*. Policy regarding *local manufacturing,* and its feasibility, may also influence the choice.

8. *Cost* is a major selection criterion. Cost comparisons between drugs, and between drugs and non-drug treatments, should include the total cost of treatment, and not only the drug costs.

9. Local health authorities should decide the level of *expertise* required to prescribe each drug or group of drugs, including the competence to make particular diagnoses.

10. Essential drugs should be formulated as *single* compounds. Fixed ratio combinations are justified only if they meet the requirements of a defined population group, and have a proven advantage in terms of therapeutic advantage, safety, compliance, and cost, compared to single compounds administered separately.

11. Essential drug lists should be *reviewed* at least annually. New drugs should be added only if they offer clear advantages over those previously selected. Drugs on the list should be removed if new information clearly shows they no longer have a favorable benefit/risk ratio, and/or that there are safer replacements (including non-drug treatment).

The choice in developing countries is not between optimal but high cost drug treatment and marginally less effective but much cheaper drugs, but between the optimum for a few and nothing for others. For example, a year's leprosy treatment with dapsone costs less than $1, but some cases are resistant to dapsone. Rifampicin is more effective but costs close to $1 per day. Evidently it is much more cost-effective to use dapsone as the standard treatment and reserve rifampicin for resistant cases rather than use rifampicin immediately. Similar reasoning applies to the choice of expensive dosage forms such as injectables and drinkable ampoules, where much cheaper tablet and syrup forms are just as effective, and to the choice of generics rather than more expensive branded products. In the latter case some allowance must be made for the problem of bio-equivalence (i.e., the fact that though a generic has the same chemical composition as its branded equivalent it may not be absorbed by the body to the same extent or at the same rate). However, significant differences in equivalence are relatively infrequent and for many drugs the range of dosages used is far greater than the differences in bio-equivalence, so they have little clinical significance.

In parallel with these developments, an international consumer and public interest movement formed to address environmental and health problems in developed and underdeveloped countries, particularly issues like the marketing practices of infant food and drug companies. In 1979, a joint WHO/UNICEF report on the feeding of infants and young children recommended a marketing code for breast milk substitutes (WHO, 1979). Following a highly polemical and controversial debate, the World Health Assembly adopted the "International Code of Marketing Breast Milk Substitutes" in 1981 (Jayasuriya et al., 1984). Although this code had no legal status, it was accepted by most of the large manufacturers and was incorporated in various forms into the legislation of a growing number of developing countries over the next few years.

The consumer groups were simultaneously pressing for a similar code for the marketing of drugs. The International Federation of Pharmaceutical Manufacturers Associations (IFPMA) forestalled this by introducing its own Code of Pharmaceutical Marketing Practices as a self-regulating measure in 1981. Although criticized by consumer groups and some industry spokesmen as insufficient and unclear, it has nevertheless had a positive impact in correcting unacceptable marketing practices, and the IFPMA publishes regular reports of the cases investigated and their results (SCRIP, 1981; Health Action International, 1982; Mahler, 1982; Bakke, 1984; Agarawal, 1978).

Many countries that have formally adopted EDLs have lacked the will or the capacity to implement them systematically, e.g., to develop EDLs for each level of health care according to its responsibilities and the training of its staff. Furthermore, most EDLs have been confined to the public sector, whereas in many developing countries the private sector accounts for a far larger share of consumption. The problem here is threefold. First, whereas the public sector clearly has a duty to ensure that essential drugs at least are available, and if necessary, to limit purchase of less- or non-essential drugs to achieve this objective, the extension of this argument to the private sector is more controversial. It encounters strong resistance, both as an unwarranted restriction on trade, and as a limitation of the right of choice of private physicians and patients. Nevertheless, the example of Norway, which has a need clause for the registration of new drugs, demonstrates that the number of drugs on the market can be restricted without any meaningful reduction in choice or effectiveness (Bakke, 1984).

Second, it is generally not in the interest of private sector suppliers to concentrate on essential drugs and generics, for branded specialty products, and low cost, high profit non-essentials such as vitamins and tonics, are more profitable. Price controls and fixed profit margins have paradoxically reinforced this tendency. For example, a branded drug sold at $3 including a 50 percent markup yields $1 profit whereas a generic equivalent sold at $1 yields only 33 cents. In addition, buyers generally prefer heavily promoted attractively packed branded drugs to anonymous generics sold in basic packaging or loose from large packs.

Third, many developing countries lack the institutional capacity to develop and implement a limited drug list for the private sector. For example, Pakistan introduced the Generic Names Ordinance in 1973 which banned brand name drugs but was unable to assure the quality of generics. Furthermore, the government took no action to persuade either the medical profession or the public of the merits of the program. The continuing heavy demand for branded products quickly gave rise to a parallel market in illegal imports, including low quality imitations, which the authorities could not hope to control. Branded drugs continued to be used but at a hefty price premium to allow for their scarcity and for the risks and costs of smuggling. The program had to be abandoned.

Similar considerations applied to the Drugs (control) Ordinance introduced by Bangladesh in 1982. This law required all drugs to be registered; set safety, efficacy and usefulness criteria as prerequisites of registration; scheduled some 1,700 drugs to be modified or withdrawn within three to eighteen months; empowered the government to fix the prices for finished products and intermediates, and to review licensing agreements between local manufacturers and foreign companies; limited the retail sale of modern drugs to outlets under the personal supervision of a pharmacist; required labels and promotional material to be approved by the licensing authority; required WHO's Good Manufacturing Practice (GMP) recommendations to be observed; and prohibited import and sale of sub-standard drugs. Praiseworthy as these measures were, they took little account of the institutional capacity to apply them. For example, the drugs scheduled for withdrawal were selected by a small committee working in great haste and secrecy, with no consultation with the medical profession or with manufacturers. The limitation of retail sales of modern drugs to outlets personally supervised by pharmacists took no account of the limited number of pharmacists in the country. The drug administration's skilled manpower was "grossly inadequate" to undertake the inspections and follow-ups required, and both the national drug testing laboratories were in poor condition. Furthermore, only the eight multinational companies in the country had good quality control; among the local manufacturers, ten of the twenty-five medium sized companies had "fairly satisfactory" systems, the remainder had "poor systems," as did twenty-five of the 130 small local companies who had any quality control worth mentioning (DANIDA and SIDA, 1985).

Despite these institutional limitations, the government reports that the program is successful. On the other hand, a recent report commissioned by the IFPMA and the U.S. Pharmaceutical Manufacturers Association reported a fall in the quality of drugs previously locally produced by multinationals or imported, and now produced by medium or small local companies. Thirty percent of samples tested by the drug administration were sub-standard in 1982–83, and all of the rejects were from local manufacturers. In addition, they found a substantial black market in illegal imports of banned drugs and spurious copies at up to ten times their previous price; use of brand names and pack designs similar to those of well known prohibited products; and a loss of foreign investment in drug production (Jayasuriya, 1985).

The lessons from both these experiments is not that their aims were necessarily misguided, but that they cut off certain products and sources of supply while not in a position to assure the market of credible substitutes.

Finally, in the majority of developing countries which have not extended the essential drug concept to the private sector, demand for drugs is heavily influenced by drug company marketing, which is generally the main source of information to both the medical profession and the public (Funkel et al., 1983). While the content and activities allowed in marketing are now controlled by the IFPMA pharmaceutical marketing code, the amounts spent remain unrestricted. Substantially more is spent on marketing than on research and development. Promotional spending by foreign companies have been estimated at 25 percent in Argentina (where large local companies spend a still higher percentage), 22 percent in Brazil and 26 percent in Colombia (Centre on Transnational Corporations, 1983; ABIFARMA, 1983; Krieger and Brieto, 1977; Chudnovsky, 1979).

Conclusions and Policy Implications

Considerable work remains to be done to extend the EDL concept to specific levels of care according to the morbidity treated and staff capabilities.

There is large scope for extending the EDL concept to the private sector, but such extensions must take account of institutional capacity and preparation of public opinion.

Developing countries could reduce the undesirable effects of heavy promotion on demand, and contribute to lowering prices, if they placed a ceiling on the proportion of turnover which may be spent on marketing, as is done in countries like the United Kingdom.

Quantification

Quantification of drug requirements in the private sector is basically left to the normal processes of the market; wholesalers and retailers simply order what they think they can sell, based on experience. In the public sector, though larger orders usually have to be placed well in advance, because of the heavy dependence on imports, quantification is done in much the same way. It is based on past consumption and subjective impressions, tempered by crisis buying when quantities are underestimated or there are unforeseen increases in demand. In principle, such estimates could be progressively refined over the years to fit the precise needs of the health services to treat the morbidity presented by the population. In practice, the lack of systematic procedures based on morbidity and health service use, and of a consensus on the most cost-effective drug treatment regimes, make such progressive improvement very difficult.

Six common symptoms which often indicate poor quantification are:

1. Chronic and widespread shortages of commonly used drugs despite adequate funding, procurement, and distribution

2. Large surpluses of otherwise appropriate drugs

3. Inequitable distribution of drugs between different levels of care

4. Excessive quantities of expensive drugs or dosage forms where cheaper ones would suffice

5. Inability to make a case for a minimum acceptable drug budget and arbitrary across-the-board cuts rather than prioritized adjustments to accommodate budget shortfalls

6. Irrational prescribing, such as shortening of treatments to the point of ineffectiveness to stretch inadequate supplies, or substitution of available but inappropriate drugs for those in scarce supply

Conclusions and Policy Implications

Considerable improvements in drug supply could be achieved by better quantification of requirements. Surprisingly, there was until recently no practical guide on how to perform quantification calculations. This gap is being filled by a WHO manual, now being tested, which explains two quantification methods. The two methods are the "adjusted consumption method," and the "patient morbidity/standard treatment method."

The adjusted consumption method estimates drug requirements on the basis of actual consumption in a sample of "standard" facilities where drug consumption levels and patterns are considered acceptable—after adjustment of any drug whose consumption is considered inappropriate. This is the simpler of the two methods, and it is particularly useful where patient morbidity data are unavailable or unreliable, and where standard drug treatments are lacking or difficult to agree upon. This method has been successfully used for mission hospitals in Ghana (Griffiths et al., 1985). The basic steps of the adjusted consumption method are (Griffiths et al., 1985):

1. Select the type or types of facility for which the quantification is to be done.

2. Obtain/draw up the essential drug list for the type of facility concerned.

3. Select the "standard" facilities whose consumption is to serve as the norm for the drug quantities to be supplied to all facilities of the type(s) concerned.

4. Select the period for which consumption is to be calculated.

5. Calculate the consumption of each drug.

6. If necessary, adjust the consumption from step 5: increase to allow for periods out of stock or underuse, or decrease to allow for avoidable losses or overuse.

7. Divide the adjusted consumption quantities from step 6 by the total number of new cases of all kinds (or total cases if new cases are not recorded) expressed in thousands, to obtain the average consumption of each drug per 1000 new cases.

8. To find the total quantity required of each drug, multiply the quantities per 1000 new cases from step 7, by the estimated number of new cases, expressed in thousands, at all the facilities to be supplied.

9. To find the number of packs, divide the total quantity requirements of each drug from step 8 by the quantity per unit pack.

10. To find the total cost of the drugs required, multiply the number of packs required of each drug from step 9 by the unit price per pack, and add to obtain the total cost.

11. Reconcile quantities to available budget—e.g., reduce quantities of less essential or very expensive drugs.

The patient morbidity/standard treatment method, as its name implies, estimates drug requirements on the basis of the number of new cases requiring each drug, multiplied by the quantity of drugs required for an agreed average standard treatment. This method is more precise and has the additional advantage of laying the groundwork for the standardization of prescribing at the clinical level. This method was recently tested in Burundi by a small team from the WHO Drug Action Programme, working with local staff. Without any previous preparation, and using routine national morbidity data from dispensaries and health centers, the team completed a detailed estimate for the primary care level of the health service in a little more than one working week. The basic steps of the patient morbidity/standard treatment method are (Hogerzeil, 1985):

1. Define an average standard drug treatment regime for each health problem to be treated at the type or types of facilities concerned.

2. Tabulate national data on the number of new cases of each health problem or, if not available, conduct a sample survey to obtain the necessary data.

3. To obtain the total quantity of each drug needed for each health problem, multiply the number of new cases by the quantity of drugs specified in the corresponding standard drug treatment.

4. To obtain the total quantity required of each drug, reorganize the quantities from step 3 by drug. Where a drug is indicated for more than one condition add the quantities required for each condition to obtain the total.

5. Increase the quantities to allow for expected losses in transit or in storage (damage, deterioration, date expiration, loss, theft).

6. Continue as for steps 9–11 of the adjusted consumption method. If the total quantity of each drug is divided by the total number of new cases expressed in thousands, the standard quantities required per 1000 new cases are obtained. These can be used to allocate the required drugs according to the workload of each facility, or to make up standard drug kits for a given number of new cases.

Procurement

Good procurement aims to ensure regular supplies of quality drugs at competitive prices. The price of a particular drug in different countries may vary considerably for perfectly good reasons. The commonest reasons include: different manufacturers; retail and wholesale margins, import duties and sales taxes, order sizes, buyer's creditworthiness and promptness in paying; currency fluctuations; transport costs; the number of intermediaries in the distribution chain; and price controls. However, ultimately, prices charged are usually based on what manufacturers, wholesalers and retailers think the market will bear, and the inefficiency of buyers in checking alternative sources and comparing prices. For example, a recent survey of the price charged by the same suppliers for 1000 500 mg capsules of ampicillin to six different Caribbean countries showed a range from $106.08 in Montserrat to $248.50 (+ 134 percent) in Trinidad (Ledogar, 1975). Comparisons in the Andean Pact countries showed price variations of up to 600 percent, e.g., tetracycline cost $30/kg in Colombia and $144/kg in Peru (Lall and Bibile, 1977).

Transfer prices (i.e., prices charged in transactions between subsidiaries of the same company) are supposed to be charged "at arms length," as if the transaction were between two unrelated companies. In fact, they too vary enormously, depending on the commercial objectives of the company concerned, for many of the products concerned are product-specific intermediates available from only one or a small number of sources, and there is no easily accessible market price for reference. The prices are usually overstated, in order to justify higher final prices, to increase hard currency remittances to the parent companies, and to minimize taxable profits. For example, a parliamentary inquiry in Brazil found transfer prices were five to ten times higher than arm's length prices; in Mexico, one company was found to be exporting progesterone at $110/kilo while another was importing it at $2490 (UNCTAD, 1977); a survey in Argentina found multinational transfer prices to their subsidiaries were anything from one and one-half to an extreme of thirty-seven times higher than independent imports of the same products (WHO, 1985).

Most developing countries now use centralized bulk purchasing by competitive international tender for their large public sector orders. Sri Lanka demonstrated what could be achieved by such measures as early as 1972 when it established the State Pharmaceuticals Corporation (SPC) to procure drugs for the whole country, instead of relying on the private sector. In the second half of 1972 the SPC took over the importation of fifty-two well established drugs. Buying generics in bulk by international tender, the SPC attracted more offers at far more competitive prices. Though it never chose the lowest tender because the companies concerned could not provide adequate quality assurance, it nevertheless paid 40 percent less overall than the private sector procurers had paid for the same fifty-two drugs in the first half of 1972. Examples of the price savings obtained for different drugs are shown in Table 14.2.

In 1973, the SPC took over the importation of intermediates for the private drug companies in Sri Lanka. The prices of these competitive imports ranged from 85 percent to only 6 percent of the transfer prices originally paid to parent companies (Table 14.3). As can be seen from the examples of Hoechst and Beecham, multinationals were persuaded to reduce their prices significantly below their original transfer prices.

The drug industry and the medical profession put up a determined resistance to the SPC. They argued that the SPC represented an unwar-

Table 14.2
Price Savings on Commonly Used Finished Drugs Achieved by the SPC in Sri Lanka, 1972

Drug	Number of Suppliers Used by Private Sector Procurers	Number of Tenders Submitted to the SPC	Private Sector Procurement ($)	SPC ($)	SPC Price as a % of Private Sector Price	SPC Supplier
			Average Price Paid			
Tetracyline	23	44	16.92	6.33	37	Polfa (Poland)
Penicillin	1	8	11.52	5.01	43	Biochomie (Austria)
Ampicillin	1	16	8.30	2.47	30	Beecham (UK)
Arthromycin	3	16	13.90	3.75	27	Upjohn (U.S.)
Chlorpromazine	2	10	3.70	0.52	14	Tablets (India)

ranted restriction on the freedom of choice, that it discouraged foreign investment in Sri Lanka's drug sector, and that SPC's imports were of sub-standard quality. However, little hard evidence was produced, and recalls of multinational company products received markedly less publicity than those of SPC's other suppliers. Relations with the five multinational subsidiaries were worsened still further by their prolonged reluctance to use their spare capacity to produce the country's total requirements of thirty-four widely used drugs, as requested by the government, and their refusal to buy SPCs imports of intermediates. When the Jaywardene government came to power in 1977 it gave way to the pressures against the SPC, and in 1978 the situation reverted more or less to what it had been in 1972, with companies once more allowed to import their own products directly (Centre on Transnational Corporations, 1983; Lall and Bibile, 1977; UNCTAD, 1977).

The main problems of state or parastatal drug procurement agencies are inadequate professional staffing, inadequate management systems, limited information on sources and prices, inadequate and irregular funding and access to foreign exchange, and, in many countries, a bureaucratic rather than a service orientation. The excellent service offered by the UNICEF Procurement and Assembly Centre (UNIPAC) has made an important contribution to the success of the public sector in obtaining the lowest possible prices for essential drugs of guaranteed quality, but the need to pay in advance in foreign exchange has prevented many developing countries from using the service, and they continue to use higher priced suppliers who offer more flexible conditions. Such problems, together with resistance from vested interests, explain to a large extent why few countries have attempted to emulate

Table 14.3
Price Savings on Intermediate Products Achieved by the SPC in Sri Lanka, 1973

Intermediate	Supplier Private Sector 1972	SPC 1973	Private Sector Transfer Price/Unit ($)	SPC Purchase Price/ Unit ($)	SPC Price as a % of Transfer Price
Tolbutamide	Hoechst (W. Germany)	Hoechst (W. Germany)	40.62	19.24	47
		Polfa (Poland)	40.62	2.52	6
Paracetamol	Sterling (UK)	Rhone Poulenc (F)	3.24	2.76	85
Chloropropamide	Pfizer (U.S.)	Plivs (Yugos.)	126.21	9.46	8
Aspirin	Glaxo (UK)	Polfa (Poland)	1.16	0.99	85
Ampicillin	Beecham (Singapore)	Beecham (Singapore)	569.90	95.11	17

Sri Lanka and extend their public sector purchasing arrangements to the private sector.

On the specific issue of quality assurance and control, WHO provides assistance in three important areas. First, the third revision of its International Pharmacopoeia now in publication is adapted to the need of developing countries, and includes authoritative standards for essential drugs, including methods of testing and analysis, adapted for simple control laboratories. Second, WHO's Good Manufacturing Practices (GMP) provide detailed recommendations for procedures and quality controls to be observed during manufacture. Third, the WHO Certification Scheme on the Quality of Pharmaceutical Products Moving in International Commerce, offers a guarantee by the regulatory authority of the exporting country that the drug concerned has been produced in accordance with GMP. It must be emphasized, however, the WHO has no direct involvement in the inspection process, so the value of this certificate is only as good as the regulatory procedures of each country, and of course it applies only to manufacturing and takes no account of problems which may subsequently occur in transit or storage.

Conclusions and Policy Implications

Most countries would benefit substantially from improved training and a higher caliber of personnel for their drug management systems.

Many countries are still using haphazard and inefficient management systems to run their central medical stores. A concerted program by the international agencies concerned, notably WHO, UNICEF and the development banks, to draw up a turnkey management system would be a powerful tool to improve the situation.

The information systems of developing countries concerning the sources and prices of good quality drugs are often very poor. WHO provides some services in this area, but they are relatively little known. Here again a small investment at the international level could have a significant impact on improving market transparency, and hence in reducing differentials.

Standard specifications for establishing a small first stage quality control laboratory are already available from WHO (1985). Such a facility is relatively easy to set up, say in a large hospital where basic facilities already exist. A systematic program, using foreign aid, to ensure that each country had at least a first stage quality control capacity would not be particularly difficult or expensive. Coordination and operational advice by WHO and its collaborating centers would help to create an integrated network with uniform standards. More sophisticated reference laboratories, while feasible in larger countries, are beyond the means of smaller ones. However, this problem could be solved by additional support to the more sophisticated laboratories already in existence in each region to enable them to perform a referral function for affiliated countries. Limited arrangements of this kind already exist, e.g., among the members of the West African Pharmaceutical Federation, Gambia, Liberia, and Sierra Leone, which have no national quality control laboratories, use those of Ghana and Nigeria. Another arrangement might be twinning of developed and developing countries, with the former making their testing facilities available.

Distribution

The first requirement in effective distribution is adequate drug storage, for most drugs are fragile in one sense or another: some, such as vaccines, are highly sensitive to heat and must be kept cool to retain their effectiveness; others, particularly powder forms, must be protected from dampness; sterile products must be kept sealed; and physically fragile items like some pills and liquid forms in ampoules and bottles must be protected from physical breakage or crushing. Many of the physical storage facilities in developing countries are severely inadequate for the proper storage of drugs, so that disturbingly high proportions of the already inadequate supplies are damaged or rendered ineffective.

The second physical requirement for good distribution is adequate transport. Here, the same foreign exchange problems which have adversely affected drugs have also affected transport capacity, for although vehicles are commonly provided by aid donors, spare parts and fuel require recurrent funding in scarce foreign exchange. For example, a recent survey in one central African country found three-fifths of the Ministry of Health's vehicle fleet out of service and another fifth in poor condition. Vehicles and fuel were so scarce that travel authorizations had to be approved by the chief transport officer, the chief accountant, and the permanent secretary or the chief medical officer.

At the management level, stock control procedures are often primitive. For example, too many stores are still so ill-organized that they have no running records of stock movements, and so have difficulty both initiating orders, when stocks reach their replacement order level, and ensuring that stock moves on a first-in-first-out (FIFO) basis. As a result, stock-outs and expirations are alarmingly common. Security is also a frequent problem, leading in the worse cases to very high percentages of pilferage.

In addition to these physical and management problems there is the problem of distribution outlets, and the range of drugs available at different kinds of outlets. Modern ethical drugs are potent and therefore potentially dangerous if incorrectly used. Some countries, like Bangladesh cited above, have responded by limiting the private sale of such products to outlets supervised by pharmacists. Such a decision not only applies stricter standards to the private sector than to the public sector, but severely limits the accessibility of such drugs. In practice, such a restriction is unenforceable. At the other extreme are countries where sale of a wide range of modern drugs is tolerated (even if legally prohibited) from general outlets with no qualified personnel, and without prescription. Neither situation is satisfactory.

Conclusions and Policy Implications

The physical storage of drugs could be considerably improved if donors funding aid to the health sector were more aware of the crucial importance of proper physical facilities. Standard designs, including both building and storage equipment, such as sloping back-loaded shelves (to make the FIFO rule physically easy to observe) would also help.

Drug storage managers need not only better training but a complete standard system which they can be trained to apply. WHO, UNICEF and perhaps the drug industry could easily prepare such a system.

Drug kits help to prevent damage and theft and also make supply management much easier in the public sector.

Adequate specialized transport is essential for many health service functions, but transporting public sector drugs need not always be undertaken by health service vehicles. Private transport companies may often be able to deliver drugs as or more reliably at competitive prices. Such a solution is even easier if the kit system is used, for the drugs are well packed and better protected from damage and pilferage.

Better access to generic drugs in urban areas could be obtained by obliging private pharmacies to carry a minimum range of generics and to display them prominently.

Better access to drugs in rural areas is being attempted in some countries by the establishment of community pharmacies. These are provided with an initial stock of drugs, and then restock using the proceeds from sales. Similar arrangements could be achieved by allowing public health services to sell certain drugs.

Concerning the qualifications required of dispensing staff, the consistent solution would simply be to require the same level of training in private outlets as in public ones, or to train a specific cadre of dispensing auxiliaries, or both.

Use

The success of the whole drug supply system is ultimately only as good as the standard of prescribing, dispensing and patient use of the drugs made available.

Some countries have used their EDL, and WHO's information sheets on essential drugs, as the basis for a national drug formulary. The information sheets summarize the pharmacological and therapeutic information needed by health professionals on the appropriate uses of each drug. Nevertheless, inadequate and inappropriate prescribing are a widespread and serious problem in many developing countries.

Problems include:

1. Prescription of inappropriate drugs, e.g., chloroquine for respiratory infections, antibiotics for many conditions for which they are not indicated.

2. Prescription of unnecessarily potent drugs and needlessly expensive dosage forms, e.g., use of broad spectrum antibiotics where penicillin would do and of injectables and drinkable ampoules rather than simple tablet and syrup forms.

3. Failure to allow for different dosage strengths—resulting in subclinical or dangerous doses.

4. Prescription of inadequate quantities for an effective course of treatment, e.g., 2–3 day curative courses of antibiotics, which may

in some cases lead to superinfections. This behavior is often but not always dictated by drug shortages and the desire to stretch the available supply as far as possible.

5. Polypharmacy, with multiple drugs per prescription, without due regard to contraindicated combinations, e.g., use of drugs which counteract or alter one another's actions in undesirable ways.

6. Failure to give patients clear instructions on how to take the drugs prescribed and to ensure that instructions are understood. These problems are compounded by inadequate dispensing, often by unqualified personnel, e.g., dispensing of the wrong drug or the wrong strength; substitution of inappropriate alternatives when the prescribed item is not available, and failure to pass on instructions written on prescriptions.

Conclusions and Policy Implications

These problems could be substantially reduced by the introduction of standard treatment manuals, at least for non-medical prescribers. Such manuals could relatively easily be developed from the standard treatment schedules used for quantification purposes already referred to and they would be useable both for training and day-to-day reference.

In addition, more attention needs to be given to the training and supervision of dispensing staff. This need is present in both the public and the private sectors, but particularly the latter, where a large volume of dispensing is done by staff with little or no training, and who often advise patients on the choice of drugs for self-medication.

References

ABIFARMA (Brazilian Association of the Pharmaceutical Industry). "Profile de industria farmaceitica brasiliera," ABIFARMA, 1979, quoted in United Nations Center on Transnational Corporations, *Transnational Corporations in the Pharmaceutical Industry of Developing Countries.* New York: UNCTC, 1983.

Agarawal, A. *Drugs in the Third World.* London: Earthscan, Publication no. 10, 1978.

Avramovic, M. *Cost of Drugs in Developing Countries: Some Determinants and Possibilities for Reduction.* The Hague: Institute of Social Studies, mimeo, 1985.

Bakke, O. M. "Drug Selection in a Regulated Society: The Norwegian Experience," *Hospital Formul* 19 (1984): 411–421.

Chudnovsky, D. "The Challenge of Domestic Enterprises to the Pharmaceutical Corporation's Domination: A Case Study of the Argentine Pharmaceutical Industry," *World Development* 7 (1979).

Cline, W. R. *International Debt and the Stability of the World Economy*. Washington: Institute for International Economics, 1983.

DANIDA and SIDA (Danish and Swedish International Development Agencies). *Quality Control of Drugs in Bangladesh*, 1983, quoted in J. C. Jayasuriya, *The Public Health and Economic Dimensions of the New Drug Policy of Bangladesh*. Washington: Pharmaceutical Manufacturers Association, 1985.

Dunlop, D. W., and M. Over. *Foreign Exchange Constraints in Financing Health Care in Poor Countries: The Evidence and Policy Alternatives*. Paper presented at the Joint UK and Nordic Health Economics Study Group, Vadstene, Sweden, July 3–5, 1985.

Funkel et al., "Tecnologia e competico na industria farmaceutica brasileira," FINEP, 1978, cited in United Nations Center on Transnational Corporations, *Transnational Corporations in the Pharmaceutical Industry of Developing Countries*. New York, NY: UNCTC, 1983.

Griffiths, A., et al. *Quantification of Essential Drug Requirements: A Draft Practical Manual*. Geneva: WHO, Action Programme on Essential Drugs, 1985.

Health Action International. *International Code of Pharmaceutical Marketing Practices*. Penang, Malaysia, 1982.

Hogerzeil, H. V. "Standardised Supply of Essential Drugs in Ghana." MD thesis, University of Numegen, 1985.

Hugon, P. "Les origines de la dette du Tiers Monde," *Revue francaise des finances publiques* 12 (1985): 5–25.

Institut de l'Entreprise. *Pour un vrai partenariat industriel avec l'Afrique. Bilan et perspectives de l'industrie Africaine*. Paris: Cen Nord/Sud, 1985.

International Market Survey. *Drug Marketing Manual*.

International Monetary Fund. *Recent Economic Developments in IMF*. Washington: IMF, 1984.

International Monetary Fund. *World Economic Outlook*. Washington: IMF, 1985.

Jayasuriya, D., A. Griffiths, and R. Rigoni. *Judgement Reserved: Breast Feeding, Bottle Feeding, and the International Code*. Sri Lanka: Asian Pathfinders, 1984.

Jayasuriya, J. C. *The Public Health and Economic Dimensions of the New Drug Policy of Bangladesh*. Washington: Pharmaceutical Manufacturers Association, 1985.

Krieger, M., and N. Brieto. "Comercio exterior, sustitution de importacionnes y tecnologia en la industria farmaceutica argentina," *Desarollo Económico* 17:66 (1977).

Ledogar, R. *Hungry for Profits: US Food and Drug Multinationals in Latin America*. New York: IDOC/North America Inc., 1975.

Lall, S., and S. Bibile. "The Political Economy of Controlling Transnationals: The Pharmaceutical Industry in Sri Lanka 1972–76," *World Development* 5:8 (1977).

Mahler, H. Address to the IFPMA meeting, Washington, D.C., June 8, 1982.

Management Sciences for Health. *Managing Drug Supply*. Boston: MSH, 1982.

Marvell, G. D. "Pharmaceutical Marketing," in C. M. Lindsay, ed., *The Pharmaceutical Industry: Economics, Performance, and Government Regulation*. New York: J. Wiley, 1985.

Pharmaceutical Manufacturers Association. *The Pharmaceutical Industry: International Issues and Answers.* Washington: PMA, 1979.

Organization for Economic Cooperation and Development. *Trade in High Technology Products.* Paris: OECD, Directorate for Science Technology and Industry, 1984.

Rigoni, R., A. Griffiths, and W. Laing. *Pharmaceutical Multinationals, Polemics, Perceptions, and Paradoxes.* Institute for Research and Information on Multinationals, Multinational Reports. New York: Wiley, 1985.

SCRIP. "Criticisms of the IFPMA Code by the Swedish Pharmaceutical Manufacturers Association and Proposals to Revise it Along the Lines of the Swedish and British Codes," *SCRIP* 650, 652 (December 9 and 16, 1981).

Togo, General Budget, various years.

United Nations, Centre on Transnational Corporations. *Transnational Corporations in the Pharmaceutical Industry of Developing Countries.* New York, NY: UNCTC, 1983.

United Nations Children's Fund (UNICEF). *Within Human Reach.* New York, NY: UNICEF, 1985.

United Nations Conference for Trade and Development. *Case Studies in the Transfer of Technology: Pharmaceutical Policies in Sri Lanka.* Geneva: UNCTAD, 1977.

World Bank. *World Development Report 1984.* Washington: World Bank, 1985.

World Health Organization. Drug Action Programme. Unpublished internal data, 1985.

World Health Organization. *Joint WHO/UNICEF Meeting on Infant and Young Child Feeding.* Geneva: WHO, 1979.

———. "Report of the WHO Expert Committee on Specifications for Pharmaceutical Preparations," *Technical Report Series 740.* Geneva: WHO, 1985.

———. "The Selection of Essential Drugs," *Technical Report Series 615.* Geneva: WHO, 1977.

———. "The Selection of Essential Drugs," *Technical Report Series 641.* Geneva: WHO, 1979.

———. "The Use of Essential Drugs," *Technical Report Series 685.* Geneva: WHO, 1983.

———. "The Use of Essential Drugs," *Technical Report Series 722.* Geneva: WHO, 1985.

Zambia, Recurrent and capital estimates, various years.

15

Selecting Medical Technologies in Developing Countries

Seymour Perry and Flora Chu

The last several decades have been witness to remarkable technological innovations in medicine encompassing drugs, devices, and procedures. In large part as a result of these advances, there has been a dramatic increase in the ability of health care providers to prevent, diagnose and treat a wide variety of medical conditions and diseases. However, these advances have also been associated with serious scientific, economic, legal and ethical questions. Among the most prominent and disturbing has been the unprecedented and extraordinary increase in health care costs. International economic difficulties, high debt loads and continued population growth have placed added pressures on the economic well-being of developing countries—with important implications for the advancement of human health and welfare. Thus, it has become critical for these countries to exercise the utmost care and wisdom in selecting appropriate medical technologies consistent with their resources and their most important needs. The key question is: How can health care technologies be developed (or modified), selected, and rationally allocated to improve quality of care and to enhance access in developing countries?

A comprehensive strategy for matching technologies more closely to the health needs of the populations of developing countries has yet to be realized. This paper will present examples of good and poor choices of technologies and will describe methodologies and criteria to help select appropriate technologies. The paper will also discuss some programs to aid in appropriate technology transfer from the Western industrialized nations and will suggest policy measures to promote the development and selection of technologies.

Background

When selecting a technology or planning a health policy to be used in a developing country one has to consider more than the country's budgetary constraints and limited foreign exchange reserves. Local circumstances and the setting in which a technology will be used are critical elements which must be taken into account. These local considerations include the availability of energy sources, sanitation, adequacy of trained personnel, limitations in transportation and distribution systems, problems associated with tropical climates, cultural factors, and restricted community resources.

Developing countries are also confronted with health problems of widely divergent etiologies which require differing approaches and technologies for their management. In contrast to the industrialized countries, populations of developing nations where malnutrition, poverty, and poor sanitation are common are exposed to far higher risk of acute infectious disease. In this situation, simple measures and technologies which can be widely applied would be appropriate. On the other hand, the chronic diseases which affect the developed nations are appearing with increasing frequency among those segments of the developing nations which have enhanced their economic status and increased their life span. Accordingly, the need for appropriate medical care for these chronic diseases often coexists with the need to improve health care for those affected with infectious diseases, malnutrition, etc.

Few developing countries have the information and ability to make critical selections from the vast range of possible technologies on the basis of efficacy, cost and feasibility. If policymakers do not consciously consider these factors and the constraints at the operating level, a technology may not fulfill its potential for improving health. Some technology "misfits" appear to result from a lack of understanding of the needs and social conditions of the purchaser, as well as from a deficient or absent transfer of skills and knowledge from developed nations. In other cases, duplication of services or extravagant purchases may result from an ad hoc or fragmented approach to health care technology. In addition, a small, affluent class within a Third World country may influence that country to select certain new and expensive technologies. On the other hand, a donor country or organization may install a technology which is neither relevant to prevailing health problems in the lesser developed countries nor economically feasible for continuing operation.

Most of the recent advances in medical technology have been designed and implemented for use in the industrialized world. Since the developing countries have less financial and political leverage than the developed countries, they do not exert enough market demand to motivate industry to produce technologies more relevant and appropriate to their needs. However, it can readily be appreciated that the potential market for new or adapted technologies in the developing countries is enormous and should warrant exploration and serious consideration by manufacturers.

"Poor Fit" Technologies

The following examples illustrate initially poor choices of technology transfer from the developed world, misapplication of technologies, and difficulty in maintaining their utility. In Cali, Colombia, an advanced neonatal care unit was established, based on model units in the United States (Maxwell, 1985). But after successful inpatient care, 70 percent of premature babies had died within three months of discharge because such elemental factors as nutrition and hydration were inadequately maintained. Strictly speaking, the technology itself worked well, but as is often the case in the developing world, there was insufficient attention to the "setting" for the technology—in this instance, the follow-up.

In Zaire, it has been reported that the treatment failure rate for tuberculosis in a regional hospital in the capital was 50 percent despite the presence of an expensive, $40,000 high quality radiology unit and a supply of drugs effective for multiple resistant organisms (Anderson, 1984). It was observed that patients traveling to the hospital distant from their villages could not earn enough to support and feed themselves and suffered from malnutrition. On the other hand, while undergoing treatment at the rural hospital they could continue working (see below).

Another example involves the transfer of technology to three neonatal intensive care units in Egypt (U.S. Congress, 1984). These units all experienced problems using acquired medical equipment due to poor initial specification of equipment, absence of technical advice and support, lack of service manuals and spare parts, faulty initial installation, and inadequate training of personnel.

Indeed, a frequent problem after the selection of a technology is in maintaining the equipment; this can seriously affect costs and availability of the services. At a conference of Latin American countries in 1983, it was reported that less than 3 percent of the hospitals in one major country had technicians trained to repair medical devices (Pan-American

Health Organization, 1983). At any given time, it has been estimated that 20 to 60 percent of all existing medical equipment in the Middle East may not be functioning (U.S. Congress, 1984). Another survey in African countries revealed that two-thirds of high output X-ray machines were inoperable because of the lack of servicing (Middlemiss, 1984). This situation reflected inadequate planning and budgeting for repair and maintenance services, which range from 10 to 20 percent of the initial capital costs of the equipment (U.S. Congress, 1984); inadequate procurement and delivery of parts and supplies; the absence of service in outlying areas; shortage of trained repair specialists; and the lack of service commitments by manufacturers not represented in the area.

Another example of a poor fit technology is growth monitoring in children, a measure intended to detect early signs of malnutrition. The simple measuring and charting of weights suffered from problems which precluded effective application of this technique (*The Lancet*, 1985). Weighing scales were not standardized in many areas, and primary health care workers sometimes had no understanding of the dynamics of growth and did not provide adequate follow-up and referral. Some mothers also appeared to be minimally interested, probably because of insufficient education about the relation between weight and health.

Policymakers sometimes overlook the most basic aspects of packaging and distribution of medication. Sometimes tablets are dispensed into a screw of paper instead of an airtight container, and sterile eye drops or lotions are placed in cans or other used containers (D'Arcy, 1984). These medications may then lose their potency or become contaminated. Another problem may occur in the transport and storage of vaccines, which need to be maintained at about freezing temperatures from the moment they leave the manufacturer to the time of actual immunization. The effectiveness of vaccines in developing countries is likely to depend upon the chain of distribution to delivery in patient care (Elliott, 1984).

A technology may be appropriate but there may be a cultural barrier preventing its use. When elaborate fiberglass chairs were installed in a mother and child center in rural Iran some years ago, the mothers assumed the chairs were there for decorative purposes, refused to use them, and instead sat on the floor with their children according to custom. Obviously, the decision to install these chairs was made by someone who did not know enough about local customs (U.S. Congress, 1984).

"Good Fit" Technologies

A good fit technology is one backed up by innovation and careful planning so that it meets local health care needs in a socially and economically acceptable fashion. For instance, for vaccine distribution and storage, a heat sensitive safety marker has been devised by the Program for Appropriate Technology in Health (PATH) to monitor the time and temperature exposure of the vaccine vials (Elliott, 1984). When the indicator turns black, the vaccine is no longer effective for use. Ongoing research efforts are aimed at developing methods to produce less fragile vaccines. The same group is also developing a reusable sterilization marker to check the adequacy of sterilization by boiling. Another innovation is the development of a solar powered refrigerator for storing vaccines and blood/plasma concentrates (Elliott, 1984).

In developing countries, it may be more cost effective to purchase multiple-use medical devices which can be simply reprocessed for reuse. For example, a disposable endotracheal tube may be safely reused if properly cleaned, sterilized and rinsed (Prior, 1984). If recognized standards for pressure-steam sterilizers are met, a simple autoclave may be adequate for use and may serve to ensure the safety of reused devices (Simpson, 1984).

Orthopedic appliances can be produced with local labor and resources using simple, standardized designs and durable raw materials (De Ruyter, 1984). Examples include crutches, walking aids, sandals made with used car tires as soles, and shoe supports. A wheelchair has been developed to be sturdy, maneuverable and sufficiently lightweight to be appropriate for rough and variable terrain in developing countries (Appropriate Technology International, 1984). It is of simple construction and can be produced in most developing countries with available resources at one-eighth to one-fourth the cost of imported wheelchairs.

In contrast to Zaire's capital's relatively expensive, unsuccessful tuberculosis program, a physician in the same country had better results with a simple radiology unit costing only $7000 and cheaper, second-line drugs. He had stopped referring patients to the distant center when he learned they were dying of malnutrition because they had spent all their money on expensive X-rays and medication. The physician attributed his success to his emphasis on better history taking, physical examination, and better nutritional management of patients (Anderson, 1984).

Another example of a good fit technology involved a controlled trial to determine appropriate delivery of care and subsequent planning and implementation to produce efficient and effective use of existing resources. This program was called the "Simplified Surgery System" and was established in Colombia to improve the delivery of surgical services (Velez Gil et al., 1983). First, policymakers conducted a trial of selected surgical procedures to compare their safety and effectiveness when performed on an ambulatory basis with that when performed on an inpatient basis. Then they assessed all the operations performed in a total study population of 2.5 million. The results indicated that 75 percent of the surgical interventions did not require hospitalization and that ambulatory surgery would save 100,000 hospital days. Subsequently the government instituted a nationwide program of ambulatory surgery and established several simplified surgical units (Yankauer, 1983).

In some cases, health problems may be solved by the most simple approach. In many developing countries the ambient temperature is warm enough so that neonatal units do not need incubators. In addition, an infant affected with neonatal jaundice will most likely receive as effective phototherapy if placed near a window and exposed to sunlight as he would if placed under fluorescent lighting (Ebrahim, 1984).

An example of a successful transfer of technology was the establishment of the Diagnostic Ultrasound Center in Cairo, Egypt (U.S. Congress, 1984). Although diagnostic ultrasound is relatively complicated, careful planning and rational management have led to its successful operation and diffusion to other centers. Contributing to the successful technology transfer were:

1. thorough training of medical, operating and maintenance personnel
2. planning for equipment specification and procurement
3. adequate budgetary allocations
4. routine progress evaluations and the convening of educational and coordinating meetings
5. cooperation between the sponsor and provider of the equipment and center staff

A promising device in terms of cost savings and convenience is the lixiscope, a lightweight, portable, real-time X-ray imaging device. The United States space program developed it in 1978 to make photographic images involving minute amounts of radiation. It is battery powered and has less radiation per minute than conventional sources. Since the radiation source for imaging is iodine 125, the device could be extremely useful in outlying areas and at accident sites where there is little or no access to conventional X-ray equipment or power sources (National Center for Health Services Research and Health Care Technology Assessment, 1985). Unfortunately, at present less than 100 units have been exported to developing countries, in part because State Department approval is required and it cannot be sold to "unfriendly" or communist countries.

Definition of Appropriate Technology

Drawing from these examples of good and poor fit technology choices, a definition of an appropriate technology may be evolved. A technology represents a package of knowledge and capability which not only is embodied in the device or equipment or technique itself, but also encompasses the original intention and design, the skills and resources required for installation and operation, and the ability to oversee and organize the health service system in which it is implemented. In short, the key to an appropriate technology is the people who design it, maintain it skillfully, and use it knowledgeably.

It is obvious that a technology cannot merely be introduced and expected to fit the needs of the people without a good deal of thought and careful initiative in arranging the environment in which it is to be applied. An imported technology will not be successfully applied unless the developing country has gained the mastery, knowledge and resources necessary to operate and use it. Any evaluation of a candidate technology must realistically appraise not only the technology's potential for improving health but also the capability of local individuals to use it wisely and effectively. Any barriers to its use must also be identified, be they cultural, economic, political, etc.

Another critical consideration is education. Although the subject of this paper deals with the wise selection of medical technology during times of economic difficulties, it should be emphasized that this cannot be accomplished in isolation. Although there are other impediments, selection and use of appropriate technology can succeed only in a setting where education—particularly maternal education—is a critical element. In this regard, the existence of specially trained parahealth professionals can play a special role.

As already suggested, the transfer or the introduction of many medical technologies into developing countries has often failed because even a minimal educational basis was lacking—or at the very least, the necessary education, training and understanding of the benefit to be gained from the specific technology had not been acquired.

Certainly there are other impediments to the introduction of medical technology, e.g., political, resource allocation and organization of health care services. These are all interdependent, but in our view, education is the single most critical element.

An important current barrier is that international financial problems, particularly ever-increasing debt burdens, limit the capability of many developing countries to provide for significant capital investments and restrict the liquidity of their foreign exchange reserves. Because of this, research and development and imports of new technologies have been scaled back. In addition, local political climates may influence the allotment of funds for acquiring new medical technologies. Some of the lesser developed countries place important emphasis on health care, but others have different priorities. One country may want to take major strides in technological acquisition and purchase high technology from developed countries, whereas others may wish to depend more on indigenous sources for the manufacture of equipment (Pan American Health Organization, 1983). In addition, available resources, including energy sources, transportation and distribution systems, and local climatic conditions (as in the tropics) may limit the types of equipment which can be acquired because of the unusual durability standards or design required.

Lastly, a technology is only appropriate if it can be incorporated within the infrastructure of the nation's health care system. It also must be linked with existing scientific and technological institutions. The technical capability and sophistication of these institutions will influence the process of selecting appropriate technologies, their operation, and ultimately their success in meeting defined health objectives.

Each technology considered for selection should be carefully evaluated and should meet certain criteria for fitness through a formal and systematic assessment. A technology should be assessed in these areas: safety and effectiveness; efficiency; cost and cost effectiveness; social and cultural fit; accommodation to the infrastructure of political, technical, and scientific institutions; and meeting the needs and capabilities of the local health care delivery system. There may be additional criteria depending upon the individual country or region or some may be emphasized over others according to local needs, values, customs, or resources.

To warrant further consideration, a technology must have been proven safe and effective and of demonstrated clinical value to fulfill an identified health need of the people. The technology should also benefit a significant number of people. Accordingly, not only should it be carefully selected for the diagnosis or treatment of a specific disease or condition, but it should also be situated so as to allow for access by a reasonable number of people. Regionalization of costly and specialized technologies in general fosters more efficient use of local skills and scarce resources.

The technology must be selected for its efficiency in performance. Thus, from a choice of alternative technologies with the same diagnostic or therapeutic potential, the selected technology should be able to discharge its function efficiently without an inordinate drain on resources. It is also essential that the technology be economically feasible from an operational standpoint. Both the initial costs as well as the recurring repair and maintenance costs must be considered in budgeting for the new technology. A selection should be made only after considering the costs and medical efficacy of available competing interventions, since exercising the most inexpensive option may be a false economy.

The following two case studies are provided to exemplify some of the points made above and to illustrate the application of research and planning efforts in developing countries in order to help resolve their health care delivery problems.

Case Study: The Basic Radiological System

In the development of the Basic Radiological System (BRS), the application of technological and health planning expertise was used to promote greater access to diagnostic radiological services, especially in outlying areas.

It is estimated that 70 percent of the world's population has no access to any radiological services (Palmer, 1984). There are some countries without even one specialist in diagnostic radiology. The World Health Organization (WHO) has estimated that an average of 50,000 to 500,000 people (depending on the country) are served by one diagnostic X-ray machine in developing countries and that 2.6 billion people have little or no access to radiodiagnostic services (Lehtinen et al., 1983). For comparison, some of the countries in Western Europe have one machine for every two thousand or fewer individuals. Such services in developing countries, when they do exist, are usually located in large hospitals and large cities—relatively inaccessible to many in rural areas. The explanation for this situation lies in the equipment's cost and sophistication and the requirement for trained technicians and highly trained radiologists.

The medical need for diagnostic radiological services is as essential in developing countries as in developed countries. The relevant indications range from tuberculosis and pneumonia to traumatic fractures, gastrointestinal diseases, and bone/joint lesions. WHO has estimated that the provision of simple X-ray services without fluoroscopy at the local hospital level would fulfill 90 percent of the radiological needs of developing countries (WHO, 1984). The advantages of investing in X-ray installations in local hospitals include more rapid diagnosis, better monitoring of treatment, shorter hospitalizations, and fewer referrals to the larger and more specialized hospitals. Overloading tertiary care hospitals with referrals from local hospitals for more routine diagnostic studies constitutes an inefficient use of expensive and scarce resources.

WHO has suggested three levels of diagnostic services to help resolve the deficiency in appropriate imaging technology: the basic radiologic system (BRS), the general purpose radiological service (GPRS) or the middle level, and the specialized radiological services (SRS), or the top level. The GPRS could act as a referral center for more complex diagnostic cases and the SRS could act as the tertiary care center with the most up-to-date and specialized technology. For example, if a developing country acquired sophisticated technologies such as digital imaging, magnetic resonance imaging (MRI) devices, or even the relatively common CT scanners, it is doubtful that they would be available anywhere other than at highly specialized centers.

The BRS concept consists of two major components: (1) appropriate equipment, and (2) appropriate training for both the operator and the physician interpreting the results. In some cases the X-ray machine can be operated with batteries which are rechargeable by solar energy, and it contains a fixed source-to-image distance in order to assure simpler and more precise operation by less qualified personnel. The construction of the machine makes it easy to identify failed parts for repair and protects the safety of technicians and patients by controlling X-ray exposure in accordance with international radiation exposure standards.

Manuals for operating the equipment and for interpreting the films have been developed. The BRS technician needs only a minimal intermediate school education and can be trained in several weeks to a few months. Also, since few radiologists will be working at the local hospital level, general practitioners will likely require assistance in interpreting the radiographs. Accordingly, regional training centers for radiologists are planned to provide educational opportunities consistent with the experience and needs of the developing world. BRS units have now been sent to several areas of the world and appear to be reliable and effective. Several manufacturers of X-ray equipment are producing BRS-specified X-ray units at a price (in 1984) of $25,000–$50,000 (Palmer, 1984).

Case Study: Oral Rehydration Therapy

Oral rehydration therapy (ORT) was developed through basic and clinical research. The result is a simple, effective, technologically appropriate treatment for the alleviation of a major public health problem. This is probably the most well known and certainly one of the most successful technologies in the Third World. Infant diarrhea, often due to infection with the organism cholera vibrio, is rampant in the Third World. In 1980 WHO estimated that at least 750 million to 1 billion episodes of diarrhea and 4.6 million deaths due to diarrhea occur each year in children less than five years of age in Africa, Latin America and Asia. By comparison, in the U.S. and Canada, the death rate in 1979 due to diarrhea in infants was about twenty-two deaths per 100,000; in Latin America, it was 915 per 100,000, more than 40 times as great (Office of Technology Assessment, 1985).

The treatment for dehydration due to diarrhea is the replacement of electrolytes and water. In the 1950s and 1960s, intravenous rehydration technology was transferred from developed countries for use in developing countries. But the treatment was costly, required specially trained personnel, was generally administered in hospitals, and required importation of sterile needles, fluids and tubing. In addition, if the needles and tubing were not sterilized properly upon reuse, there was the danger of spreading infection from one patient to another. Thus this approach to treatment was infeasible for a large portion of the population, and dehydration and death remained a major health problem.

The scientific rationale for the development of an oral rehydration solution was that physiological studies showed that glucose, a simple sugar, was still actively absorbed by the intestine even during an episode of diarrhea and could promote the concurrent absorption of sodium and water. In the 1960s and 1970s, clinical studies were begun in Asia which demonstrated that oral solutions could replace the fluid and electrolyte losses in cholera patients. Subsequent studies in many other areas of the world confirmed the effectiveness of this relatively simple treatment regardless of the etiological agent, generally replacing the deficit in fluids and electrolytes within twelve to eighteen hours.

Oral rehydration methods have been devised to allow simpler composition of solutions which can be formulated in local settings using locally available resources, tools, and ingredients such as sugar and salt. Additional advantages of these techniques over intravenous rehydration are that they are less expensive, they require no sterilization or specially trained personnel, they allow a shorter hospital stay, and they permit the mother or another family member to help administer treatment. Among the agencies involved in its dissemination are the Pan American Health Organization, the WHO, the U.S. Agency for International Development (AID), and the U.N. International Children's Emergency Fund (UNICEF). These agencies have provided technical assistance, developed treatment manuals, supported regional workshops and awarded research grants to clinical investigators to study various aspects of the problem.

Methodologies and Programs for Maximizing the Wise Selection of Technologies

At the National Level

Each developing country should develop a capacity for technology assessment and a coherent policy for the selection, monitoring and operation of health care technologies. An initial step could be to establish a clearing house to collect and analyze information about technologies and the results of their evaluation (see below). A small staff at an academic institution charged with reviewing the available literature would be a simple and useful beginning. A second but more sophisticated approach to aid in the decisionmaking process for the selection and acquisition of health care technologies lies in the use of medical information systems. For example, a prototype system for the allocation of technologies in perinatal care has been developed and presently is being tested in Brazil (Panerai and Attinger, 1986). The system encompasses major technologies used in perinatal care and describes them according to their characteristics and attributes in terms of health benefits, risks, interactions with other technologies, and impact upon community and socioeconomic structures. In this manner, different countries or localities can identify limiting factors (such as a shortage of trained manpower) or set criteria for the selection and use of technologies. The program ranks technologies according to their impact on the solution of a selected problem and assigns the appropriate technology to the regional level in which its effective utilization is feasible. This concept could also be used to match the characteristics of technologies with the health needs and circumstances of a community in areas other than medical information.

Developing countries could also take measures to improve the operation and maintenance of equipment. The standardization of products in a given facility or region would not only increase bargaining power in purchasing. It would also allow spare parts to be interchanged, allow personnel to move among related facilities or departments without requiring reorientation to each piece of equipment, and optimize the operational potential of the equipment. Preventive maintenance schedules, provisions for extra parts at the time of initial purchase of the equipment, and planning for the budgeting and procurement of spare parts are all useful strategies to lower the costs of maintenance and to enhance the efficiency of operation (Lawrance, 1984).

Developing countries are seeking to raise their standards of living and to expand their base for industrial production for future growth.

Thus, there is a strong desire to produce some of the technologies which are currently imported or not acquired because of high prices and to develop greater training and technical capability. Local innovation should be encouraged, and the assessment of existing resources for use in production of more relevant technologies can be promoted (Pan American Health Organization, 1983). Labor-intensive technologies of simple construction which use readily available raw materials would be feasible candidates for local production. In a developing country, the government could provide concessions on tax and import policies to support the establishment of these industries.

At the Regional Level

There are a number of activities that could be established regionally if countries in a given geographic region were willing to pool their resources and collaborate, particularly since they may have common needs and objectives. One such proposal several years ago envisioned the creation of a clearing house in Latin America for information on medical technologies and on the results of technology assessments (Perry, 1983).

Countries in a given region could also join to establish programs for the evaluation of candidate technologies. The sites for such programs could be determined by mutual agreement and would be based on local expertise, experience, and resources—but with all the participating countries contributing a proportion of the necessary funds. A similar program was instituted several years ago under WHO auspices in Europe.

Undoubtedly, there are other activities which could most profitably be regional in nature and such programs could supplement parallel programs at the national level.

At the International Level

While developing countries can do more at the national level or regionally, the cooperation, resources, expertise and experience of international agencies, organizations and industrialized nations are needed to apply technologies to manage the health problems of developing countries. Some of what is being proposed here has been addressed by WHO, but its efforts need to be intensified and supplemented, perhaps by other bodies.

The World Bank is currently sponsoring a broad program of studies and training on the scientific and technological aspects of development (Kamenetsky et al., 1985). This program provides for two activities: (1) a country-wide study of the scientific and technological infrastructure aimed at developing a plan for long-term development, and (2) a training program for policymakers to make them aware of the implications of choices among technologies and the effects of interrelated policies such as tariff barriers or procurement policies on incentives to develop or select technologies.

Many of the basic concepts and analyses embodied in this program may also be applicable in health care, and a similar program could be established for strengthening decision making and problem solving processes for health care delivery systems. Such a program could offer educational courses for policy makers and support studies of examples of appropriate technology transfer. It could incorporate the concept and perspectives of comprehensive assessments of technologies, including clinical safety, efficacy, costs, and cost-effectiveness.

An international institute or organization could be established within the WHO or it could be free-standing with support from private foundations which have already provided a great deal of assistance to developing countries for a variety of activities. The proposed agency would have responsibility for the program mentioned above and for acting as a clearing house to promote the transfer of information from industrialized countries to developing countries and the flow of information among developing countries. This dissemination could be in the form of handbooks or guides for the selection and use of common hospital and medical equipment, written material provided by manufacturers including training and maintenance manuals, and results of current technology assessments and health services research.

The proposed agency could also conduct surveys on request to assess important health needs and identify successful policies for managing medical technologies and provide such information to other similarly situated nations. A list of appropriate technologies or adaptations which have been effective could be drawn up and publicized, based on experiences in the field by health care personnel and policymakers. Medical professional societies in the developed countries could be encouraged to provide their expertise and experience to counterparts in developing countries, for the training of health care personnel and for the development of appropriate technologies, and to exchange their ideas on essential and effective technologies. A few such programs have been implemented in Latin America involving medical schools and institutions in the United States and Europe.

The repair and maintenance of equipment is often a weak link in the sequence of successful technology selection and application. Strategies to strengthen government commitment and planning for health care technical services and to train competent staff to determine selection criteria and technical specifications and manage the engineering tasks are needed. The WHO Program for Support to Countries in the Field of Repair and Maintenance of Hospital Equipment is considering regional workshops for training technicians, identification of priority needs for spare parts, involvement of technical colleges for translating and distributing manuals, and establishment of national inventory systems and specialist committees to select and procure equipment and parts (Malloupus, 1985).

It obviously would not be feasible in most instances to produce the more sophisticated medical technologies locally, given the complex mix of facilities and infrastructure, financial base, and training required. In addition, manufacturers may be disinclined to set up factories in these areas because of fear over newly generated competition, poor profit potential, required investment outlays, or the shortage of skilled and experienced workers. However, it is conceivable that multilateral assistance programs could be developed to enhance self-reliance and to support national or regional production enterprises in the area of medical technologies. The United Nations Industrial Development Organization (UNIDO) has identified the manufacture of drugs as an important priority for support in developing countries (D'Arcy, 1984). In other areas, the WHO, the World Bank and other international organizations have collaborated to help developing countries with industrial projects and it is possible that similar assistance could be provided for at least limited manufacture of appropriate medical technologies.

An important model for a strategic program aimed at directing international scientific and technical research efforts towards the public health problems of the developing countries is the UNDP/World Bank/ WHO Special Programme for Research and Training in Tropical Diseases (TDR) (Black, 1980; WHO, 1985). The two main objectives of this program are (1) to create and improve methods for the control of major tropical diseases, mobilizing academic, industrial and scientific institutions on a global basis, and (2) to strengthen the scientific research and development capacities of the developing countries (WHO, 1985). The proportion of funding given to the developing countries was 58 percent of the total in 1983–84, supporting training courses and research activities for various institutions and scientists in the tropical countries. The program has resulted in a number of promising and tangible products, including potential vaccines against malaria and leprosy, new antimalarial drugs and other drug agents, new diagnostic tests for Chagas' disease and schistosomiasis, and tests to measure the drug sensitivity of various parasites. This model could be extended to address additional health priorities of the developing countries.

The Role of Industry

Although there are difficulties such as cultural and language differences and the expense of establishing appropriate links, the potential of a combined market demand of the developing countries for appropriate technologies is enormous. An important step toward making this potential a reality would be to promote greater involvement of manufacturers in the process of innovation and development, training of personnel, service and maintenance of equipment, and marketing goods within user countries. Manufacturers should be urged to establish service and training programs for specific devices, provide service representatives on a permanent basis, and develop manuals and service diagrams in the native language. As mentioned previously, in many instances in which sophisticated technologies have been acquired in lesser developed countries, service and maintenance have not been adequately provided for.

Foreign producers, users and policymakers should cooperate in identifying the market demands, planning, production and procurement of appropriate technologies. International manufacturing organizations could provide expertise and training for the manufacture of medical devices analogous to the program of the International Federation of Pharmaceutical Manufacturers Association, which advises not only on distribution, procurement, and quality control but also on drug manufacture (D'Arcy, 1984). Trade fairs exhibiting various brands and models of major equipment, including simpler or older designs and demonstrations, could be held in various regions. In the negotiations over the purchase and installation of the equipment, contractual agreements could be included for training personnel, for providing spare parts and for routine maintenance and repair.

The Role of Industrialized Nations

Industrialized countries could provide financial incentives for research and development of medical technologies to address the priority health problems of the developing countries. For example, the Office of Technology Assessment (1985) has suggested some options for enhancing progress in tropical disease research: (1) include drugs and vaccines for control of tropical diseases under the Orphan Drug Act, awarding tax credits and exclusive marketing rights along with funding for clinical trials; (2) encourage federal agencies to assist interested manufacturers in clinical trials and guaranteeing purchase of products; and (3) create a quasi-public corporation to research and develop such technologies until they achieve sufficient commercial value.

In addition, the industrialized countries should reassess their export policies for medical technologies to identify areas where judicious selection may expedite or at least remove disincentives to the delivery of needed technologies. However, as mentioned previously, many developing countries share a lack of resources and mechanisms which could rigorously assess imported drugs and devices for safety and effectiveness. Thus, safeguards implemented at the level of the exporting countries may be needed. In the United States, drugs and devices already approved by the FDA are allowed to be exported, whereas nonapproved drugs have generally been barred from export. Manufacturers wishing to export nonapproved medical devices must submit statements of acceptance from the importing country to the FDA for authorization of export (FDA, 1983). Currently, legislation has been proposed to lift the ban on nonapproved drugs. The drug manufacturing industry, anxious to increase its competitive share of the market abroad, backs this legislation and claims that there would be more domestic jobs and that the drain of biotechnology expertise would be diminished (Sun, 1986).

One program to strengthen the maintenance of scientific equipment is a cooperative agreement between the Biomedical Engineering and Instrumentation Branch of the National Institutes of Health and the Egyptian Academy for Scientific Research and Technology (Metz et al., 1985). In this program, an Instrument Technology Unit (ITU) was developed as a national equipment maintenance center to provide specialized training, equipment repair services, technical literature, and spare parts. Technical assistance and guidance were also provided for centers at universities throughout Egypt. A number of engineers were trained at the ITU and then assigned to various centers in the country. Similar programs instituted in other countries or perhaps involving several countries simultaneously would seem highly desirable. Medical schools and other academic institutions in some countries already have cooperative assistance programs with their counterparts in the third world. Professional medical societies should also be encouraged to increase their activities in developing countries. For example, they could guide the selection of appropriate technologies and their application.

Conclusions

Developing countries face serious constraints and difficult economic adjustments in their ability to respond to pressing public health problems. Present circumstances impose even greater pressures for the development of rugged, relatively simple and cost-effective health care technologies and for their acquisition by these countries. In addition to limited capacities for local innovation and production of technologies, developing countries generally have made insufficient efforts to establish national policies and institutions which would define their objectives in health care, select appropriate medical technologies and assessment methods, and operate and maintain these technologies. In addition, these countries do not possess sufficient market power to attract innovators from other areas of the world. All these factors have contributed to the often inefficient or haphazard selection and purchase of technologies and to the difficulties in maintaining beneficial technologies in local environments.

In summary, there is a critical need for strong national and international technological planning and cooperative efforts in health care to assist developing countries. This requires a comprehensive understanding of the contribution of a given medical technology to a defined outcome—particularly to meeting local health needs and to working in the local social, economic and institutional context. Such an understanding is essential if technology is to promote health effectively in developing countries. Institutions in these countries need to be able to acquire information, and these countries need to be able to make appropriate decisions about technology based on criteria of safety, efficacy, costs and feasibility.

There is also an important need for clearing house functions in the developing world to collect, share and synthesize information about important relevant technologies and technology assessments. With the aid of decision making capability, informed choice, and international cooperation from public and private sources, developing countries can maximize technology selection consistent with discriminate use of scarce resources.

Various individuals and organizations have previously voiced many of these same recommendations for enhancing technology selection in developing countries (Evans et al., 1981; Hope, 1982; Banta, 1984; McCord, 1978). The World Health Organization's Global Strategy for Health for All by the Year 2000, emphasizes country-wide health programs and reforms in national health systems to help ensure that the objectives of these programs are achieved efficiently and that they are effective (Pan American Health Organization, 1981, p. 45). The plan of action to implement the regional strategies adopted by WHO in 1981 addresses the need for formal health technology policies in order to search systematically for the most appropriate technologies for priority health problems (Pan American Health Organization, 1980, p. 56).

The proposals and initiatives mentioned in this paper and identified elsewhere may be too idealistic for the current cynical global climate, but they appear to be feasible provided there is political and financial commitment by both the industrialized countries and the developing countries as well as the international political bodies which represent them. Most of the proposed activities are not particularly expensive, but such programs are essential in guiding the effective mobilization of technology for the promotion of health in these countries. The need is even greater in times of economic crises, else health care delivery and health status in the developing world will erode even further. The deterioration will continue unless there is the will and determination to change.

References

Anderson, S. H. Letter: "Appropriate Technology," *British Medical Journal* 288 (June 16, 1984): 1829–1830.

Appropriate Technology International. "Wheelchairs for the Third World." Washington, D.C., 1984.

Banta, D. "The Uses of Modern Technologies: Problems and Perspectives for Industrialized and Developing Countries," *Bulletin of the Pan-American Health Organization* 18:2 (1984): 139–150.

Black, D. A. K. "Technology in Clinical Medicine," *The Journal of Medical Engineering and Technology* 4:3 (May 1980): 119–121.

D'Arcy, P. D. "Appropriate Technology: Essential Medicines in the Third World," *British Medical Journal* 289 (October 13, 1984): 903–904.

De Ruyter, K., and O. Lelieveld. "Appropriate Technology: Orthopedic Aids at a Low Cost," *British Medical Journal* 289 (September 22, 1984): 749–751.

Ebrahim, G. J. "Appropriate Technology: Care of the Newborn," *British Medical Journal 289* (October 6, 1984): 899–902.

Elliott, K. "Appropriate Technology: Immunization, Rehydration and Transfusion," *British Medical Journal* 288 (May 5, 1984): 1364–1366.

Evans, J. R., K. L. Hall, and J. Warford. "Shattuck Lecture—Health Care in the Developing World: Problems of Scarcity and Choice," *The New England Journal of Medicine* 305:19 (November 5, 1981): 1117–1121.

HOPE. Conference Report: Appropriate Health Care Technology Transfer to Developing Countries. Millwood, Virginia: Project HOPE Center for Health Information, 1982.

Kamenetzky, M., R. Maybury, and C. Weiss. "A Program of Studies and Training on the Scientific and Technological Dimension of Development," *Bulletin of Science, Technology and Society* 4:2 (1982): 101–217. Washington, D.C.: U.S. Government Printing Office, September 1985.

The Lancet. Editorial: "Growth Monitoring: Intermediate Technology or Expensive Luxury?" *The Lancet* II (December 14, 1985): 1337–1338.

Lawrance, P. "Appropriate Technology: A Plain Man's Guide to Maintenance," *British Medical Journal* 288 (May 19, 1984): 1525–1526.

Lehtinen, E., N. T. Racoveanu, and G. N. Soukevitch. "Future of Radiation Medicine in Developing Areas." Presented at a WHO Conference, Bangkok, Thailand, November 17, 1983.

Malloupus, A. "Background Document—WHO Programme for Support to Countries in the Field of Repair and Maintenance of Hospital and Medical Equipment." WHO Document, High Technical Institute. Nicosia, Cyprus, 1985.

Maxell, R. J. "Resource Constraints and the Quality of Care," *The Lancet* II (October 26, 1985): 936–939.

McCord, C. "Medical Technology in Developing Countries: Useful, Useless, or Harmful?" *The American Journal of Clinical Nutrition* 31 (December 1978): 2301–2313.

Metz, H., E. El-Savha, and M. Shaltoot. "Report to the 16th JCC Instrument Technology Scientific Equipment Maintenance Project No. 263–0016." National Institute of Health Document, November, 1985.

Middlemiss, Sir Howard. "Radiology of the Future in Developing Countries." Presented at the Mayneord Symposium, London, England, February 19, 1982. *British Journal of Radiology* 57:681 (September 1984): 852–853.

National Center for Health Services Research and Health Care Technology Assessment. Portable Hand Held X-Ray Instrument (Lixiscope) Health Technology Assessment Reports, November 15, 1985.

Office of Technology Assessment, U.S. Congress. "Technology Transfers in Medical Services," in *Technology Transfer to the Middle East.* Washington, D.C.: Office of Technology Assessment, OTA ISC-173, September 1984.

———. *Status of Biomedical Research and Related Technology for Tropical Diseases.* Washington, D.C.: Office of Technology Assessment, OTA-H-258, September 1985.

Palmer, P. E. S. "Radiology in the Developing World. Proceedings of the British Institute of Radiology," *British Journal of Radiology* 57:681 (September 1984): 853–856.

Pan American Health Organization. "Global Strategy for Health for All by the Year 2000." WHO Official Document. Geneva, 1981.

———. Inter-American Conference on Health Technology Assessment, Report Brasilia, Brazil. November 1983.

Pan American Health Organization and World Health Organization. "Health for All by the Year 2000: Plan of Action for the Implementation of Regional Strategies." PAHO Official Document 179. Washington, D.C., 1980, p. 56.

Panerai, R. B., and E. O. Attinger. "Information System for Appropriate Allocation of Health Care Technologies." Communication with the author, January 9, 1986.

Perry, S. "Use of Technology Assessment in Policy Formulation." Presented at the Inter-American Conference on the Assessment of Technology in Health. Brasilia, Brazil, November 17, 1983.

Prior, F. N. "Appropriate Technology: Anaesthetics," *British Medical Journal* 288 (June 9, 1984): 1750–1755.

Simpson, R. "Appropriate Technology: Priorities For Hospital Cleaning, Disinfection, Sterilization and Control of Infection," *British Medical Journal* 288 (June 23, 1984): 1898–1900.

Sun, M. "Inviting the Dumping of Unsafe Drugs," *New York Times,* March 1, 1986, p. 24.

U.S. Department of Health and Human Services, Food and Drug Administration. "Import/Export Regulatory Requirements for Medical Devices." HHS Publication FDA 85-4160, (June 1985).

Velez Gil, A., M. T. Galarza, et al. "Surgeons and Operating Rooms: Underutilized Resources," *American Journal of Public Health* 73:12 (December 1983): 1361–1365.

World Health Organization. "Basic Radiological System—The WHO Approach to Better Population Coverage with Diagnostic Radiology." Presented at WHO Regional Committee for the Eastern Mediterranean, July, 1984.

———. "Recent Developments in Tropical Diseases Research—Progress Report by the Director-General." World Health Organization, Executive Board, 77th Session, November 27, 1985.

Yankauer, A. "Lessons in Surgery for the Third World," *American Journal of Public Health* 73:12 (December 1983): 1359–1360.

16

User Fees and Health Financing in Developing Countries: Mobilizing Financial Resources for Health

Donald S. Shepard and Elisabeth R. Benjamin

Economic crises and the ensuing adjustments have exacerbated the "recurrent cost" problem in the health sector in many developing countries. This problem is the public sector's lack of the funds to operate health facilities and programs in the manner in which they were designed. Economic crises may be brought about by such factors as declines in earnings from major exports, sharp rises in prices or quantities of basic imports, major crop failures, increased military or other government expenditures, or escalating debt service payments. They often require governments to curtail further budgets already inadequate for the commitments made.

The first section provides an overview of current health expenditure levels, possible solutions to the 'recurrent cost' problem, and options for generating additional revenue. We examine user fees especially, the

*The authors are indebted to David de Ferranti, whose thoughtful writings and discussions have contributed to their understanding of this subject, and to Guy J. Carrin and Prosper Nyandagazi who collaborated on the empirical analysis in Rwanda. They thank David Bell, Michael Reich, and John Akin, for constructive comments on earlier drafts, Guy Carrin for delivering this paper at the Symposium, and Nona Yarden for editorial assistance. Data collection on the Rwanda study was supported by the Resources for Child Health (REACH) Project and the Program for Combatting Childhood Communicable Diseases (CCCD) of USAID. All views expressed are those of the authors.

option we generally consider most promising. In the next two sections, these topics are addressed in detail—descriptively through health expenditure studies and analytically through demand studies. Next we review a 1986 case study of Rwanda using original data, and in the last section we offer our conclusions.

Overview

Current Expenditure Levels

Table 16.1 shows the pattern of real per capita health expenditures from 1973 through 1979, the period that saw the first shocks of higher oil prices, in forty-seven developing countries for which data could be obtained. Despite considerable variation among countries, more countries registered increases (thirty-seven countries) than decreases (ten countries) over this period.

Several factors belie this apparently rosy picture, however. First, public sector health expenditures were generally falling as a percentage of total public expenditures. They declined in thirteen out of fourteen low-income countries, nine out of twenty-two lower middle-income countries, and nine out of eleven upper middle-income countries (de Ferranti, 1985). Public expenditures have traditionally supported preventive services and care for the poor.

Second, demand was increasing as per capita income rose; the number of facilities and providers was expanding, their range of services was being extended, and important preventive services, such as immunizations and improved water supply, were being added.

Third, even where health expenditure has increased, it is often outstripped by larger increases in government budgets in other sectors and by mounting public expectations about health services.

Fourth, if comparable recent data become available, they will probably reflect declines in public sector health expenditures in more countries due to such factors as lower coffee prices and worldwide recession.

Possible Solutions

The recurrent cost problem in health is amenable to four types of solutions. A government may (1) reduce its expenditures for health services by curtailing services or achieving efficiencies, (2) seek additional revenues, (3) redistribute available revenues to the most important services, or (4) provide services more efficiently. For reasons discussed below, the authors feel that obtaining additional revenues is generally

Table 16.1
**Annual Percentage Change in Real per Capita Health Expenditures
in Selected Developing Countries, 1973–79**

Country	Rising Expenditure	Falling Expenditure
Low Income Countries		
Ethiopia	19.4	
Nepal	9.5	
Burma		−6.1
Malawi	4.4	
Burundi	2.6	
Burkina Faso		−0.5
Rwanda	4.0	
India	0.1	
Somalia		−3.6
Tanzania	4.2	
Sri Lanka	6.1	
Niger	13.5	
Sudan		−16.9
Ghana		−16.1
Lower Middle-Income Countries		
Kenya	2.1	
Yeman Arab Republic	34.1	
Liberia		−6.3
Honduras	3.0	
Bolivia	9.6	
Zambia		−5.6
Egypt	10.5	
Thailand	9.0	
Philippines	5.6	
Papua New Guina	7.2	
Morocco	2.4	
Nicaragua	13.5	
Nigeria	19.7	
Cameroon	1.7	
Guatemala	8.6	
Peru		−0.2
Ecuador	7.8	
Tunisia	15.5	
Costa Rica	17.9	
Syrian Arab Republic	24.0	
Jordan	8.2	
Paraguay	6.4	
Upper Middle-Income		
Korea	12.1	
Malaysia	5.4	
Panama	3.7	
Brazil	12.1	
Mexico		−1.6
Argentina		−8.3
Chile	1.7	
Uruguay	1.5	
Venezuela	2.0	
Israel	4.5	
Singapore	7.9	

Source: Derived from expenditure data in de Ferranti (1985), Table A-2, deflated by
consumer price index. Compound rates of change derived from the first and last years
for which data were published 1973–1980. Countries listed in order of increasing per
capita GNP. Data combine public and private expenditures. Countries are categorized
by the World Bank classification based on per capita GNP.

the more feasible option in health. Thus, this paper examines a way in which governments can cope with the effect of economic crises on their public health programs through seeking additional revenues.

This strategy has been chosen for several reasons. First, political and humanitarian concerns make it hard to cut back substantially on public sector services in general, or to redistribute funds away from some types of services. Indeed, the policy of Health for All by the Year 2000, adopted by the World Health Organization (WHO) member states at the World Health Assembly in 1978, is a major policy statement towards increasing access to services. Second, current proposals by international donors and commentators in health efforts also increase expectations and demands for services. For example, Walsh and Warren (1979) propose selective primary health care; U.S. Agency for International Development (AID) promotes "child survival"; UNICEF is advocating "GOBI" (a program of special emphasis on growth monitoring, oral rehydration therapy, breastfeeding, and immunizations); and WHO promotes the Action Programme for Essential Drugs. Although all these initiatives purport to be cost-effective, their goal is not to cut costs but to expand services. Third, the policy of encouraging more government revenues for health services—particularly non-tax revenues—is consistent with the current policies of a number of international donors in health. The World Bank, AID, and WHO are all encouraging governments of developing countries to make the health (and other service) sectors financially more self-sufficient. Fourth, strategies to improve efficiency often require additional resources. For example, Gray (1986) recommended that public sector health programs in Mali need more non-personnel expenditures relative to personnel expenditures. Politically, it is easier to add to non-personnel budgets than to fire civil servants or cut their salaries.

Options for Increasing Revenues for Health

A developing country's principal sources of funds for health are grants and loans from donors, general domestic tax revenues, and private payments by households (termed community financing). The uses, advantages, and limitations of these approaches have been discussed in the literature (Cross, 1986; Donaldson and Dunlop, 1986; Lerman, Shepard and Cash, 1985; Musgrove, 1986; Nichter, 1986; Parker, 1986; Ray, 1975; Sorkin, 1986; Viveros-Long, 1986; Wang'ombe, 1983). Here we will comment briefly on each approach.

Donor contributions would appear to be an especially attractive source of revenues, but they face a number of limitations. Usually donor funds are tied to new initiatives (e.g. expanding rural, preventive, or family planning services) and support services that might not otherwise be obtained (e.g. foreign commodities or technical assistance); they are limited in duration to the maximum life of the donor's project (e.g. usually five years for USAID); and their availability (particularly for bilateral assistance) depends heavily on the political relationship between the donor and host governments. Sometimes, international agencies such as the World Bank or International Monetary Fund provide structural adjustment loans which provide more general recurrent cost financing or foreign exchange. These are emergency measures, however, contingent on major public sector reforms. Thus, donor financing is not easily adaptable to solving recurrent cost crises.

Domestic tax revenues are the predominant existing source for financing health services but face severe problems in increasing their share. While complete discussion of the abilities of developing countries to raise additional tax revenues or to reallocate more revenues to health is beyond the scope of this paper, several constraints should be briefly noted. First, all major taxes (e.g. head taxes on households with cash, export tariffs, income taxes in the modern sector, import tariffs, and value-added taxes) have political and administrative limits. In periods of economic crises, the bases for these taxes may themselves shrink. Most serious, raising many taxes creates undesirable incentives. Taxes on export crops, for example, discourage their production (or foster black market exports), depriving a country of foreign exchange. Further, collection mechanisms may be weak, so that higher tax rates may engender more tax evasion without generating additional revenues.

Community financing may take the form of prepayment (i.e. payment in advance for the right to receive care when needed), collective payments, such as donations from a community, or user fees (payment at the time care is received). These are discussed in turn.

Prepayment takes the form of either insurance or a prepaid health plan (an organization which delivers care for a periodic payment). In Latin America, where insurance is particularly widespread, both employers and employees in the modern sector contribute to social security funds. The fund may directly operate health facilities that provide care to members, or may reimburse other facilities and providers. In other countries, major employers operate their own health systems. For example, the Indonesian oil producing enterprise, Pertamina, operates its own clinics and hospitals to care for its 200,000 employees and dependents.

In rural areas, insurance often takes the form of community prepayment schemes in which the households contribute towards the support of a community organization that provides medical services or drugs (see Russell, 1985). Some of the most successful examples are revenue producing organizations which have undertaken the provision of health care, such as milk cooperatives in India. In China, barefoot doctors have been employed by the production brigade, whose collective earnings finance their services. Stinson (1982) discusses other examples, such as prepayment in cash to a welfare fund. Thailand has a history of community welfare cooperatives which provide services to households for an annual membership (Myers, 1985).

Prepayment and community contributions have the potential to distribute the cost of health care broadly, and to finance a range of services. They provide for payment by persons who are well rather than those who are ill. They can fund preventive and promotive services, for which private demand is often limited, as well as curative services. Finally, they avoid a liquidity problem, in which a temporary shortage of cash would cut off health services. Potentially, tax revenues may allow a progressive shifting of costs, as better off persons generally pay more taxes. Unfortunately, these approaches also have a number of limitations.

With no financial deterrent to seeking care, individuals might seek more care than is economically justified. For example, they may demand sophisticated treatments whose benefits may not justify the investment of resources. Also, tax supported services may disproportionately benefit the better off members of a society. The types of health services which cost the government most to produce are generally those provided in the referral hospitals. As these hospitals are usually located in the major cities, they tend to serve urban dwellers disproportionately.

All forms of private prepayment require a high degree of community organization and cohesion. Cooperatives, brigades, or insurance companies must remain financially solvent so that a family that prepays at the beginning of the year can be sure that care will be available throughout the year. It must be possible to exclude free riders. And if health is tied to a productive enterprise, that enterprise must remain sufficiently solvent so that it can continue to support the health activities. These administrative concerns are best addressed by employers, unions, or tightly structured, cohesive communities. Cooperatives set up specifically for health may lack this sort of stability and legitimacy.

User Fees

User fees are charges levied for health care consultations, tests, drugs or services received. Developing country governments may find user fees to be an effective mechanism for financing public sector health care. First, such fees could cover part of the costs of providing health care and thus ease some of the government's economic burden. Second, user fees would avoid the problems of overuse sometimes caused by free care. Overuse can take many forms: obtaining drugs but not using them, obtaining services for conditions that are self-limiting or unresponsive to care, or obtaining services where the benefit is small relative to the cost of the service.

Third, the administrative requirements of user fees are much more modest than those for prepayment systems. They do not require sponsorship by a well established productive or benevolent organization, and are usually not expensive. For example, the costs of collection for several user fee experiments in Sudan averaged only 5.3 percent of gross revenues (Bekele and Lewis, 1986). Fourth, a user-fee system eliminates the need to safeguard a large amount of working capital (e.g. up to a year's prepayment for all members). User fees may thus be well suited to rural areas where population density is low and fewer organizational structures exist. Moreover, user fees inspire a sense of self-reliance and empowerment. They can also insulate health services from contractions in government budgets resulting from economic crises. Finally, Stinson's (1982) review of health projects with community financing found that user fees (i.e. fee for service payments) were the most commonly used method of community (i.e. private) financing. As user fees are the most acceptable and proven method of community financing, we shall emphasize them in this paper.

As we shall show, user fees have not been widely used in financing public health services. Tax revenues have been used instead. Taxes distributed the costs widely and were politically popular, as services appeared to be free or inexpensive. As economic crises have undermined the viability of tax support, user fees are now receiving attention in the public sector.

Household Expenditures for Health

To assess how much users can afford to pay for health care, we first examine available data on health expenditures. Figure 16.1 shows health expenditures as a percent of household income for 36 low income and lower middle income countries. The data, derived from de Ferranti (1985) use 1981 values of GNP per capita and the midpoint from the range of available expenditure studies which range from 1966 through 1981.

Health expenditures average 2.5 ± 1.9 percent (mean ± 1 standard deviation) of household income for low income countries and 3.0 percent ± 0.9 percent of household income for lower middle income

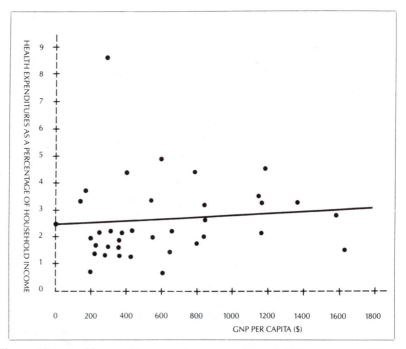

Figure 16.1. *Health expenditures as a percentage of household income versus GNP per capita.*

countries. Figure 16.1 also shows the regression line of health expenditure against per capita GNP. Although the slight upward slope (0.36 percent of household income per $1000 rise in GNP per capita) suggests a tendency for expenditure to rise with increases in the GNP, the slope is not statistically significant. The outlying point in Figure 16.1 is Haiti ($300 GNP per capita), for which 1970 data reported that health expenditures were 8.6 percent of household income. As de Ferranti acknowledged, the data come from a variety of sources and are not necessarily entirely consistent. Nevertheless, the stability is striking—health expenditures range from 1 to 4 percent of household income across a range in per capita GNP from $140 (Bangladesh) to $1630 (Paraguay).

A quite different standard of comparison, time, also shows that the resources devoted to health are modest. Ayalew (1985) found that about 5 percent of rural families' time (i.e., nineteen days per year) in the Tigrai region of Ethiopia was devoted to ill people receiving medical care and being sick. Chernichovsky (1985) has applied similar methods to Botswana. The analogous concept for income—medical expenditures plus earnings or production foregone because of illness—would undoubtedly be higher than the 1 to 4 percent range for medical care above.

As another way of describing health expenditures, Table 16.2 shows the private share of total health expenditures. Although de Ferranti (1985), who compiled these data, acknowledged possible inconsistencies in definition and coverage in the data, the range is still enormous. It is striking that the private share exceeds the public share in almost half of the countries (seventeen out of thirty-seven). Furthermore, the countries with large private shares include a number of the poorest developing countries such as India ($260 GNP per capita), Bangladesh ($140), and Afghanistan ($190). As fee-for-service is the predominant method of financing private health expenditures, this table provides indirect evidence of the willingness and ability of populations of poor countries to finance substantial parts of their health care with methods other than taxes.

Levels and Effects of User Fees

Effects on Demand for Medical Care

Economic theory suggests that as the price of a good or service increases, holding other factors constant, then the demand for the service will generally decrease. The strength of this relationship is measured by the price elasticity of demand. If demand is highly elastic (elasticity algebraically lower than -1), then an increase in price is a substantial deterrent to utilization. This elasticity is a matter of considerable policy importance. If demand is elastic lower prices can be used to encourage especially beneficial services and discourage less important ones.

Some types of primary health services such as immunizations, prenatal care, malaria prophylaxis and treatment for diarrhea can be considered "merit goods." They are technologies that many health officials would like to see more widely used, as they tend to be highly effective and cost effective. On the other hand, sophisticated hospital care, such as that in an intensive care unit of a referral hospital, is the least cost effective, as Rees et al. (1978) showed in Kenya. Thus, if elasticity of demand were high in magnitude, user fees would be socially disadvantageous for primary health services (especially for children), but helpful for referral hospital care. If elasticity of demand were low, user fees could be applied to all services, as they would generate revenues without affecting utilization.

Unfortunately, available empirical studies on price elasticity of demand are few in number and seemingly conflicting in results (Lewis,

Table 16.2

Private Health Expenditures as a Percentage of Total Health Expenditures, Selected Developing Countries

Country	Percent Private		Country	Percent Private
Lesotho	12		Swaziland	50
Zimbabwe	21		Lebanon	50
Tanzania	23		Peru	53
Malawi	23		Mali	54
Tunisia	27		Venezuela	58
Togo	31		Indonesia	62
Mexico	31		Honduras	63
Brazil	31		Haiti	65
China	32		Argentina	69
Colombia	33		Pakistan	71
Rwanda	37		Ghana	73
Senegal	39		Philippines	75
Spain	39		Syria	76
Jamaica	40		Thailand	79
Jordan	41		India	84
Sudan	41		South Korea	87
Sri Lanka	45		Bangladesh	87
Botswana	48 Median		Afghanistan	88
Zambia	50			

Source: Derived from de Ferranti (1985), Table A-4. Countries are ordered by increasing private shares. As years, methodologies, and quality of data vary among studies, results should be considered only general indications.

1985). The three best demand studies, conducted in Malaysia, the Philippines, and Kenya, are all based on household surveys that assessed utilization, travel time, prices, and other factors. The samples in Malaysia and the Philippines were randomly chosen, with upper income households deliberately overrepresented. The sample in Kenya was intentionally focused on lower income individuals. Although the studies estimate the effects of price, income, travel and waiting time on demand, it is the price elasticity that is most pertinent to the discussion of user fees.

The Malaysia study (Heller, 1982) is based on a survey of 1465 respondents in eleven states of peninsular Malaysia. That country is in the lower-middle income range ($700 GNP per capita) and has an extensive system of free care. Heller found that prices did not seem to matter in the choice about whether or not to seek care. Prices did, however, affect the choice of providers.

The Philippines study by Akin et. al. (1982, 1986) used the 1978 Bicol Multipurpose survey of 17,000 individuals in the Bicol region. With a per capita GNP of $790, the Philippines is also a lower-middle income country. The authors found that perceived quality was a significant determinant of choice of provider, but that price had no important effect in determining visit choices.

The Kenya study by Mwabu (1983, 1986) was based on 867 individuals in twenty-four villages in one Kenyan district. The author designed the study specifically to examine demand. He conducted all interviews himself and analyzed the findings with a relatively recent technique—discrete choice multiple logit. Mwabu found that demand fell very little in response to higher money prices and higher time "prices" (particularly in the wet season). His study was sufficiently precise, however, that his low elasticities did achieve statistical significance. Russell and Zschock (1986) cite work in progress from Peru that also finds very small, albeit statistically significant, price effects.

We can speculate on the reasons why price is statistically significant in some studies but not in others. Perhaps price matters more in the lower income population (Kenya, with a per capita GNP of $420) than among better off people in Malaysia and the Bicol region. The effects of price might be culture specific. Or price may really have a small negative effect in many settings, but measurement problems and limited sample sizes may mean that it is not statistically significant. For example, Russell and Zschock (1986) commented on the problems on imputing price and time in Heller's and Akin's studies. Even if price has a statistically significant effect on demand, its magnitude is small.

In view of the uncertainties in the literature about the effect of price on demand, a prudent design of user fees would be to try to set such fees relatively low for highly cost-effective outpatient services, particularly those oriented towards children. In addition, health communications, such as radio broadcasts, can be used to encourage demand for important services. Using such communications in the Gambia, for example, an AID-assisted project increased the use of home-mixed ORT from virtually zero to over 50 percent in two years at a cost under $1 per child per year (Shepard and Brenzel, 1985). Higher user fees can be imposed on services which are less cost effective.

Ability to Generate Revenues

Table 16.3 reviews recent experiences with user fees in a number of settings. This summary, like Stinson's (1982) earlier review, suggests that user fees tend to be most successful in financing drugs and curative services. These goods and services are tangible and address an immediate need.

The current level of revenues generated by user fees in the public sector is quite modest. For the thirty-four countries for which de Ferranti

Table 16.3
Recent Experiences with User Fees for Drugs and Health Services

Site and Author	Type of Costs Covered	Degree of Success
Indonesia, 4 subdistricts (Shepard, Lerman, Cash, 1985)	Consultation and drugs	15–17% of clinical costs.
Fiangha, Chad (Carrin, 1986a)	Drug costs	Recovered 100% of drug costs.
Sine Saloum, Senegal (Gray, 1983, 1986; AID, 1980, 1984)	Consultations and drugs	Problems with accounting. Recovered 6–7% of designed drug costs.
Koro, Mali (Gray, 1982)	Village Health Worker drug distribution	Little or no cost recovery.
Jikjeam Baptist Health Centre, Cameroon (Carrin, 1986b)	Drug costs including immunizations, antimalarials	Communities cover 99% of recurrent costs.
Salvation Army Rural Health, Care, Central African Republic (Carrin, 1986b)	Consultations and drugs	40% of recurrent costs financed by the community.
National Program of Auto-Encadement Sanitaire, Niger (Carrin, 1986b)	Drugs	Difficulties for VHW to manage funds.
Vanger Hospital Community Medicine Program, Zaire (Carrin, 1986b)	Consultations and drugs	Fees cover 39% recurrent and 59% drug costs.

developed estimates (Table 16.4), the average (unweighted) contribution of user fees is only 7 percent. De Ferranti (1985) estimates that this amount could be increased to 20 to 25 percent of total public health expenditures with widespread implementation of user fees.

As a guide towards establishing the level of fees, de Ferranti has compared the official fee for an initial adult outpatient consultation to the prevailing daily agricultural wage in the area (Table 16.5). A metric such as this adjusts for differences in ability to pay among countries.

To show that this level of fee is not unreasonable, we shall make a number of simplifying assumptions. We began with data from the districts of Kitui and Kirinyaga in Kenya and found that these rural populations averaged from 0.9 to 2.0 visits to government facilities per person per year (Irving and Shepard, 1983). Assuming that each adult had to support one child under fifteen (mirroring the country's approximate age distribution), and that there was no additional charge for revisits, then each adult would have to work 1.8 to 4.0 days to pay for outpatient care. Assuming a work year of 250 days, this effort would constitute 0.7 percent to 1.6 percent of the work year. This share is well below the current share of household income for medical care and would seem quite affordable. Yet only three of the thirteen countries have fee levels that equal or exceed one day's wage.

Table 16.4
Revenues from User Charges as a Percentage of Recurrent Expenditure on Government Health Services in Selected Developing Countries

Country	User Charges Percentage
Botswana, 1978	3
Burundi, 1982	4
Columbia, 1980	28
Ghana, 1976/77	3
Indonesia, 1982/83	16
Jordan, 1982	13
Lesotho, 1980/81	6
Malawi, 1982	3
Pakistan, 1980/81	3
Peru, 1981	8
Philippines, 1981	7
Rwanda, 1982	7
Sri Lanka, 1982	1
Sudan, 1980/81	1
Togo, 1979	6
Tunisia, 1982/83	2
Zimbabwe, 1980/81	2

Note: The following seventeen other countries have user fees that are believed to be under 2 percent of recurrent expenditures: Angola, Bangladesh, Bolivia, Cameroon, Egypt, Gabon, Guatemala, Honduras, Jamaica, Liberia, Libya, Mali, Morocco, Nigeria, St. Lucia, Yemen, and Zambia.
Source: Derived from de Ferranti, 1983.

Another factor that suggests that a day's wage is approximately the right magnitude is that users currently experience a time cost of about this magnitude to seek care. Travel, waiting, and treatment time in a government clinic can easily total to a half a day per visit, or a whole day for an episode of illness that requires one follow-up visit. Thus, the total price of care already exceeds the money price suggested by de Ferranti.

Fees for an inpatient hospitalization were found to be close to those for an initial adult visit (de Ferranti, 1985). Yet compared to the total price of hospital care, where an adult family member must remain with the patient throughout most of his stay, the money price is relatively low. Using the same principle, the fee for inpatient care should be several days' agricultural wages. In fact, only two countries (Burundi and China) had inpatient fees which amounted to even one day's agricultural wage.

Data for Rwanda, discussed further below, can illustrate the potential revenue that would be generated by linking user fees to agricultural wages. Suppose that the fee for an initial adult outpatient visit were set

Table 16.5
Health Service Fees and Agricultural Wage Rates

Country	Year	Initial Adult Outpatient Visit	Daily Agricultural Wage		Ratio to Wage
Botswana	1977	$.30	Pula 7.4	$8.78	0.03
Burundi	1983	$.22	F 100	$1.11	0.2
Cameroon	1983	CFA 600	CFA 600	$1.83	1.0
China	1982	Y 2.2	Y 2	$1.17	1.1
Indonesia	1983	$.36	Rp 425	$0.64	0.6
Lesotho	1980	$1.20	R 2.8	$3.60	0.3
Malawi	1981	free	K .59	$0.52	0.0
Mali	1982	MF 1250	MF 850	$1.26	1.5
Niger	1981	free	CFA 712	$2.17	0.0
Pakistan	1982	Rs 1	Rs 12.02	$1.01	0.1
Philippines	1982	Pesos 2.6	Pesos 18.53	$2.35	0.15
Rwanda	1977	FRW 20	FRW 92	$1.00	0.2
Burkina Faso	1982	free	CFA 425	$1.11	0.0

Note: The midpoint has been used where ranges were specified for China, Indonesia, Mali, the Philippines, and Burkina Faso.
Source: de Ferranti, 1985, Table 5.

at $1 (one day's wage) and a hospitalization were set at $3 (three days' wages). These are five times the current fees for these services in government health centers. Since Rwanda currently recovers 7 percent of government health expenditures through user fees, a fee structure 5 times as high would generate some 35 percent of government expenditures.

Rwanda: A Case Study in User Fees

Background

To illustrate the potential and constraints of user fees, we present recent data from Rwanda, a low-income, landlocked country in Eastern Africa. Its per capita GNP was $270 in 1983. The population of about six million persons lives primarily in scattered farms over the hilly terrain. The rural population supports itself primarily from subsistence agriculture, though coffee is an important export crop. Rwanda is the most densely populated country in Africa. The average rural household has 5.5 persons and a farm of only about one hectare.

Rwanda's willingness to examine higher user fees stems from two factors. First, the government has been finding it increasingly burdensome to operate public sector health facilities. Facilities are forced to accept budget cuts; for example, Rwanamanga district hospital saw its budget for drugs halved from 1984 to 1986, a pattern they considered common in government facilities. In addition, a facility may not be allowed to spend all that is budgeted. Second, with donor support, Rwanda is expanding family health and child health services, but both donors and government recognize the need for new services to be financially self-sufficient in the long run. As part of its agreement to participate in the CCCD (Combatting Childhood Communicable Diseases) funded by AID, Rwanda committed itself to find domestic sources of financing for these activities.

In April and May, 1986, two health economists (Drs. Donald Shepard and Guy Carrin) visited Rwanda at the invitation of its Ministry of Public Health and Social Affairs to examine approaches for strengthening the financing of health care in general, and treatments for diarrhea and malaria in particular. Collaborating with the Ministry's Director of Finance and Administration, Mr. Prosper Nyandagazi, they carried out household surveys and visited health facilities to contrast the fee systems in government with those in mission health centers.

Design of the Study

Facilities in two of Rwanda's provinces were selected for study. Kigali province, site of the national capital (Kigali), has a relatively sound infrastructure and good soil. Both its urban and its rural dwellers enjoy above average standards of living. Gikongoro province, a few hours drive south of Kigali, is one of the country's poorer regions. Crop yields are low due to acidic soil; poor roads hamper communication.

Within each of these provinces, one government and one mission health center were chosen for study. These reference centers were sufficiently distant from other facilities that most of the population they were intended to serve could be expected to travel to the reference center. (The household surveys, described below, confirmed this pattern of use.) All of the health facilities contained busy outpatient departments and a few rooms (with about twenty-four beds) for inpatients.

Operating Costs

Table 16.6 identifies the health centers and presents salient data on their costs and financing. Government health centers are supported primarily by the national government, which pays staff salaries and provides drugs and supplies. Local governments (communes) contribute to the upkeep of the building and the vehicle. Government facilities collect user fees according to a schedule unchanged since 1975. These fees formerly reverted to the national treasury but now are remitted to

Table 16.6
Costs and Financing at Four Health Centers in Rwanda, 1985

	Kigali Province		Gikongoro Province	
	Musha (Gov't)	Rwankuba (Mission)	Ngara (Gov't)	Kaduha (Mission)
Operating Expenses				
FRW 1000[a]	1871	1092	2369	4661
$	21,500	12,600	27,200	53,600
Distribution of Expenses (%)	100	100	100	100
Salaries	68	62	48	49
Medications	6	15	31	32
Other Expenses	26	22	21	19
Sources of Revenues (%)	100	100	100	100
User Fees	28	59	14	26
Government	72	25	86	13
Mission	0	16	0	61
Outpatient Episodes	30,000	10,000	10,833	24,495
Cost/Episode				
FRW	44	47	109	142
$	.51	.54	1.25	1.63
Basic Fee/Episode[b]				
FRW	20	40	20	50
$	.23	.46	.23	.57
Ratio of Basic Fee to Cost (%)	39	85	18	35
Inpatient Days	5056	1287	1650	9890
Cost/Day				
FRW	110	153	316	76
$	1.26	1.76	3.67	0.88
Basic Fee/Day				
FRW	10	10	10	20
$	.11	.11	.11	.23
Ratio of Basic Fee to Cost (%)	9	10	3	26
Overall Cost Recovery[c]	28	59	14	26

[a] FRW = Rwandan franc. US $1.00 = 87 FRW (1986).

[b] Basic fee includes consultations in all facilities and medications in government facilities. Laboratory examinations cost from 5 FRW for malaria slides to 40 FRW for some stool examinations in most facilities. All medications except antibiotics were free in Rwankuba.

[c] User fees from inpatient and outpatient care, medications, laboratory examinations, and ambulance as percent of total cost.

Source: Shepard, Carrin, and Nyandagazi, 1986.

the commune. The standard fee for a new outpatient episode is 20 FRW (Rwandan francs, equivalent to about $0.23 at $1.00 = 87 FRW). For inpatient care, patients pay $0.11 (10 FRW) per day, with additional modest supplemental fees for laboratory examinations. Persons certified as indigent by the authorities of their commune, along with pupils and civil servants, are exempted from fees.

Mission facilities establish their own charges, which tend to be about twice as high as those in government clinics. They can also set their own policies for exemptions for indigence. Mission facilities are financed by user fees, in-kind contributions from the national government for drugs and personnel, and support by the parent mission in Rwanda or overseas.

Within each province, mission and government facilities used the same amount of resources to treat one episode of care on an outpatient basis. They have similar staffing, each being headed by a medical assistant.

We wished to compare the present outpatient fees with the cost of resources used to treat one average episode. We allocated costs among outpatient consultations, inpatient care, and preventive and promotive services (e.g. organizing vaccinations) based on the estimated proportion of time spent by the senior medical officer on each type of activity. The comparison of fees with costs shows that mission facilities are considerably more self-sufficient than government facilities. It is remarkable that the Rwankuba (mission) health center approaches financial self-sufficiency, generating 85 percent of the costs of ambulatory care. User fees cover a much lower share of inpatient costs than they do of outpatient costs.

Household Surveys

Approximately one hundred randomly chosen households from the target population of each health center, grouped in twenty-five clusters, were visited by an interviewer. Heads of households and adults who reported illnesses during the reference period were questioned in Kinyarwanda by Rwandan interviewers, based on a written questionnaire. Although the questions were written in French, duplicate interviewing at the start of the survey confirmed good agreement among interviewers. The interviewers were men in their twenties or thirties with at least secondary school education. The team leaders were medical assistants (equivalent to nurse practitioners) with previous survey experience.

Table 16.7 gives key results from household surveys. The annual incidence of illness (extrapolated from the four-week recall) is surpris-

Table 16.7

Per Capita Health Expenditures in the Catchment Areas of Four Health Centers in Rwanda

	Kigali Province		Gikongoro Province	
	Musha (Gov't)	Rwankuba (Mission)	Ngara (Gov't)	Kaduha (Mission)
Sample Size (no. of):				
Households	101	102	100	100
Persons	572	556	565	535
Persons per household	5.66	5.45	5.63	5.35
Number of completed illnesses in sample (4 Weeks)				
Total	68	57	48	56
Percent with any treatment	87	86	92	89
Percent treated at Reference Center	57	33	48	39
Mean health expenditure per episode ($)	1.95	2.48	2.90	3.32
Mean values per person per year				
Number of illness episodes	1.55	1.33	1.10	1.36
Health expenditure ($)	3.01	3.31	3.20	4.52
Cash income (from employment and cash crops) ($)	41.04	36.24	15.99	22.80
Total income (incl. value of subsistence farming) ($)	186.53	115.23	117.16	113.30
Health expenditure as percentage of				
Cash income	4.7	11.3	13.3	15.2
Total income	1.0	3.6	1.8	3.1

ingly low. Illness rates for the two centers within each province are similar, as intended.

A useful indicator of whether higher fees affect demand is the likelihood that an individual seeks any treatment for his illness. Surprisingly, the rates of illnesses receiving any treatment are almost the same among all four areas, despite the five-fold differences in fees among facilities. On the other hand, the varying percentages of illnesses treated at the reference health center shows that highest fees do discourage utilization somewhat. After correcting for other characteristics of the patient (duration of illness and gender) the price of care was statistically significant, though small in magnitude. The elasticity of demand with respect to price was found to be -0.25. Doubling the fees at government health centers would reduce the proportion of illnesses treated there from 53 to 50 percent—a small reduction.

It is noteworthy that the 1.0 to 3.6 percent share of household income allocated to health is within the range previously identified in the literature. When health expenditures are compared to just the cash income, the share is dramatically higher. For the poorest area, Kaduha, health consumes almost 15 percent of cash of the meager income ($22.80 per person per year).

There are noticeable differences in quality between mission and government centers that may reduce any deterrent from higher fees. In each of the facilities, the head of the center was asked about the availability of basic drugs on the day of the interview, the preceding month, and the preceding twelve months. Averaging results across all three periods showed that each of the ten most frequently used drugs were in stock 79 percent of the time in Musha and only 53 percent of the time in Ngara. In the mission facilities, all ten of these drugs were available all the time. Amenities also differed between the two types of facilities. The mission facilities enjoyed more spacious buildings; they provided clothing for newborns and offered showers, flush toilets, and some laundry service for hospitalized patients. The high per person expenditure in Kaduha ($4.52 per year) suggests that people are willing to pay a lot for a service they regard highly. Since the Kaduha health center exempts 40% of users from fees because the Catholic sisters consider them indigent, the high expenditure at Kaduha is striking.

Attitudes Towards Fees

Heads of households were asked a number of questions about their attitudes towards user fees. Table 16.8 presents responses to the following question: "Suppose that the government found that it needed to raise medical fees to assure the availability of medications. Which do you prefer, the current situation or the proposed modification?" It is striking that the preference for the higher fees necessary to assure a reliable supply of medications was overwhelming among all households in all four areas. To see whether income affected responses to higher fees, households were categorized into two income groups. Low-income households were those with cash incomes under 1000 FRW ($11.50) per person per year. These households supported higher fees as much as those with higher incomes.

The head of each household was asked whether current medical fees prevented members of the household from receiving care (Table 16.9). Despite their acceptance of higher fees for a stable drug supply, present fees do create some problems, particularly among low income households in Kaduha. While the higher fees in areas served by mission

Table 16.8

Percentage of Households Willing to Accept Higher Fees to Improve Drug Availability, by Income

Income Category	Kigali Province		Gikongoro Province	
	Musha (Gov't)	Rwankuba (Mission)	Ngara (Gov't)	Kaduha (Mission)
All households	88	88	93	89
(No. of households)	(100)	(101)	(99)	(100)
Low-income	81	95	96	86
(No. of households)	(31)	(41)	(48)	(80)
Normal income	91	83	90	100
(No. of households)	(69)	(60)	(51)	(20)

facilities are associated with more frequent problems, the difference between the lowest percentage (19 percent in Musha) and the highest (32 percent in Kaduha) is only a modest thirteen percentage points.

To identify ways to make higher fees more affordable, respondents were asked about their interest in a form of prepayment. Would they buy a card which cost 1000 FRW ($11.50) per household per year and offered a 50 percent discount in government or mission facilities? Interest was strongest among the population served by government facilities. One possible explanation is that respondents see less need for prepayment at mission facilities, because indigent exemptions are more freely available. As mentioned, 40 percent of the patients at Kaduha health center were considered indigent and exempted from charges.

The results in Tables 16.8 and 16.9 suggest that even though some households occasionally have trouble paying for medical care, they value availability of drugs sufficiently to pay more, and they are willing to consider prepayment plans that might ease the burden.

Based on the field work in Rwanda, Shepard, Carrin, and Nyandagazi proposed a demonstration project on user fees at government facilities. They suggested that the community, a mission, or the local government establish a revolving drug fund. The fund should sell drugs at the cost of acquisition plus distribution. This proposal would effectively double fees but would still leave them below the level of mission facilities and would not seem to put them beyond the population's means. As one example, the Program for Combatting Childhood Communicable Diseases (CCCD) in Rwanda could institute a nominal charge of 5 FRW (about $0.06) for a series of chloroquin tablets. Malaria is one of the most frequent illnesses, accounting for 19 percent of illnesses reported in the household survey, and yet the health facilities sometimes run out of chloroquin.

Table 16.9
Effects of Current Fees and Interest in Prepayment

	Kigali Province		Gikongoro Province	
	Musha (Gov't)	Rwankuba (Mission)	Ngara (Gov't)	Kaduha (Mission)
Percentage of households indicating problem with paying medical fees, by income (%)[a]				
Low income	25	28	30	36
(N)	(34)	(44)	(59)	(82)
Normal income	16	20	22	14
(N)	(62)	(58)	(41)	(18)
All households	19	24	27	32
(N)	(96)	(102)	(100)	(100)
Would buy health card for gov't health center (%)				
No	18	44	24	40
Yes	82	56	76	60
Total	100	100	100	100
Would buy health card for mission health center (%)				
No	49	66	46	59
Yes	51	34	54	41
Total	100	100	100	100

[a] Households reporting that they "sometimes" had a problem were assumed to have a problem half the time.

Conclusions

Economic crises create strains on governments and individuals. In the health sector, one symptom of the strain is the recurrent cost problem— facilities and programs lack the funds for normal operation. As drug budgets are considered the most flexible category, they are often the first to be cut when funds are tight. In rural areas such as those studied in Rwanda, where the nearest pharmacy may be several hours walk, drug shortages substantially undermine the usefulness of a health facility.

This chapter has argued that user fees often provide an attractive solution to the recurrent cost problem. Available data on the share of household income devoted to health, household expenditures for health, and attitudes towards drug availability all suggest substantial willingness to pay for health care.

Undeniably, user fees for medical care may present political and administrative risks. Some countries, such as Kenya, traditionally made free medical care a fundamental matter of national policy or a constitutional right. Charging user fees appears to be a major retrenchment. The urban populations that generally have the best access to medical services, may claim to be adversely affected and oppose the change. Inevitably, user fees will create hardship for some ill persons. The change in funding may diminish the power of national officials relative to local ones. Sound administrative procedures must be established and enforced to assure that the fees are used as intended. Administrative personnel must be found, trained, hired, and paid. Other problems that may impede drug supply, such as inadequate logistic systems, must be remedied as well.

These concerns should not be ignored, but they can be overcome. By linking user fees with improvements in quality or access to care, they should become politically acceptable. Exemptions for indigent persons, such as those found at both government and mission health centers in Rwanda, help assure that the truly needy are not denied care. Good administrative mechanisms have functioned for over a decade in a country with good infrastructure, such as Thailand (Myers, 1985). But user fees—especially fees for drugs and revolving drug funds (Cross, 1986)—are relatively easy to administer and generate funds that can be used specifically for drug resupply. Without user fees, however, economic crises mean that public services will continue to decline in many countries. Most patients would rather pay a modest price than have no service available at all.

References

Agency for International Development (AID). *The Sine Saloum Rural Health Care Project, Project Evaluation Report No. 9,* October, 1980.

———. "Prospects for PHC in Africa: Another Look at the Sine Saloum Rural Health Care Project in Senegal," *AID Evaluation Special Study No. 2,* April, 1984.

Akin, J. S., et al. "The Demand for Child Health Services in the Philippines," *Social Science and Medicine* 16 (1982): 267–284.

———, et al. "The Demand for Adult Outpatient Services in the Bicol Region of the Philippines," *Social Science and Medicine* 22:3 (April 1986).

Ayalew, Solomon. "Time Budget Analysis as a Tool for PHC Planning," *Social Science and Medicine* 21:8 (1985): 867.

Bekele, Abraham and Maureen Lewis. "Financing Health Care in the Sudan: Some Recent Experiments in the Central Region," *International Journal of Health Planning and Management* 1 (1986): 111–127.

Carrin, Guy. "Self-Financing of Drugs in Developing Countries: The Case of the Public Pharmacy in Fianga (Chad)." Boston, MA: Takemi Program in International Health, Harvard School of Public Health, 1986a.

———. "The Economics of Drug Financing in Sub-Saharan Africa: The Community Financing Approach." Boston, MA: Takemi Program in International Health, Harvard School of Public Health, 1986b.

Chernichovsky, Dov. *The Household Economy of Rural Botswana: An African Case*, Staff Working Paper No. 715. World Bank, 1985.

Cross, Peter, et al. "Revolving Drug Funds: Conducting Business in the Public Sector," *Social Science and Medicine* 22:3 (April, 1986).

de Ferranti, David M. *Paying for Health Services in Developing Countries: An Overview*, Staff Working Paper No. 721. World Bank, 1985.

———. "Health Sector Financing: An Overview of the Issues," Mimeo, Washington, D.C.: World Bank, 1983.

Donaldson, Dayl, and David Dunlop. "Financing Health Services in Developing Countries," *Social Science and Medicine* 22:3 (April, 1986).

Gray, Clive. "Pharmacies Villageoises dans le Cadre du Projet de Sante Rurale, Mali." Cambridge, MA: Harvard Institute for International Development, May, 1982.

———. "Community Financing of PHC in Rural areas of Senegal's Sine Saloum." Cambridge, MA: Harvard Institute for International Development, October, 1983.

———. "State-Sponsored PHC in Africa: The Recurrent Cost of Performing Miracles," *Social Science and Medicine* 22:3 (April, 1986).

Heller, Peter S. "A Model of the Demand for Medical Health Services in Peninsular Malaysia," *Social Science and Medicine* 16 (1982): 267–284.

Irving, Susan, and Donald Shepard. Health Statistics in Kenya: Teaching note. Boston: Harvard School of Public Health, 1983.

Lerman, Steven J., Donald S. Shepard, and Richard Cash. "Treatment of Diarrhoea in Indonesian Children: What It Costs and Who Pays for It," *Lancet* 2 (1985): 651–654.

Lewis, Maureen. "Comments on Willingness to Pay for Health Services in LDCs: What do we Know, What do we Mean?" Paper presented at the NCIH Conference. Washington, D.C., 1985.

Musgrove, P. "What Should Consumers in Poor Countries Pay for Publicly-Provided Health Services," *Social Science and Medicine* 22:3 (April, 1986): 329–334.

Mwabu, Germano. "Conditional Logic Analysis of Household Choice of Medical Treatments in Rural Villages in Kenya," paper presented at African Studies Association Conference, Dept. of Economics, Boston University, December, 1983.

———. "Health Care Decisions at the Household Level: Results of a Rural Health Survey in Kenya," *Social Science and Medicine* 22:3 (April, 1986).

Myers, Charles N., Dow Mongkolsmai, and Nancyanne Causino. "Financing Health Services and Medical Care in Thailand." Cambridge, Mass: Harvard

Institute for International Development, Development Discussion Paper No. 209, September 1985.

Nichter, Mark. "Paying for What Ails You: Socio-cultural Issues Influencing the Ways and Means of Therapy Payment in South India," *Social Science and Medicine* 22:3 (1986): 957–965.

Parker, R. "Health Care Expenditures in a Rural Indian Community," *Social Science and Medicine* 22:1 (1986).

Ray, Anandarup. *Cost Recovery Policies for Public Sector Projects*, Staff Working Paper No. 206. World Bank, July, 1975.

Rees, P. H., et al. "Medical Care in a Tropical National Reference and Teaching Hospital: Outline Study of Cost-Effectiveness," *British Medical Journal* 2 (1978): 102–104.

Russell, Sharon, et al. *Community Financing*. PRICOR Monograph Series Issues Paper No. 1, May, 1985.

Russell, Sharon, and Dieter K. Zschock. Health Care Financing in Latin America and the Caribbean. Report under USAID Contract 0632-C-005137-00. Stony Brook, NY: Department of Economics, State University of New York, 1986.

Shepard, Donald S., and Logan Brenzel. Cost-Effectiveness of the Mass Media in Health Practices Project. Prepared for the Institute for Applied Communications, Palo Alto, CA. Mined: Institute for Health Research, Harvard School of Public Health.

Shepard, Donald S., Guy Carrin, and Prosper Nyandagazi, "Self-Financing of Health Care at Government Health Centers in Rwanda." Prepared for the Resources for Child Health Project, Arlington, VA. Mined: Harvard Institute for International Development, January, 1987.

Stinson, Wayne. *Community Financing of PHC*. American Public Health Association, PHC Issues Series, No. 4, 1982.

Sorkin, Alan. "Financing Health Development Projects: Some Macro-Economic Considerations," *Social Science and Medicine* 22:3 (April, 1986): 345–350.

Viveros-Long, A. "Changes in Health Financing: The Chilean Experience," *Social Science and Medicine* 22:3 (April, 1986): 379–386.

Walsh, Julia A., and Kenneth S. Warren. "Selective Primary Health Care: An Interim Strategy for Disease Control in Developing Countries," *New England Journal of Medicine* 301 (1979): 967–974.

Wang'ombe, J. K. "Economic Evaluation in PHC: The Case of Western Kenya Community Based Health Care Project," *Social Science and Medicine* 18:5 (1983): 375–385.

INDEX